Phenomenal Qualities

Phenomenal Qualities

Sense, Perception, and Consciousness

EDITED BY

Paul Coates
and Sam Coleman

OXFORD
UNIVERSITY PRESS

OXFORD
UNIVERSITY PRESS

Great Clarendon Street, Oxford, OX2 6DP,
United Kingdom

Oxford University Press is a department of the University of Oxford.
It furthers the University's objective of excellence in research, scholarship,
and education by publishing worldwide. Oxford is a registered trade mark of
Oxford University Press in the UK and in certain other countries

First Edition published in 2015

Published in the United States of America by Oxford University Press
198 Madison Avenue, New York, NY 10016, United States of America

British Library Cataloguing in Publication Data
Data available

Library of Congress Control Number: 2014960245

ISBN 978–0–19–871271–8

To Tigran and Joanna Coates
and
To Mike and Cinny Coleman

Acknowledgements

This book is the fruit of the *Phenomenal Qualities Project*, an investigation into the nature of phenomenal qualities—from a number of different perspectives—through a series of seminars, workshops, and conferences organized over several years between 2009–14 thanks to a generous award by the Arts and Humanities Research Council, to whom we would like to express our gratitude. The papers in this collection derive from the Project's final conference that took place at the University of Hertfordshire in Hatfield, UK in 2012. Also included is a paper by David Rosenthal, who contributed to one of the earlier conferences. The overall Project attracted widespread interest and support, and we would like to take this opportunity to thank everyone involved for their enthusiasm and lively contributions, all of which helped to make it such a success.

We would like to acknowledge the support of the *Institute of Philosophy* at Senate House, University of London, which, through Barry Smith, kindly hosted three of our one-day conferences. We are also grateful to the two anonymous referees for excellent advice on the general form of the collection as well as on individual papers, and likewise to Peter Momtchiloff at OUP, whose warm encouragement of the *Phenomenal Qualities Project* from the outset and support throughout publication have been much appreciated. Thanks are due also to David Chalmers and Galen Strawson for advice on the introduction.

We owe a particular debt to Jenefer Coates for the invaluable editing of the whole volume, and to Florence Curtis for preparing a first-rate index.

Contents

List of Contributors xi

Introduction: The Nature of Phenomenal Qualities 1
Paul Coates and Sam Coleman

Section I. The Ontology of Phenomenal Qualities

1. Quality Spaces and Sensory Modalities 33
David Rosenthal

2. Neuro-Cosmology 66
Sam Coleman

3. Phenomenal Qualities: What They Must Be, and What They Cannot Be 103
Howard Robinson

4. Real Acquaintance and Physicalism 121
Philip Goff

Section II. Perception and Phenomenal Qualities

5. Moore's Dilemma 147
M. G. F. Martin

6. Projection, Revelation, and the Function of Perception 181
Paul Coates

7. Real Direct Realism: Reflections on Perception 214
Galen Strawson

Section III. The Kinds and Character of Phenomenal Qualities

8. A New Argument for Realism from Perceptual Content 257
E. J. Lowe

9. Can We Really See a Million Colours? 274
David Papineau

10. The Nature of Pain and the Appearance/Reality Distinction 298
Michael Tye

11. The Life of the Mind 322
Michelle Montague

Section IV. Phenomenal Qualities and Empirical Findings

12. A Function-Centered Taxonomy of Visual Attention 347
Ronald A. Rensink

13. Can Sounds Be Red? A New Account of Synaesthesia as Enriched Experience 376
Ophelia Deroy

14. Technical Issues in Naive Sense-Datum Theory 400
John M. Nicholas

Index 423

List of Contributors

PAUL COATES is Professor Emeritus of Mind and Metaphysics, Department of Philosophy, University of Hertfordshire, and Principal Investigator of the AHRC Phenomenal Qualities Project.

SAM COLEMAN is Senior Lecturer, Department of Philosophy, University of Hertfordshire, and Chief Co-Investigator of the AHRC Phenomenal Qualities Project.

OPHELIA DEROY is Senior Researcher, Centre for the Study of the Senses, and Associate Director of the Institute of Philosophy, School of Advanced Study, London University.

PHILIP GOFF is Lecturer in Philosophy, Liverpool University, and was Post-Doctoral Researcher in the AHRC Phenomenal Qualities Project.

MICHAEL MARTIN (M. G. F. MARTIN) is Professor of Philosophy at University College, London University, and Mills Adjunct Professor, Department of Philosophy, University of California, Berkeley.

MICHELLE MONTAGUE is Associate Professor of Philosophy, University of Texas at Austin.

JOHN M. NICHOLAS is Professor Emeritus, Department of Philosophy, and Faculty Member, Rotman Institute of Philosophy, Western University, Ontario.

DAVID PAPINEAU is Professor of Philosophy at King's College, London University and at the Philosophy Program, Graduate Center, City University of New York.

RONALD A. RENSINK is Professor in the Departments of Psychology and Computer Science, University of British Columbia.

HOWARD ROBINSON is University Professor, Department of Philosophy, Central European University, Budapest; Senior Fellow, Rutgers Center for the Philosophy of Religion, New Brunswick; and Recurrently Visiting Scholar, Fordham University, New York.

DAVID ROSENTHAL is Professor of Philosophy and Coordinator of Cognitive Science, Graduate Center, City University of New York.

GALEN STRAWSON is holder of the President's Chair in Philosophy, University of Texas at Austin.

MICHAEL TYE is the Dallas TACA Centennial Professor in Liberal Arts, Department of Philosophy, University of Texas at Austin.

Very sadly, one of our contributors, JONATHAN LOWE (E. J. LOWE), did not live to see this volume appear in print. He was Professor of Philosophy at Durham University, and will be dearly missed by all who knew him.

Introduction

The Nature of Phenomenal Qualities

Paul Coates and Sam Coleman

1 Phenomenal Qualities: Preliminaries

You are at this moment conscious of phenomenal qualities. In reading these words you are seeing black shapes against a white field, or you are hearing the sounds of the words being read aloud, or perhaps feeling them on a page of braille. Whichever way, there are certain qualitative features present to you in your experience—the colours and shapes associated with the written text, or the particular auditory qualities arising when the words are spoken aloud, or the lumpy texture of the braille characters. Perceptual experiences of these kinds—visual, auditory, tactile—are paradigmatic bearers of phenomenal qualities. Plausibly, several other sorts of conscious experience also possess them. Phenomenal qualities thus feature in much (if not all) of human mentality, and provide the immediate basis of a good deal of what goes on in daily life (for instance, the purchase of foods on account of their taste). Yet, for reasons soon to be broached, ascertaining the precise nature of phenomenal qualities, as well as their exact place in the structure of the world, has proved very difficult. The chapters in this volume, one way or another, all address these difficulties, which we explicate in outline form below.

Recent work in philosophy has seen an upsurge of interest in questions about the nature of perception and conscious experience, and the phenomenal qualities they involve. At the same time there has been an increasing awareness of the contributions made by different perceptual traditions, and also of the relevance of empirical work in cognitive science and neighbouring disciplines to such questions. Our focus in this collection is on the *metaphysical* aspects of phenomenal qualities; that is, on such matters as their phenomenological and cognitive status, their location, their fundamental ontological nature, and on the way they relate to the entities postulated in the sciences. States with phenomenal qualities have both subjective and objective aspects. Getting clear about the nature of phenomenal qualities involves, *inter alia*, understanding how such qualities fit into the physical world. Since the mind is related to reality through experience, there are very good reasons for regarding the topic of phenomenal qualities as central to issues in the philosophy of mind, metaphysics, and epistemology.

What are phenomenal qualities? Central to our thinking about consciousness is the idea that conscious states have a certain kind of *phenomenal character*. Paradigm cases of conscious states to which it is appropriate to attribute a phenomenal character include—in addition to the experiences of reading mentioned above—the perceptual experiences we have in smelling the scent of a rose, tasting a mint, seeing a ripe yellow lemon, hearing a musical chord played on the piano, or touching a hard, hot railing on a summer day. Other states which it is appropriate to consider in respect of their phenomenal character include hallucinatory experiences, such as having a red after-image, or having a ringing noise in the ear, and bodily sensations such as feeling a sharp pain, having an itchy sensation on one's knee, or experiencing an orgasm. Thoughts, or cognitive episodes more broadly, for example the sudden realization that the wet washing is still in the machine, are also candidates for bearers of phenomenal character. For states with phenomenal character there is an answer to the question 'What is it like?', although this may elude full expression in words. Contrastingly, there is nothing it is like merely to have the myelin sheathes of one's neurons growing, or to instantiate an unconscious urge to kill your father. What-it-is-like-ness or phenomenal character, then, is something revealed to us in conscious awareness.[1]

The relation of phenomenal character in general to phenomenal qualities is roughly that of a determinable to its determinates. In describing experiences as exhibiting different phenomenal characters, we are implicitly noting the kinds of ways in which experiences can be compared as similar or dissimilar. Without thereby drawing conclusions about the underlying logical form of claims about experiences, we can express the same point by stipulating that, in being conscious of the different characters of our various experiences, we are immediately aware of the different phenomenal qualities exhibited in them. Thus we can speak, for example, of the reddish appearance of a ripe tomato and of an after-image, or of the sweet flavour of a wine one tastes, or of the painful experience of stubbing one's toe. In having such experiences, the subject is immediately aware of the phenomenal qualities of redness, sweetness, and painfulness. It is arguable that the awareness of phenomenal qualities also occurs in other kinds of mental states or episodes, such as desires, thoughts, and emotions.[2] We embrace here no particular policy about the individuation of phenomenal qualities: one's total phenomenal character at a time might be considered itself a sort of maximal phenomenal quality—a complete qualitative state not part of any larger experience. On the other hand it seems natural to distinguish elements

[1] See Nagel (1974) for influential discussion of the connection between the phenomenal character of experiences and what-it-is-like-ness.

[2] See Pitt (2004) for an important argument that such states have phenomenal qualities, which are proprietary and individuating.

within such states on account of their felt differences, such as the two elements you are plausibly experiencing now of *perceptual qualities relating to these words*, and *the sensation of your clothes against your skin* (the latter you are now aware of even if you weren't a moment ago—assuming you are indeed clothed). Such component elements are also naturally understood as phenomenal qualities, and the term is routinely employed to pick them out.[3]

When an experience has a certain phenomenal character, the subject is aware of phenomenal qualities in an especially intimate way. We will speak of a phenomenal quality being (phenomenologically speaking) immediately *present* to consciousness, in order to single out the distinctive features of this particular form of awareness (which may usefully be highlighted by considering the difference between being aware of someone else's orgasm, and the manner in which you are aware of your own). The notion of *presence* highlights a subjective aspect of experience, and is intended to be neutral between representational and non-representational theories of consciousness.[4]

With the notions of phenomenal character, phenomenal qualities, what-it-is-likeness and conscious awareness now in play, we can make the following useful conceptual distinction. It seems that phenomenally conscious episodes can be separated (by the mind at least) into two aspects. There is, first, what might be more appropriately labelled '*that-it-is-for-ness*': this is the sheer awareness on the part of the subject of a given phenomenal character (a determinate phenomenal quality); the fact *that* it—*viz.* what she is conscious of—is like something for her at all.[5] Possession of that-it-is-for-ness is what would distinguish a conscious sensory episode from an unconscious sensory episode, if there could exist unconscious sensory episodes.[6] Second, there is the strict *what-it-is-like-ness* of the conscious episode, which is determined by which phenomenal qualities the subject is aware of in consciousness.[7] A full state of phenomenal consciousness, then, includes that-it-is-for-ness and what-it-is-like-ness aspects. Whether this conceptual distinction has a metaphysical counterpart is an interesting question.[8]

[3] The aspects of experience that we are here referring to as 'phenomenal qualities' are sometimes termed 'the sensory qualities' of experience.

[4] Though not a position we favour, it is important to see that *presence* also leaves open the view that phenomenal qualities are not genuinely *instantiated* properties. Even if phenomenal qualities are taken to be purely intentional properties, subjects are still capable of being in different sorts of conscious state, with respect to what it is like to be in those states. As we use the terms, such states will exhibit phenomenal character, and different phenomenal qualities.

[5] Some authors label this aspect of consciousness 'subjective character' or 'for-me-ness', e.g. Kriegel (2009: Ch. 1). See also Levine (2001: 6–7).

[6] For instance, some theorists consider that blindsighters have perceptual states instantiating sensory qualities of which they are unaware, as regards phenomenal consciousness (see e.g. Rosenthal 2010).

[7] Along with the way the qualities are structured: see Kriegel (2009: Ch. 5) for an account of the structural aspect of phenomenal character.

[8] Sam Coleman's chapter in this volume takes it that phenomenal character can come apart from consciousness. Michelle Montague explicitly denies this, and Michael Tye seems to agree, at least for the

The chapters in this volume deal both with questions about the general nature of phenomenal qualities, and also with questions concerning their specific characteristics. Amongst the first group are questions about the *ontology* of phenomenal qualities: how they fit together with the kinds of physical properties that belong to the sentient creatures and inanimate objects that we take to make up the world, and, in particular, with the kinds of properties that figure in the mature sciences. These questions are connected with a further issue, which we call the *location problem*: do phenomenal qualities always belong, in some sense, on the side of the subject, or should they at least in some cases—in veridical perception and normal sensation—be identified with objective properties belonging to the physical objects perceived, or to events in the subject's physical body? Or might they belong to entities that cannot straightforwardly be identified under either category? These questions are further complicated by issues concerning the relation of phenomenal qualities to the intentional aspects of experience. It is arguable that most, if not all, experiences also involve some kind of intentionality. When I perceive an object, the world seems to me to be a certain way; likewise, if I have a sensation, such as a pain in my knee, it seems to me as if there is some kind of disturbance in part of my body. Experiences have content, and represent things as being in certain states.[9] But the manner in which the intentional component of experience is connected with the phenomenal aspect is by no means clear.

2 Phenomenal Qualities, Representation, and the Structure of Experience

Motivated in part by the phenomenological fact that the phenomenal qualities present at the sensory level in veridical, illusory, and hallucinatory experiences are subjectively indistinguishable, philosophers such as Bertrand Russell and G. E. Moore at the start of the twentieth century introduced the notion of *sense-data*. Sense-data were held to be the bearers of phenomenal qualities, particular entities known through an act of acquaintance. Much of the early discussion about the nature of sense-data and phenomenal qualities was dominated by a focus on perception. It was left open, in principle, by some early advocates of sense-data theory, whether, in veridical perception, sense-data could be identified with the physical objects we perceive around us, or parts thereof.[10] In practice, sense-data were typically interpreted as different in kind from physical objects, as ordinarily understood. For those who accepted the sense-data approach, physical objects were usually conceived of either as causes of the sense-data that represented them—as in

case of pains. Note that, as we use the terms, it is not definitional that phenomenal character/what-it-is-like-ness always occurs consciously.

[9] See the arguments presented in Byrne (2001); however, for a contrary view, see Travis (2004).

[10] In his contribution, Michael Martin explores some of the ramifications of this point.

Russell (1912) and Grice (1961)—or as constructions out of sense-data—e.g. Russell (1918) and Ayer (1940).

The theory of sense-data came to be associated with the following claims:

(1) Sense-data are entities that are immediately given in experience. They are known directly through a unique act of *acquaintance*, which constitutes a type of *non-propositional knowledge* of things, not of facts;
(2) Awareness of sense-data involves a *two-term relation* between the subject and a sense-datum, a *real entity* logically distinct from the subject;
(3) Sense-data have the properties that they *appear* to have—they instantiate the phenomenal qualities that the subject is immediately aware of in experience;
(4) Sense-data are entities that are *distinct from* the ordinary mind-independent physical objects that we normally take ourselves to be perceiving in the external world.

Thus, a first account of the nature of phenomenal qualities is the one entailed by the traditional sense-data view: they are qualities belonging to non-physical items located in a realm existing somewhere between the experiencing subject and the objective physical world.[11]

The idea of sense-data was trenchantly attacked from a number of different standpoints. In response, various alternative positions concerning the nature of phenomenal qualities were arrived at by modifying some or all of the four central tenets listed above.

One of the main criticisms of the sense-data theory focused on the lack of clarity of the central relation appealed to, the notion of acquaintance.[12] According to a second account, the *inner experience* view, we should abandon the first and second tenets of the theory, but aim to do justice to the intuitions that gave rise to the third and fourth claims. Phenomenal qualities do not belong to particular entities, *distinct* from the subject, which are the objects of perception. In having a perceptual experience of an object, the subject normally focuses her attention on some objective mind-independent thing taken to be in her physical surroundings, without inference. However, such attention is mediated by a non-conceptual awareness of inner states, states involving phenomenal qualities.[13] This position is frequently, but misleadingly, described as 'indirect realism'; a more informative label is the one adopted by its original proponents, 'critical realism'.[14] On this view phenomenal qualities belong, non-relationally, to the subject. In veridical perception, phenomenal consciousness is

[11] See especially Moore (1913) and Russell (1914).

[12] See, in particular, criticisms of the classical notion of acquaintance in Parts I–VI of Sellars (1956).

[13] This view originated with criticisms put forward in Ducasse (1942); see also Chisholm (1957) and especially Sellars (1978) and (1982).

[14] The critical realist position was initially set out in papers edited in Durant Drake (1920), by Arthur Lovejoy, Santayana, Roy Wood Sellars, and others, and developed subsequently in the work of Wilfrid

always logically independent of any particular object in the perceiver's external environment, just as it is in hallucination. The difference between the two types of experience is extrinsic. Hence this position is also sometimes referred to as 'conjunctivism', or the 'common-factor' view.[15] *Perceptual* experiences are properly identified as such because they are caused, in the appropriate manner, by the external, mind-independent objects perceived. In the case of sensations, phenomenal qualities are construed likewise as belonging to subjective states, independent of the subject's body (or at least, of the rest of her body apart from her brain, or whatever portion thereof supports her mind). It remains as a further question whether they can be reduced to the subject's neurophysiology.

The inner experience theory is open to question. Suppose someone veridically sees a red apple, in normal circumstances. It cannot be assumed, without additional argument, that the phenomenal quality of redness present in her experience belongs to an inner state, one logically independent of any feature of the external object seen.[16] We introduced the notion of phenomenal qualities as those which we are immediately aware of in various paradigm experiences. Taken by itself, this does not entail that all phenomenal qualities are properties of *inner* states, belonging to the subject conceived of in isolation from his or her surroundings. There is therefore a third possible general position. This involves abandoning the third and fourth tenets, whilst retaining a version of the idea that the normal experience of objects involves some kind of two-term acquaintance relation.

This third account is referred to by a confusing array of different titles, including 'direct realism', 'naive realism', 'disjunctivism', and 'the relational view'. Here we take 'direct realism' to refer to the general position, although the use of that label is not without its problems.[17] According to such accounts of perceptual experience, the phenomenal qualities we are immediately aware of in veridical experiences are not qualities of our inner states. They are possessed by external, mind-independent objects.[18] The red quality the subject is aware of when she sees the apple belongs, in some manner, to the external object that she is related to in having her visual

Sellars (1956) and (1978); essentially the same position is defended by Grice (1961), Mackie (1976), Millar (1995), Lowe (1996), and Coates (2007).

[15] One main reason for accepting the inner experience view is the causal-scientific argument elaborated by Valberg (1992) and Robinson (1994).

[16] Compare Clark (1993), Levine (2001), and the various papers in Haddock and Macpherson (2008), and Byrne and Logue (2009); see also the discussion in Alex Byrne (2011).

[17] In Strawson's contribution to this volume *real direct realism* is interpreted somewhat differently, and comprehends a view opposed to the version of direct realism that is allied to the disjunctive account.

[18] The idea that we should relax the restriction on the kinds of object with which the subject can be acquainted is defended in McDowell (1986). The claim that we can be acquainted directly with external physical objects is implicit in the versions of disjunctivism advocated by Snowdon (1981), Campbell (2002), Martin (2002), and Fish (2009). McGinn's (1996) *impressionism* also seems to be an account of this kind. Hinton's work in the late 1960s is often taken as the inspiration for the disjunctivism, but the underlying metaphysics of the view was already developed in some detail in the work of the new realists, in particular that of Holt and Perry; see Holt et al. (1912).

experience of the apple. The phenomenal character of her experience is (at least partly) constituted by the way that things are, objectively, in the physical environment.[19] As Paul Snowdon summarizes the central defining feature of the position, in veridical perception the experience 'in its nature reaches out to and involves the perceived object'.[20]

Stated in this form, the direct realist view leaves open questions about the status of the phenomenal qualities present in hallucination. As many have pointed out, hallucinatory experiences involve a felt reality. The subject has a sense that there is something sensory going on. However, according to some versions of the direct realist view, there is little or nothing of a positive nature that we can say about the phenomenal aspects of hallucinations. According to Martin, all I can say about a visual hallucination of a red apple is that it is indiscriminable through reflection from a genuine veridical visual perception of a red apple.[21] According to Fish's extreme view, although subjects may form beliefs that there are phenomenal qualities present in hallucinatory cases, in actual fact they lack phenomenal character altogether.[22] Arguably, it is more plausible to say that the reason why a subject is able to describe her hallucinatory experience in terms such as 'indiscriminable from seeing a red apple' is because she is antecendently able to identify the separate phenomenal features which are present in her experience, and which contribute to its being the type of hallucinatory experience it is. It is because of this ability to attend to the different phenomenal qualities comprising an overall hallucinatory experience that a subject is able to accurately describe novel hallucinatory experiences—for example, migraine visual auras—when she encounters them for the first time.[23]

A qualified version of direct realism has been defended by Johnston, who allows that hallucinations do involve the awareness of phenomenal qualities.[24] Hallucinations involve the presentation of genuine items, but these are universals; there is no acquaintance relation with any particular entities. When we are aware of them in veridical perception, the phenomenal qualities present are instantiated by the external objects directly perceived, but nothing instantiates them in the hallucinatory case. Both types of experience involve the awareness of a complex relational and qualitative structure, which Johnston refers to as a 'sensible profile' or a 'complex of sensible

[19] Note that, on the question of whether phenomenal qualities can exist unconsciously, direct realism might seem to be a position on which they can, since on this view it is an external object that contributes phenomenal qualities to a subject's experience, e.g. apple redness, yet the apple plausibly exists just as redly whether perceived or not. This result can be avoided by the terminological stipulation that 'phenomenal qualities' picks out those qualitative properties present upon, and only upon, a subject's conscious perceptual engagement with the external object in question. But this doesn't touch the substantive question: can these qualitative properties, supplied *ex hypothesi* by, and belonging to, the perceived item, survive unexperienced?

[20] Snowdon (2005: Section III). [21] See Martin (2006). [22] Fish (2009).

[23] One indirect test of such accuracy is the general agreement in standard reports of migraine experiences. See, more generally, the discussions in Valberg (1992), Siegel (2008), and Robinson (2013), in addition to the works by Martin and Fish cited.

[24] Johnston (2004: Sections 7 and 8); he refers to them as sensible qualities.

properties'. Hallucination can therefore provide us with *de re* knowledge of qualities. We should distinguish between the primary and secondary objects of hallucinations. The primary objects are just the phenomenal qualities that are immediately present to the subject in experience. On Johnston's account the phenomenal qualities in hallucinations do exist for periods of time. They are present as features of experience in a manner that merely intentional objects are not. Hallucinations also involve a secondary object, which is determined by how the primary object, the sensible profile, strikes the subject, and gives rise to perceptual beliefs relating to particular things that may, perhaps, no longer exist. Such beliefs account for the intensional contexts that talk of hallucinations can give rise to.

One argument that motivates the direct realist account is based upon the view that perceptual experience is transparent. It appeals to two connected intuitions about the phenomenology of experience. The first involves a claim about the directness of perception. In normal perception I am not aware of any inner entities as mediating my perception of mind-independent physical objects. I recognize sensible qualities of external objects directly, without inference. The second involves a claim about the intrinsic contents of experience: when I introspect my experience, and try to switch my attention to the nature of my experience as it is in itself, I don't discover any new entities in my consciousness, in addition to the objects and their qualities that I perceive to be in the external world. These points are taken to show that there are no qualities belonging to experiences on their own account, independently of the perception of mind-independent objects. Hence no inner entities instantiate the phenomenal qualities I am aware of in perception.[25]

But there is arguably something odd about this attempt to enrol transparency and similar phenomenological considerations in support of direct realism. Recent empirical work on hallucination makes it clear that realistic-seeming hallucinatory phenomena (that is, Charles Bonnet hallucinations) are not philosophers' inventions, but instead are widely prevalent. Their occurrence must be taken into account in any theorizing about the structure of perceptual experience.[26] In a Macbeth-type case, the subject of a deceptive hallucination will have exactly the same sorts of phenomenological reasons for holding that the qualities immediately present to experience are the sensible qualities of mind-independent physical objects, as it is claimed apply in the veridical case. Yet, by the nature of the case, the features immediately present in hallucinatory experience are independent of any particular objects perceived. It follows that, no matter how we account for the phenomenon of transparency, it cannot be taken on its own to establish the correctness of the direct realist view. The fact that, in the usual case, I am not aware of any additional inner entities *as* mediating my perception of external, mind-independent, physical objects does not

[25] The idea of transparency is also employed by those who uphold externalist versions of the intentionalist view: see Tye (2009).

[26] See in particular the papers by Bental, and by ffytche, in Macpherson and Platchias (2013).

contradict the claim that there actually are inner entities bearing phenomenal qualities which play this mediating role, inner entities that I do not normally conceptualize as such.

The issue of transparency does raise problems, but it is hard therefore to see how it constitutes an argument for direct realism in its own right. For someone not antecedently persuaded of the view that we are directly aware of the sensible qualities belonging to objects external to the mind, it carries little weight against theories that hold that hallucinatory and veridical experiences are intrinsically on a par. The smooth and effortless nature of our ordinary perceptual grasp of the objects around us has undoubtedly been a strong motive for direct realist and related views of perception (such as the enactive account); yet it remains the case that the phenomenology of perception is quite compatible with the inner experience theory.[27]

We noted earlier that there are reasons for holding that experiences have some form of intentional content, and represent the things and events that we perceive. It is arguable that even the most attenuated forms of experience essentially involve some kind of representational state. In having a conscious experience of the world about me, I *take* there to be, minimally, self-contained individual objects of some kind situated somewhere in egocentric space: although the point is contentious, the idea would be that this *taking* already involves the employment of sortal concepts of a broad kind.[28] However, there are several different positions about the relation of intentionality to experience that need to be distinguished.

One position is the dual-component conception of experience that derives from Kant, and which is defended, in rather different ways, in the philosophical systems of Husserl and Wilfrid Sellars. Both are versions of the inner experience account introduced above. According to Husserl, who, with Brentano, was largely responsible for introducing the idea of intentionality into mainstream philosophy in the twentieth century, experiences involve two fundamentally different types of consciousness. In virtue of its intentional component, an experience as a whole has a content, whereby it is directed onto something; this accounts for the subject's experience being *as of* an apple. But visually experiencing a red apple is very different from merely thinking about a red apple. In the former case the intentional directedness is accompanied by a sensory component, an aspect that accounts for the phenomenal character of the experience. Husserl refers to this phenomenal aspect of experience

[27] Compare also the position of Amy Kind (2003), who argues that perceptual experiences are at most *weakly transparent*: it is hard, but not impossible to attend to one's own experiences *as such*. A plausible suggestion is that in attending to our experiences, we need to conceptualize what is immediately present in a different way from in ordinary veridical experience. The phenomenal qualities present do not change in introspection, but the overall phenomenology can by virtue of a shift in the categories employed. The transparency issue is discussed in Galen Strawson's contribution to the present volume.

[28] We understand the notion of a *concept* broadly in this introduction, to include what some writers refer to as 'low-level concepts', and also what others have in mind by their use of the expression 'nonconceptual content'. Jonathan Lowe discusses issues connected with sortal concepts and non-conceptual content in his contribution to this volume.

as its 'sensory content', sometimes employing the technical term 'hyletic-data'. On Husserl's account, phenomenal qualities accompany the intentional states that endow our experiences with meaning. But phenomenal qualities themselves are not *about* anything, nor are they the *objects* of perception. The phenomenal red that is present when I see a red apple must therefore be distinguished from the physical redness of the apple that my experience focuses on, by virtue of its intentional component.[29]

Despite their very different concerns, there are similarities between the positions held by Husserl and Wilfrid Sellars. Sellars also maintains that a perceptual experience is incomplete without the addition of a low-level intentional or conceptual component (understood broadly), which he refers to as the 'perceptual taking'. This intentional component is caused and guided by an underlying sensory state that involves the consciousness of phenomenal qualities. As on Husserl's theory, the phenomenal qualities involved account for the difference between perceiving and merely thinking.[30] They are not to be confused with the objects of perception. The phenomenal and intentional aspects of experience can vary independently of each other, yet are intimately connected through the activity of the productive imagination.[31] The phenomenal colour and shape caused by the apple she sees in front of her prompt the subject to exercise some form of recognitional capacity in respect of the apple, the exercise of which guides further implicit expectations of how her future experiences relating to the apple will develop as she acts upon it. According to the dual-component views of Husserl and Sellars phenomenal qualities belong to inner states of the subject, in accordance with the second account canvassed above. They are distinct from the physical properties belonging to the external objects we perceive and otherwise interact with.[32]

It is worth noting that an analogous dual-component version of experience is also available to the direct realist. Thus, the direct realist can agree that fully-formed perceptual experiences, and perhaps also sensation experiences, essentially involve the exercise of low-level concepts. It is through their exercise that we are able to consciously grasp something of the nature of what we perceive or feel. Yet this would not preclude a theorist from adopting the direct realist's non-inner conception of experience and claiming that the phenomenal component of experience comprises the immediate awareness of qualities that belong to the external mind-independent objects perceived; by adopting this variant of the dual-component model the direct realist can account straightforwardly for the intentionality of perception.

[29] See Husserl (1913/1931: Third Section) and McIntyre and Woodruff Smith (1989).

[30] Although it is still possible to argue that there is a distinctive kind of non-sensory phenomenal quality that attaches to conscious thoughts in their own right, as Michelle Montague argues in her contribution. (We bracket this point in the ensuing discussion of perceptual experience.)

[31] For an elaboration of these ideas see Sellars (1978.)

[32] Paul Coates, in his contribution, examines reasons for favouring this account of experience.

In more recent times, however, starting with the work of Anscombe, a number of writers have argued for a closer connection between the phenomenal and the intentional aspects of phenomenal consciousness.[33] *Intentionalism* (or *representationalism*), as understood in recent work, takes the intentional and the phenomenal aspects of an experience to be more intimately related than on the dual-component view. Experiences are construed as unitary, in which the phenomenal character and representational content arise from a single state of consciousness. According to Jackson, experiences are exhaustively representational, in the sense that the content of a perceptual representational state, plus the fact that the experience represents that that content obtains in the manner distinctive of some mode of perception, together determine the experience's phenomenal character without remainder.[34] According to a closely related alternative version of intentionalism, the phenomenal character of an experience is the more fundamental element, and is what grounds its representational content. Either way, there is a logical—rather than merely causal—link between the two aspects. Intentionalism rejects the sense-data theory by focusing its attack on the first and second tenets of that theory, and denies that a real relation connects the subject to the entities immediately perceived.

The intentionalist approach to the nature of experience and phenomenal qualities gives rise to a number of different variants, and has generated a great deal of discussion in recent times. We make no attempt here to explore the full range of options open to the intentionalist.[35] It can be noted, however, that the general approach is compatible with different views on the location issue. One version, sometimes characterized as 'weak intentionalism', holds that the phenomenal character of an experience supervenes upon its intentional content, without being reducible to it. In perceiving, as opposed to cases of pure intentional states like thought, the intentional properties of experience involve further higher-order non-intentional phenomenal qualities. Phenomenal qualities therefore only exist through being instantiated by the intentional properties of experience. They can be interpreted as belonging to inner states of mind, only contingently connected to their distal causes, that is, to the physical properties of the external objects perceived. These qualities are located on the side of the subject, allowing for a unified treatment of the phenomenal character of veridical and hallucinatory experiences.[36]

On the alternative, *strong*, form of intentionalism, for a perceptual experience to involve the presence of phenomenal qualities is just for that experience to intentionally represent certain properties of the object perceived. Roughly speaking, the phenomenal character of an experience just is its intentional content. It seems natural

[33] For just a few examples of this currently popular view, see Anscombe (1965), Lycan (1987), Harman (1990), Tye (2000) and (2009), Byrne (2001), and Crane (2001).

[34] See Jackson (2007: Section 5).

[35] There are different versions of weak intentionalism, and different conceptions of the kinds of content involved; for some discussion see Crane (2001), Tye (2009), and Byrne (2011).

[36] Compare the view defended by Chalmers (2004).

to associate this interpretation with an externalist treatment of content. On Tye's version of the theory, in veridical experience phenomenal character is out there in the world (or in the body, in the case of pains and other sensations). The only qualities of which we are aware when we attend to the character of our veridical experiences are the qualities of external things, outside the mind. Hence, despite their differences, strong intentionalism can end up in a very similar position to direct realism, in locating phenomenal qualities in the world outside the experiencing subject.

Whether intentionalism is of the right form to capture the occurrent nature of phenomenal experience, and its *presentational* aspects, is open to question. One central problem for the intentionalist view worth noting is the one emphasized by Wilfrid Sellars: it is difficult to account for the radical contrast between the different ways that the same content can be represented, either perceptually, when the subject is immediately aware of phenomenal qualities, or through pure thought alone, when there is no consciousness of experiential qualities of the kind involved in perceptual experiences.[37] More recently, David Papineau has argued that the representational aspect of an experience relates the subject only to abstract objects, and cannot account for its here-and-now conscious experiential character. A number of writers have urged that there are essential differences between the logical features of representational episodes and those of sensory states, rendering the former unfit to capture all of the essential characteristics of the latter. A representational state involves a pseudo-relation to an intentional object that need not have any existence; in virtue of its essential nature, it points away from itself to something else, something that may or may not exist. In contrast, a sensory state plausibly involves the actual presence of monadic properties to consciousness.[38]

3 Phenomenal Qualities and the Physical World

In addition to the question of their location (and connected matters), there is a further major issue associated with phenomenal qualities that is treated in this volume. Whether phenomenal qualities are held to supervene on inner or outer goings-on, there arise intriguing, deep, and difficult questions about their ontological nature, in particular concerning their relationship to physical properties. Their being physical (in some acceptable sense) seems to be a condition on their being naturalized. And given the particular vigour with which phenomenal qualities present themselves to us—we are aware of them to some degree in every moment of waking life—there are strong motivations for wanting to naturalize, thus physicalize, them.

[37] See Sellars (1975). It is arguable that responses to this difficulty that appeal to some notion of non-conceptual content, or to differences in modes of representation, presuppose the very notion of phenomenal presence that they seek to explain: see Block (2003) and (2005); but contrast Tye (2000) and Tye's contribution to the present volume.

[38] For more on this issue see the discussions in Bennett (1974), Sellars (1981), Valberg (1992), Robinson (1994), Coates (2009), and Papineau (2013).

To fail in this enterprise would entail that an especially salient aspect of our world defies integration into the otherwise pleasingly unified picture pieced together thanks to the last several centuries of painstaking science. Other high-level properties of organisms and their environments seem on the whole to be susceptible of explanation (at least in principle) in terms of the activity of massive conglomerations of physical particles under the influence of the physical forces.

The physicalization of phenomenal qualities, however, has proved a singularly arduous theoretical endeavour. Organismic physical properties, such as neuronal spiking-frequencies, no less than external world physical properties, such as surface reflectance triples, seem *prima facie* inadequate as realizers for phenomenal qualities like *phenomenal baby blue*. Familiarly, there is a troublesome and persistent 'gap' apparent between the realized and would-be realizing properties in these sorts of cases.[39] This gap manifests in several interconnected ways. No story told in terms of surface reflectance triples seems *a priori* to 'snare' baby blueness in the external world, in the following sense. One never grasps a description of surface reflectance triples and *just thinks* 'Ah, that's baby blueness instantiated there'. By contrast, and to illustrate the sort of conceptual necessity one might hanker for in physical-phenomenal cases, a description of a pocket of fleshy membranes rhythmically taking in and expelling atmospheric gases, all the while exchanging carbon dioxide for oxygen in the blood passing through it, *does* plausibly *a priori* snare the property of 'breathing': one *just thinks* 'That's a lung breathing'.[40] The shortfall in the physical-phenomenal cases does not seem simply to be a product of a relative lack of knowledge about surface reflectance triples and their physical ilk. Turning to the brain side of things: even those steeped in neuroscience, with extensive knowledge of the plausible neurological correlates of conscious experiences (e.g. feedback loops in the visual cortex), don't find that phenomenal qualities are *a priori* snared by any descriptions utilizing such concepts.

The recalcitrance of this conceptual gap in the face of much scientific and philosophical innovation supports the hypothesis that phenomenal qualities are *in principle* physically inexplicable—descriptions framed in physical concepts just will never manage to *a priori* snare phenomenal qualities.[41] And because physical descriptions cannot *a priori* snare phenomenal qualities, this ensures that any physical description, however elaborate, will always seem to be consistent with asserting the absence of phenomenology in a given case.[42] The conceptual gap—the

[39] See Levine's (1983) influential expression of the 'gap' idea.

[40] Though see e.g. Block and Stalnaker (1999) for the case against the possibility of such conceptual explanations, or the need for them in scientific accounts.

[41] This intuition is classically captured in Jackson's knowledge argument (Jackson 1982). Though even most physicalists now accept it, some still demur, holding that consciousness might be reductively explained in physical terms. See e.g. Jackson (2003) and Kirk (2006).

[42] This idea is ably expressed by Chalmers's zombie argument (Chalmers 1996). See also Leibniz's Mill (1714: Section 17).

fact that no array of physical descriptions seems able to *a priori* snare phenomenal qualities—is of the essence of the difficulty we encounter in understanding how phenomenal qualities could be of a piece with the rest of (what appears to be) a pretty plain physical world. Yet, elsewhere, we have very good reasons to take it that phenomenal qualities *are* in fact integrated with the physical order: they seem to cause physical happenings for one thing, like the purchase of baby blue t-shirts, and physical happenings always seem to have a physical provenance.[43]

We are thus in a state of tension. An ideal naturalistic solution would show how phenomenal qualities are just physical, whilst at the same time doing full justice to their qualitative nature as disclosed in our awareness of them—their 'conscious feel'. This would enable us to understand how the qualities we are aware of in consciousness have the effects in the world that they seem to common sense to have—such as pains causing us to withdraw from painful stimuli, and visual experiences as of baby blue t-shirts causing their purchase. What consciousness discloses in the first-person mode would then be fully integrated with what the physical sciences tell us about the world from their third-person perspective. This represents the Holy Grail of solutions to the problem of phenomenal consciousness, hitherto elusive.

Meanwhile, other options have presented themselves. One notable theory, of increasing popularity at the time of writing, is that phenomenal qualities are in fact illusory; the erroneous, though perhaps useful, upshot of the representation of the physical world by our perceptual (or introspective) systems.[44] Another widespread view has it that the manner of the physical snaring of phenomenal qualities is simply metaphysically brute, and thus not capable of further explanation beyond an *a posteriori* identity based in correlations.[45] Then again, perhaps, as another faction maintains (one variant of this view is to be discussed further below), the manner of phenomenal qualities' physical snaring is merely unintelligible *to us* for some more or less contingent reason, usually held to concern the vagaries of the human psychological endowment.[46]

On the other side of the debate, some writers have come to the conclusion that phenomenal qualities are non-physical after all—possibly they are even causally inert, at least as regards the physical realm.[47] Or, alternatively, every time someone buys a baby blue t-shirt on account of its perceived colour the laws of physics are broken—as interactionist dualists have it.[48]

[43] See Papineau (2002: Ch. 1) for an elaboration of this 'causal argument' for physicalism.

[44] See e.g. the first half of Pereboom (2011) for this view. If the world *entirely* lacked qualities, we might wonder about the capacity of our perceptual/introspective systems to represent properties that nowhere exist, for whence does the representational content derive? Pereboom seems unworried by this sort of point, however.

[45] This is the way that Block and Stalnaker (1999) recommend snaring consciousness in the physical world. See also Tye (2009).

[46] See McGinn (1989) for an early incarnation of this variety of view.

[47] See Jackson (1982) for an influential argument for this view, also Chalmers (1996).

[48] See Foster (1991) for a sophisticated recent defence of this unfashionable Cartesian position.

Through consideration of these major existing attempts to relieve the tension produced in us by the physical-phenomenal gap, a further aspect of this tension becomes evident. It seems that the more the physicality of phenomenal qualities is emphasized—their integration in the objective order—the harder it is to accept at face value their qualitative nature as apparent in consciousness, and conversely. Purported resolutions of the tension, accordingly, always seem either to forgo the physicality of phenomenal qualities in favour of preserving their literal appearances, or else to deflate, or otherwise trim away at, their qualitativity, in order to reconcile them with a physical grounding. It might well appear, then, that the Holy Grail of complete physical-phenomenal integration—doing full justice to both sides of the equation—more than being merely elusive, is unattainable as a matter of principle.

Returning to the physicalist side, a particularly promising approach, developed in the last couple of decades, appeals to our allegedly special modes of conceptualizing phenomenal qualities in order to account for the inability of physical science to *a priori* snare consciousness.[49] There are many variants of this 'phenomenal concept strategy',[50] but the common theme is that, for whichever reason of choice, our conceptual framework may be so constituted that physical-to-phenomenal entailments are never *a priori* for us, in which case the physical will always seem to fail to *a priori* snare the phenomenal. Perhaps we just have two families of concepts, unhappily dislocated in conceptual space, where nonetheless a subset of one family (certain of the physical concepts, e.g. some of the neurological ones) co-refers with the other family (the phenomenal concepts). This conceptual predicament would explain, so say proponents, why purely physical descriptions cannot communicate what it is like to see a colour—since no amount of physically conceptualized information by itself suffices to activate our phenomenal conceptualizations. In order for those conceptualizations to come into play we have actually to enjoy the relevant conscious experiences, or to think about them directly in respect of their quality. For a similar reason zombies will remain stubbornly conceivable: Given a purely physical description of some (in actual fact sentient) creature, no conceptual pressure will be put upon us to think of this being in phenomenal terms as well—i.e. to conceive of it as enjoying phenomenal qualities. In this spot, it is alleged, the tendons of our conceptual scheme are severed right through, and we exert our thought to no explanatory avail.

What is of course attractive to physicalists about these conceptual-level explanations of the physical-phenomenal gap, and of our powers of conceiving, is that they have no obvious metaphysical ramifications. The gap is on this understanding a matter of irreducibly different varieties of concept, or conceptual scheme, rather than irreducibly different varieties of ontological item as referred to by the two classes of concept. We might for all we know be in receipt of such an unfortunate conceptual

[49] For one prominent account of this sort see Papineau (2002). The modern originator of this strategy is taken to be Loar (1990).

[50] The name is due to Stoljar (2005).

scheme (it sounds like something Descartes's demon would gleefully arrange), and yet for all that consciousness could be perfectly physical: each phenomenal concept necessarily co-refers with some physical concept. Naturally, *given* our conceptual scheme it will forever seem a mystery quite how this could be so, at the level of extension. Thus ontological dualism will always remain a temptation for those unable to hold on to the deflationary explanation in terms of a merely conceptual dualism of phenomenal and physical concepts. The strength of this strategy lies in its broad acceptance of the data adduced by the anti-physicalist—the seeming gap between physical and phenomenal—even as it removes the metaphysical import of this gap by means of the merely epistemological explanation.

4 The Ontology of Phenomenal Qualities

In their chapters in this collection, Howard Robinson and Philip Goff both concentrate, each in his own way, on this phenomenal concept strategy. Neither finds it satisfactory as a physicalist defence mechanism. Robinson argues in Chapter 3 that the phenomenal concept strategy glosses over a deeper problem for physicalism, distinct from the issue of the conceptual gap, but plausibly closely related to the matter of the second aspect of tension remarked upon above: the fact that solutions to the physical-phenomenal gap seem inevitably to emphasize one of the two elements at the expense of the other. Robinson claims that, beyond the mere appearance of a *gap* between them, the manifest natures of physical and phenomenal properties *positively clash*—they actually seem to be different sorts of properties, and so cannot be the same (by Leibniz's law, hence this being the 'Leibniz Law Problem'). Thus, beyond simply mounting an explanation of why we seem unable to *a priori* snare the phenomenal in the physical workings of the world, as the phenomenal concept strategy aims to do, a full defence of physicalism, for Robinson, would require overcoming the natural antagonism between the physical and the phenomenal. If correct, this would leave the phenomenal concept strategy looking somewhat beside the point: it would at best serve to mask, or distract attention from, the real issue of substance. A major component of Robinson's argument concerns the central role of phenomenal qualities in construction of the manifest world of common sense.

For his part Goff—rather boldly—argues in Chapter 4 that the phenomenal concept strategy positively implies a variety of dualism. His argument relies on the claim that we have a peculiarly direct form of epistemic access to phenomenal qualities—that supplied by a Russell-style cognitive acquaintance with them,[51] which Goff labels 'real acquaintance'. Given real acquaintance, the conceptual gap described above implies an ontological gap: irreducibly different sorts of concept will signal irreducibly different sorts of property. And since phenomenal properties disclose no physical aspect in

[51] See for example Russell (1912).

introspection, Goff claims, property dualism is entailed. Much of Goff's chapter, unsurprisingly, is devoted to defending the thesis of real acquaintance, in the form of an argument to the best explanation of our special knowledge of the phenomenal.

Goff mentions in passing one interesting way of avoiding the alleged property dualist consequence of the phenomenal concept strategy, which connects with Sam Coleman's chapter (Chapter 2), and to another general position on the problem of consciousness that is steadily gaining in popularity and attention at the time of writing. This position involves the adoption of a Russell-inspired model of the respective modes of reference of physical and phenomenal concepts, a model we can approach by first considering its more orthodox counterpart. Since the central state materialism of the 1960s, it has been common to think of physical concepts like the neurological concept C-FIBRES FIRING—which we will for the moment (counterfactually) take to be a candidate to co-refer with the phenomenal concept PAIN—as disclosing the *categorical natures* of their referents. This is what enabled the mind-brain identity theory to have its reductive physicalist character in spite of the strict egalitarian nature of the identity relation. When it was suggested that C-FIBRES FIRING co-refers with PAIN, the metaphysical upshot was that pain was reduced to c-fibres firing: a stand was taken on the categorical nature of pain. The way for this reductive result was paved by the important thesis that phenomenal concepts such as PAIN *refrain* from taking any stand on the particular nature of their referents—they were said to be 'topic neutral' concepts.[52] Given the alleged neutrality of phenomenal concepts, there was no bar to their referents being identified as ultimately physical items. Against this background, the incommensurability that many anti-physicalists intuit between the physical and the phenomenal can be captured by ascribing to them the view that phenomenal concepts *do* in fact take a stand on the nature of their referents, revealing them to cognition in unclothed form, and as devoid of any physical aspect. Since the corresponding claim is made by physicalists with respect to physical concepts, a clash is produced if both conceptual theses are taken seriously. It seems that we have on the face of it quite distinct, perhaps irreconcilable, categorical natures being revealed, respectively, by families of concepts that purport to refer, in a direct manner, to just the same thin slices of reality.[53] The anti-physicalist stances adopted by Robinson and Goff can be taken as expressing a rejection of the physicalist claim that physical concepts get to the heart of phenomenal properties.[54]

[52] It's worth saying that the philosophers of the time didn't put the idea in quite these terms: Smart (1959: 149), for example, makes the claim that *statements* reporting experiences can be translated without remainder into topic neutral vocabulary: 'When a person says "I see a yellowish-orange after-image" he is saying something like this: "*There is something going on which is like what is going on when* I have my eyes open, am awake, and there is an orange illuminated in good light in front of me".' This 'something going on' is of undetermined, and so possibly physical, character.

[53] See e.g. Demircioglu (2013) for an account of this sort of difficulty, and its possible implications for physicalism.

[54] Robinson and Goff differ subtly on the nature of the clash between physical and phenomenal conceptualizations: Robinson maintains that phenomenal conceptions positively exclude, i.e. are

The Russell-inspired model of physical/phenomenal conceptual relations is the converse of that adopted by the physicalist identity theorists of the 1960s.[55] Put in simple terms, the idea is that physical concepts in fact refer to their targets in a somewhat *indirect* way, as the fillers of certain causal/relational roles, as specified in the physical sciences (especially by physics). C-FIBRES FIRING, then, refers to that feature of the brain, whatever its ultimate nature, which fills the requisite role in neurological theory (crudely: 'activated by this, activates that, fires at this rate, etc.') and which plays the role of mediating between damaging stimulus and protective behaviour. This physical concept, however, remains (as it were) silent about the 'in-itself' nature of the role-filler that it picks out. Physical theory—the 'hard sciences'—thus sets out a *structure* of interrelated and interdefined entities and their properties, but without settling the categorical nature of the items that fill in the structure. For an example at the lower level of physics, we might consider the concept NEGATIVE ELECTRICAL CHARGE. Russellians hold that this concept picks out its referent in relational terms—mostly in terms of the dispositions the property bestows upon its bearer: to affect other charged items (i.e. to repel fellow negatively charged things and to attract positively charged ones), or to effect a magnetic field when the bearer moves.[56]

On the Russellian model, then, it is physical concepts that are topic neutral, in effect. In the case of C-FIBRES FIRING, we can therefore go on to ask what it is that plays the relevant neurological role. The elegant Russellian answer is that this slot is in fact filled by a *phenomenal* nature, a pain quale in this case. Thus C-FIBRES FIRING picks out the quale of pain by virtue of its location in the structural description of the physical sciences. It can be seen that the Russell-inspired model achieves physical-phenomenal conceptual co-reference—as demanded by physicalism—for C-FIBRES FIRING and PAIN will (applied in a given case) pick out just the same worldly goings-on.[57] Pain is thus in a sense physicalized. But this comes at the cost to the physicalist of rendering her world quite different to the one she originally envisaged. For pain, the quale, is not *reduced to* anything physical on this scheme. Rather, the 'physicality' of the pain quale, its being the 'same thing' as c-fibres firing, really boils down to the fact of the quale playing a certain (largely causally specified) relational role which it is the remit of science to set down. Ontologically speaking, the quale, as the locus and bearer of the relational properties and tendencies recorded by neuroscience, is in a good sense primary.

incompatible with, physical conceptualizations. Goff seems merely to hold that phenomenal conceptualizations don't include physical aspects. But this isn't to say that, at the conceptual level, they *could not* do so, due to the sort of positive incompatibility Robinson claims to detect.

[55] See e.g. Russell (1921) for the inspirational view in question.

[56] See McGinn (2011) for a thorough survey of the relational view of the basic physical concepts, with some interesting metaphysical conclusions drawn from this thesis.

[57] At least, if the physical concept is permitted to refer to the filler of the relevant role and not merely to the role.

The next question naturally concerns those physical concepts which don't obviously pick out phenomenal features—including the great mass of non-neurological scientific concepts. If the Russellian is right that these concepts under-specify their referents, by not taking a stand on their categorical natures, we can go on to ask what kinds of natures these are. This question is especially interesting as regards the basic concepts of *physics*, since its referents compose the physical world, and, on a non-emergentist and broadly materialist view at least, it is the properties of these fundamental items that fix the character of everything at higher levels.

There are three broad Russellian schools of thought on this issue, all of which represent promising avenues of future philosophical research. First is an option that envisages the smallest possible gap between the categorical natures Russellians hold to be picked out by neurological concepts like C-FIBRES FIRING, and those referred to by the rest of the concepts of the physical sciences. On this view—panpsychism—the entire physical world is ultimately phenomenal in character. The concept ELECTRON, then, would in a given case pick out some intrinsically conscious, phenomenally qualitied item, something for which there is an answer to the question 'What is it like to be this X?', and so on, for all other fundamental physical items. Panpsychists may justifiably feel that their theory, of all theoretical positions on the mind/body problem, makes the puzzle of how the material world can be arranged so as to support human consciousness most tractable: since consciousness is in place from the ontological outset. But they face serious objections of their own—not least, concerning the apparent metaphysical laziness of planting your *explanandum* into the very roots of your conception of the *explanans*; not to mention the difficult question of how very many tiny conscious things could unite into single-perspective consciousness of the sort we each enjoy.[58]

A second option as regards the unspecified categorical nature of the physical world is to hold that it is some resolutely non-mental nature, presently unknown—perhaps unknowable, if science is limited to relational characterization of its referents—but suitably unexciting as to merit the epithet 'physical'. This would be a sort of 'Russellian physicalism', which admits that our physical concepts fall in a sense short of their targets, but rejects the notion that anything more colourful than an unknown physical nature is needed to plug the hole.[59] The mysterious physical nature in question is conceived of as tailor-made to generate the phenomenal given the correct combinations of physical things (i.e. as comprising the relevant portions of brain/world). An obvious difficulty for this view is that the physical-phenomenal gap remains unbridged, with the generation of phenomenality every bit the conceptual obstacle it was previously. All we are really offered is a promissory note on a bridge, along with the assurance that it will be physical. Russellian physicalism would

[58] See Strawson (2006) for good accounts of panpsychism's appeal and the problems it faces. For more on the combination problem see James (1890), Goff (2009), and Chalmers (2015).

[59] Proponents include Stoljar (2006) and the second half of Pereboom (2011).

thus apparently fall foul of Goff's argument, since in introspecting consciousness we do not gain access to the elusive categorical physical nature said, on this view, to constitute the phenomenal. Moreover, there must be concerns over the sense to be accorded to the claim that there is a 'physical' nature that in principle outstrips the descriptive, if not the referential, resources of the concepts of physical science. It is just not clear what the assertion that this nature is *physical* exactly amounts to. The claim would admittedly get some grounding from a denial that the nature in question is *mental*; but this move, while it might nicely prevent panpsychism from counting as physicalism, will seemingly not discount a third, intermediate, Russellian position, which physicalists tend to find almost equally distasteful.

This third position makes the categorical nature of fundamental physical entities less than fully phenomenal, but more than recognizably physical. This would be a neutral monism of the sort Russell (following James)[60] in fact endorsed, on which the categorical character of basic physical items is of a kind with the qualitative properties encountered in consciousness, but where consciousness itself only obtains in the particular context of brains, which serve to enable a special awareness relation.[61] Physical items outside the conscious reach of brains are held to be qualia-like, but unexperienced by anyone. This middle-ground Russellianism is in practice only negligibly less off-putting to sober physicalists than full-blown panpsychism, whilst panpsychists and anti-dualists in general, not to mention many physicalists, find the notion of unexperienced qualia to be incoherent.

None of this prevents Coleman from arguing in Chapter 2 that neutral monism amounts to the sought-after Holy Grail of full physical-phenomenal integration. The first half of his chapter adapts an argument of Nagel's for panpsychism, making it an argument instead for the ubiquity of *non-conscious* qualities in basic physical matter ('panqualityism'), which move helps to evade a powerful critique of Nagel's argument due to Rosenthal. The second part of the chapter elaborates the idea of physical matter as qualitative, and offers sketches of objective explanations of qualia and consciousness. The counterintuitive consequence of the way in which Coleman makes qualities the categorical nature of basic physical matter is that they thereby become intersubjectively accessible features—a significant *desideratum* of the physicalist worldview.

Robinson, Goff, and Coleman are united in denying what might be called *austere physicalism*: the claim that phenomenal qualities are nothing over and above physical goings-on as described by current scientific concepts when these are taken at face

[60] See e.g. James (1912), Russell (1921).

[61] This is compatible with claims either that the qualia which brains enable awareness of are distal features of environmental things, or that they are internal to the brain itself. Relational conceptions of conscious awareness are on the up, quite aside from associations with neutral monism: see e.g. Rosenthal (2005) and Kriegel (2009) (both are conventional physicalists). Rosenthal's work since the 1980s has been notably influential in this resurgence of a line of thought that dates back to Aristotle's *De Anima*.

value.[62] In terms of the Russellian conceptual thesis, austere physicalism would be the claim that physical concepts alone disclose the categorical natures of their referents, i.e. what phenomenal concepts disclose to cognition is in some sense second class. However, of the three only Coleman shows any interest in preserving the truth of physicalism.

David Rosenthal's chapter (Chapter 1) provides an interesting counterpoint to the line pursued by Coleman.[63] Rosenthal also emphasizes that the qualities we find in consciousness can occur non-consciously. However, while Coleman—with Robinson and Goff—accords primacy to the conception of phenomenal qualities as based on their conscious appearance, Rosenthal privileges instead the role such qualities play in perceptual discrimination, as recorded objectively through testing subjects's responses to 'just noticeable differences' between stimuli. By assigning distinct qualities to each subjective judgement of perceptible variation in stimulus, Rosenthal envisages the construction of 'quality spaces' for our mental qualities: objectively cataloguing their differences and relative locations. The picture of qualities provided by our access via consciousness is doubly defective, Rosenthal argues, in its proneness to error, and due to the fact that this first-person mode tends to obscure the causal connections qualities stand in, promoting a conception of them as ineffable. Where Coleman maintains that qualia stand in the relations they do thanks to their quality, Rosenthal encourages us to understand their quality as nothing but the product, or expression, of their relations, internal and external. In this way, Rosenthal aims to anchor mental qualities firmly in the traditionally conceived physical world. These four chapters comprise the first section of the volume, on the ontology of phenomenal qualities.

5 Perception and Phenomenal Qualities

The second set of chapters concentrates on the location problem concerning phenomenal qualities. In Chapter 5, Michael Martin examines the dilemma presented by Moore in his 1918 paper 'Some Judgments of Perception'. In that paper Moore mooted an alternative to the sense-data theory, one which became known as the Multiple Relation Theory of Appearing (the MRTA). According to this alternative account, when it seems to a subject as if they are aware of some quality in their experience, such as a certain visual shade of red, it need not be the case that they really are aware of an actually existing entity which instantiates the quality in question.

[62] This will go equally for all future physical/scientific concepts if the physical description of the world coincides necessarily with a structural/relational conception, as some believe. What the 'current' leaves room for is that we might come to employ qualitative concepts directly in the hard sciences—reversing the trend that began in earnest with Galileo.

[63] Rosenthal presented a paper at an earlier conference in the *Phenomenal Qualities Project*, while the rest of the chapters in this collection are from the *Project*'s final conference.

In criticizing alternative interpretations of Moore's views, Martin makes a case for the claim that Moore never abandoned the central thesis of the position he adopted in his 'Refutation of Idealism' paper, that experience always involves a two-term, act-object, relation of immediate awareness to an existing object. Moore's idea, in allowing the possibility of the MRTA, is that in an illusory experience a phenomenal quality can be consciously present to the subject relative to that experience, without it belonging to the object that the perceiver is immediately aware of. However, as Martin notes in reflecting upon Moore's general treatment of experience, Moore's assumption that there always is an object to which the subject is related in experience may be questioned. Moreover, in reflecting upon the nature of visual illusions, we should acknowledge the possibility that there need not be one distinctive way of experiencing a quality: there are various different kinds of circumstance under which we can confront, for example, the colour or the shape of objects. Martin's chapter indicates one strategy for avoiding the argument from illusion that is open to a direct realist about perception.

Paul Coates (Chapter 6) sets out reasons for thinking that direct realism faces an intractable problem in providing a positive, non-causal account of the perceptual relation. That view is unable to explain what it is for a perceptual experience to be *of* a particular object. He argues that the function of perception is not to reveal the intrinsic qualities of external objects, but to enable the subject to navigate around the physical environment, so as to make beneficial use of items in it. Perceptual experiences involve the non-conceptual awareness of phenomenal qualities, which guide direct knowledge, at the cognitive level, of the location of external physical objects, their spatial structure, and—very often—of their kind. Perception also enables us to examine objects, and to enjoy aesthetic experiences. None of these roles requires us to interpret the immediate awareness of phenomenal qualities as the awareness of sensible properties belonging intrinsically to external objects. Different subjects could, in theory, and perhaps do, in practice, recruit quite different inner states in order to carry out the function of discriminating and recognizing structural and other features of their environment. These considerations help to support a causal theory of perception, according to which phenomenal qualities are located on the side of the observer, and projected onto the objects we perceive in the external world.

Galen Strawson (Chapter 7) is concerned to undo many of the confusions that have arisen about the nature of the perceptual relation, in particular about what the directness of perception does and does not entail. To perceive an object is, necessarily, to represent it in some minimal way. However, this representational state does not get in the way of the subject's direct perceptual relation to that object. Strawson defends the position he describes as 'real direct realism', arguing that in normal perception we are in direct perceptual contact with the external world. Perception is essentially a transaction between perceiver and object perceived, so that what is experienced is a function *both* of the nature of the object and of the nature of the perceiver. Direct perceptual contact, on this account, is therefore compatible with an error theory of colour. Colour, as it exists in objects, should not be conflated with colour as we experience it. Although our perceptual sensations are transparent to us phenomenologically speaking, this does not mean they are transparent in a metaphysical sense. The fact that the phenomenal qualities present in experience are located on the subject's side is not inconsistent with the phenomenology of veridical experience. When I see a clear sky, I can, if I choose, attend to my sensation of blue as such, as a feature of my inner experience. Strawson therefore rejects the disjunctivist account of experience. He further argues that it is a mistake for theories of perception to be motivated by the goal of ruling out scepticism. The resulting position, he argues, is compatible with a physicalism that properly acknowledges the reality of experiential states.

6 The Kinds and Character of Phenomenal Qualities

In the third section, more specific issues connected with theories of phenomenal qualities are explored. Jonathan Lowe defends a modest form of metaphysical realism in Chapter 8. First distinguishing different kinds of non-conceptual content, he rejects an argument for realism due to Raftopoulos, which appeals to a representational form of non-conceptual content. Lowe develops a different argument for realism, based upon a more fundamental conception of phenomenal non-conceptual content. This form of non-conceptual (and non-representational) content is introspectively accessible, relating to how things appear, in the *phenomenal* sense. We have introspective awareness of the phenomenal character of visual experience—the way the visual field is divided into different chromatic regions. Lowe argues that the visual field, diachronically, has the formal spatial feature of being a central projection of a three-dimensional Euclidean space upon a *topologically* two-dimensional spherical surface. This supports an inference to the best explanation as to why visual experience takes the form it does: the cause of the visual field is a three-dimensional Euclidian manifold, containing physical structures, and a projective mechanism—something akin to light rays—in which subjects are located.

David Papineau (Chapter 9) challenges the orthodoxy that human beings possess over a million or more conscious visual responses to coloured surfaces, a view apparently supported by our ability to experientially register a million or more differences in colour shades. Though we lack recognitional concepts corresponding to the extensive range of shades we can distinguish, it might still seem that, at some level, there are phenomenal differences far exceeding our conceptual grasp. Rejecting this inference, Papineau claims that humans are only capable of a limited number of conscious colour responses to surfaces presented singly, perhaps as few as 100. Our colour-discrimination abilities, and conscious awareness of colour, are accounted for by the combination of two different colour-related processes in the brain. One is comparative, enabling the subject to detect relational differences—e.g. brighter, different in hue, etc.—between simultaneous samples. The second process is categorial, enabling the subject to classify shades as, e.g. yellow, or red. To support his two-process account, Papineau adduces considerations concerning the apparent intransitivity of colour indiscriminability, and also neurophysiological evidence.

Michael Tye offers a sophisticated representationalist account of pain experiences in Chapter 10. One especially salient feature of pains demanding explanation is that an experience as of pain in some body part need not correspond to actual damage in any actual part of the body—in the case of phantom limb pains both damage and body part are missing. This suggests to Tye that pains are experiences that *represent there to be* damage in some body part, permitting merely intentional existence of the object. A more troublesome feature to accommodate, which sets pains apart from (at least many) perceptual experiences, is that pains include negative affect. Rejecting the proposal that pains have an imperative aspect of content (something like 'Stop this bodily disturbance!') Tye argues that adding a 'badness for the subject' element to a purely indicative content suffices to capture this feature. The chapter ends with an interesting proposal about the neurological bases of these two central features of pain—representation of damage and negative affect—explaining how they can dissociate.

In Chapter 11, Michelle Montague discusses the question of what marks out a consciously entertained thought as conscious. She argues that an adequate answer must invoke phenomenological features of the thought. But any connected sensory qualities would be at best arbitrary associates of the consciously entertained thought content, and at worst would displace the thought outright, leaving it as an unconscious event with some phenomenally conscious sensory brocade. Thus sensory phenomenology does not supply what is distinctive of a conscious thought as compared with one not currently entertained. Montague also rejects the possibility that cognitive access to thoughts (so-called 'access consciousness')[64] might make the difference to their being phenomenally conscious. She concludes that conscious thoughts must possess a proprietary brand of *cognitive phenomenology*.

7 Phenomenal Qualities and Empirical Findings

We have spoken up to now of *phenomenal* qualities as those of which we are immediately aware in consciousness, and which capture the what-it-is-like-ness of experience. But such a characterization, even when supplemented by examples, leaves open the precise extension of the term. It might be assumed that the principal route to our understanding of the general nature of sensory consciousness is via the first-person perspective. It is only because of the subjectivity of consciousness that we

[64] See Block (1995) for the original distinction. Nowadays Block is given to talk in terms of 'cognitive access', instead of the dispositional talk of 'availability to cognition' which marked his earlier discussions of a-consciousness.

can arrive at a grasp of the kinds of phenomenal qualities, such as colour, that are immediately presented in each sense modality. However, as both philosophers and psychologists have noted, introspection is a relatively poor guide when it comes to questions about the detailed nature of consciousness. Two particular problems are worth mentioning here. First, it is unclear which qualities that a subject discerns in their experience can be properly said to belong immediately to the experience itself, as opposed to those arising at an interpretative level, prompted by the awareness of properties that belong more immediately. I seem to be directly visually aware of something roughly red and round; yet arguably, I am not in the same way directly aware that what I see is a ripe and juicy tomato. To speak, as some philosophers do, of what is represented in the experience itself does not advance matters. It is still unclear on what basis we should distinguish the different conceptual and non-conceptual manners in which qualities can be represented in experience.[65] The problem of what belongs strictly as a phenomenal feature of a given experience is not one that can be easily answered. A second problem concerns the question of background consciousness. If I taste a fine wine, or look at a Persian carpet, or listen to an orchestral work, I may focus my attention on one aspect of what I am aware of; yet I seem at the same time to be conscious of further aspects of experience that I feel to be present, but which I am unable to categorize directly.

One way of making some advance on these kinds of problems is to supplement our first-person approaches, which appeal to introspection and the results of phenomenology, with a consideration of the empirical work on perception and attention, and of the theoretical models that seem best to make sense of the empirical results. Such a convergence of first- and third-person perspectives may ultimately prove a fruitful way of deepening our understanding of the structure of experience.

In the final section of this collection we present chapters linking up conceptual issues relating to the nature of phenomenal qualities with experimental work on perception in psychology and the brain sciences.

In Chapter 12, Ronald Rensink investigates the relationship between visual experience and attention. He presents a function-centred taxonomy, characterizing distinct attentional processes in terms of the different perceptual effects that can be objectively characterized and form the focus of detailed experimental work. Rather than thinking of attention as one process, we should consider it as the co-ordination of several interrelated, yet distinct, processes. Visual experiences, he argues, result from three broad systems. An initial attentional sampling of sensory input—the stage traditionally associated with overt attention—leads on to further covert attentional processes. Central to the overall transformation of perceptual information is a second stage that involves the filtering (or gating) of outputs of low-level neural processing. The result is a level of fragmented experience comprising a dense and volatile spatial

[65] The difficulties in drawing this distinction are well made in Firth's seminal article criticizing the notion of sense-data (Firth 1949); see also Goodman (1968).

field with small-scale local structure belonging to *proto-objects*. Further attentional processes—binding, holding, and individuating—lead to the construction of visual objects with greater coherence over time and space, yielding what we normally think of as the perception of objective structures in our surroundings.

Rensink offers plausible suggestions about the complex interconnections that hold between, on the one hand, the representations posited in the various processing stages of the account—the proto-objects, fragmented structures, and integrated visual objects—and on the other hand, the subject's consciousness—the awareness (conceptual or otherwise) that a subject has of coloured physical objects in his or her surroundings. Representations at the second stage, following filtering, are categorized only by their spatial features and location, and being extremely volatile, are continually replaced without being stored. Nevertheless, such low-level representations still play a crucial explanatory role in accounting for changes in attention, for priming, and for our knowledge of the overall layout, and of the gist of scenes. Their occurrence may explain the sense we can have of background unattended detail in our conscious experiences when, for example, attending to some particular feature in a complex scene. Rensink examines possible connections between the results of the higher-level attentional mechanisms, and the differences between phenomenal consciousness and access consciousness. The relationship between phenomenal experience and attention turns out to be a complex one, suggesting that a full understanding of these interrelations awaits more detailed investigation of matters both experimental and conceptual.

Ophelia Deroy (Chapter 13) opposes the view that a synaesthetic experience is to be analysed as a conjunction of two distinct elements, a normal experience, together with an atypical sensory content, which is tacked on as an extra feature. Such dual-component accounts usually make two assumptions: that normal and synaesthetic experiences can share similar overlapping contents, and that such contents are in principle separable from each other. Deroy presents reasons for objecting to these assumptions on conceptual grounds, also drawing from empirical research in psychology. Strictly speaking, synaesthetic experiences are not experiences that normal subjects can imagine having. What can be discriminated as one aspect of a synaesthetic experience is not necessarily a feature that is conceptually separable and distinct from the other aspects of experience. Instead, Deroy recommends that we think of the synaesthetic concurrents in experience as analogous to extra dimensions of experience, as a form of phenomenal enrichment. Deroy further argues that synaesthetic experiences are not straightforwardly subjective; they have some objectively representational properties.

John Nicholas defends the much-maligned sense-data theory of perception in Chapter 14. On this view, when one sees an external world scene, one does so by being aware in the first instance of a mental object possessing analogues of the properties perceptually ascribed to the distal stimulus, i.e. colours, shapes, and so on. Nicholas is primarily concerned to purge the theory of its connotations of dualism—traditional exponents often located sense-data in a non-physical portion of the perceiver. On Nicholas's theory, however, sense-data are neurally implemented. He examines in depth several proposals for their location in the brain, along the way defusing neuroscientific evidence adduced against any central phenomenal 'locus', and eventually settling on the superior colliculus as a plausible site, due to the convergence there of several sensory processing channels. He makes detailed proposals about the neurophysiology of the sense-data array, and also takes the time to respond to the 'homunculus fallacy' often raised against sense-data accounts.

8 Conclusion

Both subjective and objective approaches to the philosophical issues connected with phenomenal qualities generate extremely important challenges. The concepts advanced in the sciences to make sense of perception, consciousness, and attention still leave their fundamental character unexplained. On any view about the structure of experience, there are deep—and so far unresolved—problems regarding the nature of phenomenal qualities, and their relation to physical reality. These problems have profound implications for questions about the way human consciousness fits into the world. The chapters in this collection explore these problems in detail and aim to deepen our understanding of them, and of the prospects for their solution.

References

Anscombe, E. (1965), 'The Intentionality of Sensation: A Grammatical Feature', in R. Butler (ed.), *Analytical Philosophy: Second Series* (Oxford: Blackwell), 158–80.

Ayer, A. J. (1940), *The Foundations of Empirical Knowledge* (London: Macmillan).

Bennett, J. F. (1974), *Kant's Dialectic* (Cambridge: Cambridge University Press).

Block, N. (1995), 'On a Confusion about a Function of Consciousness', in *Behavioural and Brain Sciences* 18: 227–47.

Block, N. (2003), 'Mental Paint', in M. Hahn and B. Ramberg (eds), *Reflections and Replies: Essays on the Philosophy of Tyler Burge* (Cambridge, MA: MIT Press), 165–200.

Block, N. (2005), 'Bodily Sensations as an Obstacle for Representationism', in M. Aydede (ed.), *Pain* (Cambridge, MA: MIT Press), 137–42.

Block, N. and Stalnaker, R. (1999), 'Conceptual Analysis, Dualism, and the Explanatory Gap', in *Philosophical Review* 108 (1): 1–46.

Byrne, A. (2001), 'Intentionalism Defended', in *The Philosophical Review* 110 (2): 199–240.

Byrne, A. (2011), 'Sensory Qualities, Sensible Qualities, Sensational Qualities', in B. McLaughlin and A. Bekermann (eds), *The Oxford Handbook of Philosophy of Mind* (Oxford: Oxford University Press).

Byrne, A. and Logue, H. (eds) (2009), *Disjunctivism: Contemporary Readings* (Cambridge, MA: MIT Press).

Campbell, J. (2002), *Reference and Consciousness* (Oxford: Clarendon Press).

Chalmers, D. J. (1996), *The Conscious Mind* (New York: Oxford University Press).

Chalmers, D. J. (2004), 'The Representational Character of Experience', in B. Leiter (ed.), *The Future for Philosophy* (Oxford: Oxford University Press).

Chalmers, D. J. (2015), 'The Combination Problem for Panpsychism', in G. Brüntrup and L. Jaskolla (eds), *Panpsychism* (Oxford: Oxford University Press).

Chisholm, R. M. (1957), *Perceiving: A Philosophical Study* (Ithaca, NY: Cornell University Press).

Clark, A. (1993), *Sensory Qualities* (Oxford: Clarendon Press).

Coates, P. (2007), *The Metaphysics of Perception: Wilfrid Sellars, Perceptual Consciousness and Critical Realism* (London/New York: Routledge).

Coates, P. (2009), 'The Multiple Contents of Experience: Representation and the Awareness of Phenomenal Qualities', in *Philosophical Topics: Perception and Intentionality* 37 (1): 25–48.

Crane, T. (2001), *Elements of Mind* (Oxford: Oxford University Press).

Demircioglu, E. (2013), 'Physicalism and Phenomenal Concepts', in *Philosophical Studies* 165 (1): 257–77.

Drake, D. (ed.), (1920), *Essays in Critical Realism* (New York: Macmillan).

Ducasse, C. J. (1942), 'Moore's Refutation of Idealism', in P. Schilpp (ed.), *The Philosophy of G. E. Moore* (Chicago, IL: Northwestern University Press), 223–52.

Firth, R. (1949), 'Sense-Data and the Percept Theory, Part 1', in *Mind* 58: 434–65; reprinted in R. Swartz (ed.) (1965), *Perceiving, Sensing, and Knowing* (New York: Anchor Books), 204–42.

Fish, W. (2009), *Perception, Hallucination and Illusion* (Oxford: Oxford University Press).

Foster, J. (1991), *The Immaterial Self* (London: Routledge).

Goff, P. (2009), 'Why Panpsychism Doesn't Help to Explain Consciousness', in *Dialectica* 63 (3): 289–311.

Goodman, N. (1968), *Languages of Art: An Approach to a Theory of Symbols* (Indianapolis, IN: Bobbs-Merrill).

Grice, H. P. (1961), 'The Causal Theory of Perception', in *Supplementary Proceedings of the Aristotelian Society* 35: 121–52.

Haddock, A. and Macpherson, F. (eds) (2008), *Disjunctivism: Perception, Action, Knowledge* (Oxford: Oxford University Press).

Harman, G. (1990), 'The Intrinsic Quality of Experience', in *Philosophical Perspectives* 4: 31–52.

Holt, E. B. et al. (1912), *The New Realism: Co-operative Studies in Philosophy* (New York: Macmillan).

Husserl, E. (1913/1931), *Ideas*, translated by W. R. Boyce Gibson (London: George Allen and Unwin).

Jackson, F. (1982), 'Epiphenomenal Qualia', in *Philosophical Quarterly* 32 (2): 127–36.

Jackson, F. (2003), 'Mind and Illusion', in Anthony O'Hear (ed.), *Minds and Persons* (Cambridge: Cambridge University Press).

Jackson, F. (2007), 'Colour for Representationalists', in *Erkenntnis* 66: 169–85.

James, W. (1890), *The Principles of Psychology* (New York: Dover).

James, W. (1912), *Essays in Radical Empiricism* (New York: Longmans).

Johnston, M. (2004), 'The Obscure Object of Hallucination', in *Philosophical Studies* 120 (1–3): 113–83.

Kind, A. (2003), 'What's So Transparent about Transparency?', in *Philosophical Studies* 115 (3): 225–44.

Kirk, R. (2006), *Zombies and Consciousness* (Oxford: Oxford University Press).
Kriegel, U. (2009), *Subjective Consciousness: A Self-Representational Theory* (New York: Oxford University Press).
Leibniz, G. W. (1714/1991), *The Monadology*, in *Discourse on Metaphysics and Other Essays*, edited and translated by D. Garber and R. Ariew (Indianapolis, IN: Hackett Publishing Company).
Levine, J. (1983), 'Materialism and Qualia: The Explanatory Gap', in *Pacific Philosophical Quarterly* 64: 354–61.
Levine, J. (2001), *Purple Haze* (Oxford: Oxford University Press).
Loar, B. (1990), 'Phenomenal States', in *Philosophical Perspectives* 4: 81–108.
Lowe, J. (1996), *Subjects of Experience* (Cambridge: Cambridge University Press).
Lycan, W. (1987), *Consciousness* (Cambridge, MA: MIT Press).
Mackie, J. (1976), *Problems from Locke* (Oxford: Oxford University Press).
Macpherson, F. and Platchias, D. (eds) (2013), *Hallucination: Philosophy and Psychology* (Cambridge, MA: MIT Press).
Martin, M. G. F. (2002), 'The Transparency of Experience', in *Mind and Language* 17: 376–425.
Martin, M. G. F. (2006), 'On Being Alienated', in T. Z. Gendler and J. Hawthorne (eds), *Perceptual Experience* (Oxford: Oxford University Press), 354–410.
McDowell, J. H. (1986), 'Singular Thought and the Extent of Inner Space', in P. Pettit and J. H. McDowell (eds), *Subject, Thought, and Context* (Oxford: Clarendon Press), 137–68.
McGinn, C. (1989), 'Can We Solve the Mind-Body Problem', in *Mind* 98 (3): 349–66.
McGinn, C. (1996), 'Another Look at Color', in *Journal of Philosophy*, XCIII(11): 537–53.
McGinn, C. (2011), *Basic Structures of Reality: Essays in Meta-Physics* (Oxford: Oxford University Press).
McIntyre, R. and Woodruff Smith, D. (1989), 'Theory of Intentionality', in J. N. Mohanty and W. R. McKenna (eds), *Husserl's Phenomenology: A Textbook* (Washington, DC: Centre for Advanced Research in Phenomenology and University Press of America), 147–79.
Millar, A. (1995), 'The Idea of Experience', in *Proceedings of the Aristotelian Society* 96: 75–90.
Moore, G. E. (1913), 'The Status of Sense-Data', in *Proceedings of the Aristotelian Society* 14: 355–81.
Moore, G. E. (1918), 'Some Judgments of Perception', in *Proceedings of the Aristotelian Society* 19: 1–29.
Nagel, T. (1974), 'What Is It Like to Be a Bat?', in *The Philosophical Review* 83: 435–50.
Papineau, D. (2002), *Thinking about Consciousness* (Oxford: Oxford University Press).
Pereboom, D. (2011), *Consciousness and the Prospects of Physicalism* (New York: Oxford University Press).
Papineau, D. (2013), 'Sensory Experience and Representational Properties', in *Proceedings of the Aristotelian Society* 114 (1): 1–29.
Pitt, D. (2004), 'The Phenomenology of Cognition, or, What Is It Like to Think That *P*?', in *Philosophy and Phenomenological Research* 69 (1): 1–36.
Robinson, H. (1994), *Perception* (London: Routledge).
Robinson, H. (2013), 'The Failure of Disjunctivism to Deal with "Philosophers' Hallucinations"', in F. Macpherson and D. Platchias (eds), *Hallucination: Philosophy and Psychology* (Cambridge, MA: MIT Press), 313–30.
Rosenthal, D. (2005), *Consciousness and Mind* (Oxford: Clarendon Press).

Rosenthal, D. (2010), 'How to Think about Mental Qualities', in *Philosophical Issues* 20 (1): 368–93.

Russell, B. (1912), *The Problems of Philosophy* (London: Williams and Norgate).

Russell, B. (1914), 'The Relation of Sense-Data to Physics', in *Scientia* 4; reprinted in Russell, B. (1917), *Mysticism and Logic* (London: Allen and Unwin), 108–31.

Russell, B. (1918), 'The Philosophy of Logical Atomism' reprinted in R. C. Marsh (ed.) (1956), *Logic and Knowledge* (London: Allen and Unwin), 177–281.

Russell, B. (1921), *The Analysis of Mind* (London: Allen and Unwin).

Sellars, W. (1956/1997), *Empiricism and the Philosophy of Mind*, edited by R. Brandom (Cambridge, MA: Harvard University Press).

Sellars, W. (1975), 'The Structure of Knowledge: (1) Perception; (2) Minds; (3) Epistemic Principles', in H. Casteñeda (ed.), *Action Knowledge and Reality* (Indianapolis, IN: Bobbs-Merrill), 277–347.

Sellars, W. (1978), 'The Role of Imagination in Kant's Theory of Experience', in H. W. Johnstone (ed.), *Categories: A Colloquium* (Philadelphia: Pennsylvania State University).

Sellars, W. (1981), 'Foundations for a Metaphysics of Pure Process: Carus Lectures', in *The Monist* 64 (1): 3–90.

Sellars, W. (1982), 'Sensa or Sensings: Reflections on the Ontology of Perception', in *Philosophical Studies* 41: 83–111.

Siegel, S. (2008), 'The Epistemic Conception of Hallucination', in A. Haddock and F. Macpherson (eds), *Disjunctivism: Perception, Action, and Knowledge* (Oxford: Oxford University Press).

Smart, J. C. C. (1959), 'Sensations and Brain Processes', in *Philosophical Review* 68 (2): 141–56.

Snowdon, P. (1981), 'Perception, Vision and Causation', in *Proceedings of the Aristotelian Society* 81: 175–92.

Snowdon, P. (2005), 'On the Interpretation of Disjunctivism', in *Proceedings of the Aristotelian Society* 105: 129–41.

Stoljar, D. (2005), 'Physicalism and Phenomenal Concepts', in *Mind and Language* 20 (2): 296–302.

Stoljar, D. (2006), *Ignorance and Imagination* (New York: Oxford University Press).

Strawson, G. (2006), 'Realistic Monism—Why Physicalism Entails Panpsychism', in *Journal of Consciousness Studies* 13 (10–11): 3–31.

Travis, C. (2004), 'The Silence of the Senses', in *Mind* 113: 57–94.

Tye, M. (2000), *Consciousness, Color, and Content* (Cambridge, MA: MIT Press).

Tye, M. (2009), *Consciousness Revisited: Materialism without Phenomenal Concepts* (Cambridge, MA: MIT Press).

Valberg, J. J. (1992), *The Puzzle of Experience* (Oxford: Clarendon Press).

SECTION I

The Ontology of Phenomenal Qualities

1

Quality Spaces and Sensory Modalities

David Rosenthal

1.1 Introduction

Perhaps nothing in the theoretical study of mind has occasioned more debate than the qualitative character of states such as perceptions, bodily sensations, and emotions. Such qualitative character seems to resist physicalist treatment and, moreover, to cause difficulties beyond those that affect accounts of purely intentional states, such as thoughts and desires.

But before one can usefully address the question of whether some phenomenon, mental or otherwise, can be given a naturalist or physicalist account, one must have some suitable way of fixing the phenomenon we want to account for. Many discussions take it for granted that we can do that well enough by way of our introspective or intuitive understanding of qualitative character, and that nothing beyond the deliverances of intuition and introspection is needed. Indeed, many discussions assume that there simply is nothing more to say about what it is for a mental occurrence to exhibit qualitative character or what such qualitative character consists in. We know what it is simply from our being in states that exhibit it; there is no more informative account to be had.[1]

Such an approach is unduly dismissive. First-person access is doubtless important to understanding the nature of conscious qualitative character. But we also ascribe states with qualitative character to others, and indeed often feel confident that we know, independent of others' reports, what qualitative states they are in. So we must have some understanding of what qualitative character consists in cast in third-person terms.

The idea that we know nothing of the nature of qualitative mentality except what first-person access tells us does much to undermine any promise of a naturalist or

[1] Ned Block gives vivid expression to this approach when he writes: 'You ask: What is it that philosophers have called qualitative states? I answer, only half in jest: As Louis Armstrong said when asked what jazz is, "If you got to ask, you ain't never gonna get to know"' (Block 1978: 1.3).

physicalist account of qualitative character, since any such account would have to rely on informative features of qualitative character even to get started. Our knowing that water is identical with H_2O is informative because we have some informative grasp independent of that identity of what water is; without any such independent grasp, the identity would at best seem uninformative and mysterious. We need an informative account of qualitative character before assessing whether a physicalist or naturalist account of it is possible.

Elsewhere I have argued that any approach to qualitative character that relies exclusively on intuition and introspective awareness is mistaken, and that an alternative account is available that is richly informative (e.g., Rosenthal 2005: ch. 5–7, 2010, forthcoming, and 1999). We can describe and explain mental qualities not by appeal to what it's like for us to be in conscious states that exhibit qualitative character, but instead by appeal to the role states with qualitative character play in perception. And the appeal to perceptual role covers more ground, since perceiving sometimes occurs without being conscious. So such an approach will account for subliminal as well as conscious perceiving, and indeed be independent of consciousness, intuition, and introspective awareness.

The best way to take perceptual role into consideration will rely on the ability an individual has to discriminate stimuli, since all perception involves discrimination. Proceeding this way lets us explain mental qualities as the mental properties in virtue of which an individual can perform perceptual discriminations. And since perceptual discrimination occurs in respect of various dimensions, the mental qualities that enable such discrimination can be arranged into a quality space. I'll call the resulting theory of qualitative character quality-space theory (QST). The resulting characterization of mental qualities gives the theory considerable explanatory power, enabling us to understand such things as the role of mental qualities in perceiving, the relations qualitative states bear to other mental phenomena, and the role qualitative character plays in mental representation (e.g., Rosenthal 2005: ch. 7, 2001, and Berger, under submission).

QST may seem especially inviting for mental qualities of color, since the discriminations we make among color stimuli are readily arranged along dimensions of hue, brightness, and saturation. But it arguably works no less well with complex and difficult sensory modalities, such as olfaction (Young, Keller, and Rosenthal 2014).

But apart from the taxonomy of particular types of mental quality, there is another question about qualitative character: how to individuate these various perceptual modalities themselves. This is an ancient question, discussed at length in Aristotle's *de Anima* and in contemporary times in Paul Grice's deservedly famous 'Some Remarks about the Senses'.[2]

[2] Aristotle (1993), Grice (1962), and Macpherson (2011), which reprints Grice (1962) and selections from Aristotle's *de Anima*, Books II and III, and to which Macpherson contributes an impressive, detailed preface.

There are standard answers to the question of individuating the modalities, which have received extensive discussion. Among them is some appeal to the nature of the stimuli each modality senses, the type of representation each modality subserves, the organ used in the sensing, or some combination of these.

It may seem especially tempting to individuate the modalities simply by appeal to the type of mental quality that occurs in each. It may seem clear intuitively that the mental qualities of vision, for example, differ from those of audition, and so forth. But any such account requires an independent grasp of how the mental qualities distinctive of each modality differ from those distinctive of the others, an account that does not simply appeal to the modalities being individuated. So the threats of triviality or circularity loom large for any such account.

Still, the question about modalities plainly intersects with issues about qualitative character even if an individuation of modalities in terms of types of mental state is itself not promising. However one individuates the modalities and however one taxonomizes the mental qualities, the two accounts will not only have to assign the right mental qualities to the right modalities, but will also have to fit comfortably with one another.

In what follows, I'll argue that we can use the methodology of QST itself not only to taxonomize the mental qualities, but also to individuate the perceptual modalities. This methodology yields accounts of both the mental qualities and the modalities that are theoretically sound and experimentally testable. The methodology delivers results that largely conform to pretheoretic expectations about the modalities, but nonetheless allows for principled revision to our commonsense taxonomy.

In section 1.2, I review the way QST taxonomizes mental qualities, sticking for examples mainly to mental qualities of color and making no explicit mention of differences among the modalities. In section 1.3, then, I appeal to the considerations QST uses to taxonomize the mental qualities to develop a methodology for individuating the modalities, and reply to various objections to this approach to the modalities. In the concluding section 1.4 I consider some consequences of adopting this methodology for understanding qualitative mentality.

1.2 Quality-Space Theory

There are two ways the qualitative character of perceiving, sensing, and emotions figure prominently in our mental lives. One is that qualitative character appears subjectively in our stream of consciousness; the other is the role qualitative character plays in perception and, in particular, in perceptual discrimination among perceptible stimuli. This provides two ways to approach questions about the nature of qualitative character and how to taxonomize mental qualities.

In the search for an informative account, we cannot afford to ignore what either approach can tell us. But as already noted, relying just on subjective awareness of mental qualities leads to uninformative results. This is to be expected. For one thing, we typically learn about the nature of things by appeal at least in part to causal ties they have with each other and with other phenomena. But subjective awareness of qualitative character reveals nothing about the causal ties qualitative states have with other mental states and with behavior. Indeed, subjective awareness by itself reveals nothing even about causal ties qualitative states have with relevant stimuli; we have no subjective awareness of such causal ties, but must rely instead on folk-psychological inferences from qualitative state to stimulus.

In addition, relying exclusively on subjective awareness restricts access to mental qualities to one's own case. Subjective awareness is first-person access, which can provide access only to one's own mental qualities. Indeed, that goes hand in hand with the inability of subjective awareness to reveal the causal ties that qualitative states have with anything else or one another. When we know that somebody else is in pain or has a particular visual experience, such knowledge is largely due to knowing the causal ties folk psychology tells us obtain between qualitative states, behavior, and stimuli. Subjective awareness can tell us nothing here.

The restriction to first-person access makes it seem inviting to imagine that when you and I look at a red object, the mental quality you have might be the same as the mental quality I have on seeing something green, and that such inversion would be undetectable. Only if one relies exclusively on subjective awareness to taxonomize mental qualities could one hold that such inversion could be undetectable, or even that we can conceive of such a situation's being undetectable; if any factor other than subjective awareness figures in the way we taxonomize mental qualities, such inversion would plainly be detectable. Such considerations have led some to imagine also that creatures exactly like us in every detectable respect might nonetheless lack qualitative mentality, that is, conscious qualitative mentality, or at least that this is conceivable (e.g., Chalmers 1996: 94). Only if we restrict ourselves to first-person access could we even imagine such a thing.

The restriction to one's own case, the apparent possibility of undetectable inversion, and the failure to reveal any causal ties all speak to the uninformative nature of the access to mental qualities that subjective awareness provides. But there is another important downside to the exclusive reliance on subjective awareness.

It is beyond dispute that perceiving occurs not only consciously, but without being conscious as well, in masked priming and other forms of subliminal perceiving (e.g., Marcel 1983, Breitmeyer and Öğmen 2006, and Öğmen and Breitmeyer 2006). Absent special assumptions about how to taxonomize mental qualities, the natural and indeed inevitable conclusion would be that, apart from the property of being conscious itself, whatever mental properties occur in conscious perceiving also occur in the subliminal, nonconscious case.

Those, like Thomas Nagel (1974), who take subjective awareness to be essential to qualitative character and accordingly our only access to its occurrence, would deny that subliminal, nonconscious perceiving exhibits any qualitative character, properly so called. But this overlooks a crucial aspect of the way we think about mental qualitative character. As noted above, we sometimes are completely confident from third-person evidence that another individual is in pain or perceives a particular stimulus. And if I am in pain and you know in a third-person way that I am, the state you know me to be in is a state of the very sort that I am subjectively aware of being in.

So if you had the same third-person evidence and I failed to be subjectively aware of being in pain, there should be no difference in the type of state you know me to be in except that in the second case the pain in question is not a conscious state. The only way conscious qualitative states differ from those that are not conscious is in respect of the property of being conscious. Apart from simply assuming that subjective awareness is essential to qualitative character and the only way to come to know about it, we have no reason to insist that states that lack the property of being conscious also lack qualitative character. And there seems to be no reason to adopt that assumption that is not simply stipulative.

Some have sought to preserve special status for subjective awareness by positing two types of concept we use in thinking about qualitative states, third-person concepts cast in functional terms and phenomenal concepts, whose mode of presentation is some mental quality as one is subjectively aware of it (e.g., Stoljar 2005, Chalmers 2007, and Balog 2009). But the challenge for such an appeal to phenomenal concepts is to explain how, if you assert that you are in pain and I say that you are not, I am denying what you assert. Your assertion would express your phenomenal concept, and my denial expresses my third-person concept; so what we say conflicts only if there is a suitable connection between phenomenal and third-person concepts. But since the modes of presentation of phenomenal concepts are mental qualities as one is subjectively aware of them, nothing in such concepts can ensure even that they are coextensive with third-person concepts of mental qualities.

Exclusive reliance on subjective awareness is not a satisfactory way to approach our understanding of qualitative character. And there is an alternative. Mental qualities play a distinctive role in perceiving, and in particular in perceptual discriminations. So we can take advantage of that discriminative role to understand the nature of mental qualities and develop a methodology for taxonomizing them into types. It is this approach that underlies QST.

Consider seeing colors. For colors broadly taxonomized, we all recognize that orange is closer, at least in respect of hue, to both red and yellow than it is to either green or blue. Similarly for brightness and saturation; shades of red that are quite bright or saturated resemble one another in that respect at least more than they resemble shades that are quite dark or unsaturated. These broad-stroked similarity relations allow one to construct a relatively coarse-grained space of colors, with dimensions for hue, saturation, and brightness, which capture these relations of similarity and difference.

But our arsenal of such relations can be made as fine-grained as one pleases. In the limit, we can test experimentally for just noticeable differences (JNDs), that is, color stimuli that are so close physically that were they physically any closer they would be perceptually indistinguishable.[3] So instead of a coarse-grained taxonomy of red, green, and the like, we can construct a quality space (QS) of perceptible color stimuli based on such JNDs. This yields a 3-dimensional color space with maximum fineness of grain.[4]

The JND methodology yields a space of perceptible color stimuli, though it can be applied to stimuli perceptually distinguishable by any sensory modality, and indeed to stimuli that result in bodily sensations of various types, such as pains, tickles, itches, and the like, and even to different types of pains, tickles, and itches. And this has a direct bearing on taxonomizing the mental qualities and on their nature.

For an individual to discriminate two perceptible stimuli, that individual must be able to be in two types of perceptual state, each corresponding to one of the two stimuli. If the stimuli are JND, the individual will be in perceptual states as close as the individual's discriminative ability allows for stimuli of that sort. We can think of any pair of stimuli that an individual can discriminate as separated by some number of JND steps,[5] and to be able to discriminate those stimuli from one another and from each of the JND stimuli in between, the individual must be able to be in states that differ correspondingly. So the QS that represents the stimuli an individual can discriminate will also represent the similarities and differences among the perceptual states in virtue of which such discriminations are possible for that individual.

What is it for one stimulus to be comparable to another? In virtue of what does one stimulus belong in the same QS as another? These are questions about the individuation of perceptual modalities and about which stimuli and which mental qualities belong to which modality. In section 1.3 I will argue that the methodology of QST for individuating mental-quality types provides us with answers to these questions. But for now I will simply assume a commonsense understanding of the various modalities, and postpone addressing those questions till that later section.

The QS for a particular range of perceptible stimuli serves to fix the types of perceptual state that figure in discriminating among that range of stimuli. But when

[3] The methodology of JNDs delivers results that are not transitive; one stimulus can be JND from a second and the second from a third without the first being JND from the third. An alternative methodology is that of matching: Instead of making stimuli physically closer until they're perceptually indistinguishable, start with physically identical stimuli and make them physically diverge until they become perceptually distinguishable. Matching also delivers results that are not transitive; *a* can match *b* and *b* match *c* without *a*'s matching *c*. But as Nelson Goodman (1951: 221) in effect notes, matching allows for a neater individuation of types than JNDs; we can rule that one stimulus is perceptually the same as another if, but only if, they perceptually match all the same stimuli. And that allows us in turn to handle the failure of transitivity of being JND; two stimuli are JND as soon as matching fails. But this methodological refinement will not matter for present purposes.

[4] For an example of such a color space, see *Commission Internationale de l'Eclairage Proceedings, 1931* (1932). There are many others. For more on quality spaces, see Clark (1993). For the special case of color, see Clark (1993) and also Kuehni (2003, especially ch. 6; and 2010).

[5] The lack of transitivity of JNDs introduces a complication; see n. 3. To get an accurate measure in terms of steps, one would need to use matching instead of JNDs.

we discriminate one stimulus from another, we are able to do so because our perceptual states differ relevantly in respect of their qualitative character. So the QS that captures a range of discriminable stimuli also tells us what mental qualities figure in such discriminations. Sticking with color, the QS that describes the JNDs among perceptible color stimuli also tells us what the mental color qualities are for the individual in question.

Since the QS that captures a range of perceptible stimuli also provides an account of the mental qualities in virtue of which we are aware of those stimuli, it is natural to regard each mental quality as representing the stimulus that occupies the position in its QS isomorphic to the position of the mental quality. But QST is not on that account a representationalist theory of mental qualities, at least of the form pioneered by Gilbert Harman (1990) and Alex Byrne (2001), since the representing of the stimuli is not done by intentional or conceptual content. More important, we are, contrary to Harman and Byrne, aware of mental qualities as such when we are introspectively conscious of our qualitative states. And we are aware of them not as representational states, but as mental qualities, as properties that mirror somehow the properties we are aware of in perception.

Experimental testing of JNDs must be done in circumstances that allow for optimal discrimination; so no appeal to typical circumstances of perception, often made in such discussions, is relevant here. QST relies on the most fine-grained discriminations an individual can make between very similar stimuli, since that will reveal the most fine-grained differences among the mental qualities that figure in such discriminations. QST appeals to whatever perceptual circumstances maximize fineness of discrimination.

Testing JNDs for the stimuli accessible by any perceptual modality must be done one individual at a time, and individuals differ in their discriminative ability. Individuals differ in color discrimination partly because the distribution of color-sensitive cells in the retina differs from one individual to another. In addition, extended exposure to a range of stimuli or training with respect to that range can enhance the fineness of grain with which an individual can discriminate stimuli within that range, a process known as perceptual learning (e.g., Sasaki et al. 2010). So the QSs that represent the discriminative ability in respect of a range of stimuli for some particular species, say, humans, are always an idealization, averaging over individuals.[6]

Using JNDs to establish types of mental quality has the signal advantage that it allows taxonomizing mental qualities wholly independent of whether the relevant qualitative states are conscious. Perceiving occurs subliminally, that is, without being conscious, and perceiving invariably relies on discrimination of perceptible properties. Indeed, even perceptual learning occurs subliminally (e.g., Watanabe et al. 2001).

[6] Different methods of averaging may yield different results, but such refinements are not relevant for present purposes.

So such discrimination also must occur without being conscious. Since the QSs of perceptible properties constructed from JNDs do not require the relevant discriminations to be conscious, the mental qualities fixed by those QSs need not themselves be conscious.

And there is ample evidence for nonconscious JNDs. When stimuli are degraded, subjects' JND judgments remain accurate even when subjects take themselves to be merely guessing (e.g., Cheesman and Merikle 1986, Merikle 1992, Mealor and Dienes 2012, Dienes and Seth 2010, and Dienes 2004). Forced-choice guesses about whether two stimuli differ remain accurate even when the individual guessing has little or no confidence in those guesses. And somebody's guessing about something is a good indicator that the individual is not consciously aware of it. So taking oneself to be guessing about JNDs shows that the JNDs are not conscious. Constructing the QSs that fix mental-quality types by JNDs alone allows QST to proceed altogether independently of whether the relevant perceiving is conscious.

One might object that the mental qualities must, after all, be conscious, since otherwise one would be unable to compare the QS of perceptible stimuli with that of mental qualities and determine that they are isomorphic. That misconstrues the methodology of QST. QST does not rely on comparing the two QSs. Rather, it reasons that differences in mental quality are responsible for an individual's ability to discriminate perceptible stimuli. So the QS that captures discriminable differences among those stimuli must also fix differences among the mental qualities that enable those discriminations. Imagining that QST must compare the QSs that describe discriminable stimuli with those that fix the types of mental quality rests on assuming, contrary to QST, that taxonomizing of mental qualities can occur only by appeal to the way we are subjectively aware of them.

And the methodology of QST not only explains how to taxonomize mental qualities independent of such subjective awareness; it also undermines the idea that one can rely on subjective awareness in constructing a satisfactory taxonomy. Suppose that qualitative character is invariably conscious. One might take that by itself to underwrite a technique for taxonomizing mental qualities. One could individuate mental-quality types by appeal to what it's like for one to be in particular qualitative states, by appeal, that is, to how the mental qualities in question subjectively appear to consciousness.

Perhaps the resulting taxonomy would conform to QSs constructed from JNDs. Perhaps what it's like for one to be in two distinct qualitative states would always provide just those similarities and differences that the QS-theoretic methodology reveals. But it is by no means obvious that this would be so. And there is reason to think it would not. For one thing, we can expect subjective awareness to discriminate in a less fine-grained way than discrimination that occurs without such awareness, since JND judgments are stable even when individuals take themselves simply to be guessing. And subjective awareness is doubtless subject to biases due to attention, expectation (e.g., Shankar et al. 2001), and other distorting confounds.

So some conflict between JNDs and subjective awareness is likely. And when the two techniques for taxonomizing mental qualities diverge, we must invariably go with QST. Mental qualities indisputably figure in perceptual discriminations. So whatever results derive from their role in such discriminating must take precedence over the way they subjectively appear in consciousness. Not only is there reason to be wary of factors that can lead such subjective appearances astray, but also we know that not all mental qualities even occur consciously. QST must trump subjective appearances.

QST relies on first taxonomizing perceptible physical properties, such as the physical colors, and extrapolating from that to a taxonomy of corresponding mental qualities. But one might object that this gets things the wrong way around. Indeed, color vision may seem to present a special difficulty here. Which colors humans perceive is due not to stimulation of one type of retinal receptor cell, but rather to the ratio of stimulation of the three types of daylight receptor cells. And different wavelengths can result in the same ratio of receptor stimulation, and in such cases we see those different stimuli as being the same color. Sets of different wavelengths that result in this way in color perceptions that are indistinguishable are known as metamers.

Metamerism has led some to conclude that there simply are no colors, conceived of as properties of perceptible physical objects (e.g., Hardin 1993). This plainly overshoots; we can identify the physical colors as reflectance profiles of physical objects taxonomized by appeal to their effect on an individual's visual system. We will not then identify any particular color type with a single reflectance profile, but rather with a set of such profiles that in conditions of maximal discriminability are indistinguishable. The physical colors are fixed by these equivalence sets of physical reflectance profiles.[7]

The upshot is that we need not understand the mental qualities independent of the relevant physical stimuli, though we must taxonomize those stimuli by appeal to the way particular individuals discriminate them. We need not appeal to mental qualities first; indeed, there would be no way to do so other than by way of subjective awareness, which carries with it various sources of distortion and shortcomings in respect of fineness of grain. We can instead, with QST, fix the mental qualities by the way individuals discriminate among physical stimuli, though those stimuli are identified independently of such discrimination. This point will be pivotal when we turn in section 1.3 to the individuation of the sensory modalities.

QST taxonomizes the mental qualities of each modality comparatively. What type a mental quality belongs to depends on its relative location in the relevant QS, that is,

[7] It's important, however, to note that relativity to perceptual discriminability pertains only to the taxonomy of the relevant reflectance profiles. Those profiles exist independent of any actual discrimination and, indeed, independent of any creatures with the ability to perceive those reflectance profiles. Perceptible colors are straightforwardly physical properties. For more, see Rosenthal (2001).

on its relations of similarity and difference to other mental qualities in that QS, which depend on its JNDs in respect of its closest neighbors. So the position of each mental-quality type, according to QST, rests on its discriminability relative to other mental-quality types in the relevant QS.

There is considerable reason to taxonomize mental qualities comparatively, despite some superficial pull of the idea that each mental quality is what it is just on its own. The color appearances that particular stimuli present vary, often quite dramatically, with the colors of the surround, an effect known as simultaneous color contrast.[8] Such variation is not due to the way we are subjectively aware of our color experiences, since the effect arises in the earliest stages of visual processing, prior to subjective awareness. Particular color stimuli give rise to very different mental color qualities depending on visible context and independent of subjective awareness. This by itself points to a comparative taxonomy of those mental qualities.

Still, it may seem that the way subjective awareness presents each mental quality is on its own, each independent of the others. And subjective awareness might seem by itself sufficient to determine how we should taxonomize mental qualities, regardless of such perceptual phenomena as simultaneous color contrast. So if subjective awareness does present qualitative states noncomparatively, that would undermine any comparative taxonomy.

But it is not at all clear that subjective awareness does actually present each type of mental quality independent of the others. The primary temptation for holding that it does is doubtless the idea that subjective awareness tells us what it's like for one to be in each qualitative state on its own (e.g., Nagel 1974, Chalmers 1996, and Jackson 1986), and that underwrites a noncomparative taxonomy. But this is a mistake. What it's like for one to be in a particular qualitative state tells us nothing about what type of state it is independent of other comparable states.

It is tempting to think otherwise and to see knowing what it's like as a way of knowing what kind of state one is in. But simply knowing what it's like for one to be in a particular state tells one only that one is in that state. We might cast that in terms of knowing that the conscious experience is like *that*, where the demonstrative, 'that', refers to the state in question. Perhaps such demonstrative reference could operate by way of attention; an attended state is picked out demonstratively, though it is unclear that attention actually works that way. But that issue aside, knowing only that a qualitative state is like *that* could not by itself provide any information about what type of state it is. Indeed, being in a conscious qualitative state cannot by itself even guarantee that one would be able to recognize another conscious state of that type.[9]

[8] For a good description of the phenomenon and a review of and challenge to traditional explanations, see Ekroll and Faul (2012).

[9] *Pace* Nemirow (1990) and Lewis (1990). Knowing what it's like is equivocal as between knowing what it's like to be in a type of state and knowing only that one is in a particular token state. One can know one is in that token state without knowing what type it is, and recognitional ability is being able to identify in respect of type.

Knowing what it's like to be in a token qualitative state amounts only to one's consciously being in that token state.

One might seek to hold onto a noncomparative taxonomy because subjective awareness at least gives us access to token mental qualities one by one, independent of comparisons with other token qualities. But even that is doubtful. The only way one can identify a particular token is by contrast with neighboring qualities; one picks out a token mental quality of red, for example, only by contrasts with surrounding mental qualities.[10] And even if subjective awareness did provide access to token mental qualities independent of comparisons with other tokens, that access would not by itself provide noncomparative information about what type each quality is.

Qualitative states make one aware of characteristic stimuli. And that again may seem to suggest an atomistic, noncomparative taxonomy of the mental qualities, each quality being typed by the type of stimulus it enables us to distinguish. On such a view the awareness of each stimulus would be noncomparative; a mental color quality of red would be that which makes us aware of red physical stimuli and similarly for every other type of mental quality. Tokens would each belong to their mental type noncomparatively, in virtue of the type of stimulus it makes one aware of.

But that misrepresents the way qualitative states make one aware of stimuli. Each stimulus does have a physical nature that is independent of every other. But qualitative states do not make one aware of stimuli in respect of those characteristic physical natures, but only in respect of the way we perceive stimuli of each type. And we perceive stimuli comparatively, by the ways stimuli of each type resemble and differ from other comparable stimuli, as being closer to red than to blue or closer to lilacs than to roses.[11] Which stimuli a particular type of mental quality makes us aware of cannot deliver a noncomparative taxonomy of mental qualities. Effects such as simultaneous color contrast are by no means the only reason to expect a comparative taxonomy of mental qualities; reflection on what subjective awareness actually tells us also points to a comparative taxonomy.

[10] Indeed, if one's visual field becomes thoroughly uniform in respect of color, one soon loses the ability to see anything. See, e.g., Avant (1965).

[11] That relative location in a QS is what matters to how we perceive stimuli is usefully illustrated by a case due to Jacob Berger. Berger considers the possibility of a creature with a QS for color stimuli isomorphic to ours, but with a QS in which different reflectance properties occupy locations from the reflectance properties that occupy corresponding positions in ours (personal communication). Berger suggested this as an objection to QST, since if mental color qualities are ways of being aware of each individual physical color independent of the others, that creature's mental color qualities should correspond to the physical nature of the stimulus, rather than being fixed by relative location in its QS.

But the physical nature of stimuli matters to how mental qualities make one aware of those stimuli only insofar as they affect the ability to discriminate among stimuli. This accords with common sense, on which qualitative character reflects similarities and differences among stimuli, not their physical natures independent of perception. Berger's imagined creature would experience as very different reflectance properties that we regard as barely distinguishable, which would be reflected in the JNDs from which the two QSs would be constructed.

Subjective awareness gives no substantive information about mental qualities in a noncomparative, atomistic way. But it does characterize and taxonomize conscious experiences comparatively. Just as perceiving tells us that some stimulus is closer to red than to blue or to lilac than to roses, so subjective awareness tells us that a particular sensation is closer to one mental color quality or mental olfactory quality than to another.

Indeed, subjective awareness likely gives us no information whatsoever about what type a particular qualitative experience belongs to that is not at bottom cast in such comparative terms. Even the information subjective awareness gives us about the modalities is comparative. Visual qualities are dramatically unlike auditory qualities, and likely cannot be compared in any useful way with them. But that is again a comparative matter; subjective awareness says nothing noncomparative about how visual and auditory mental qualities differ.

Since subjective awareness tells us about mental qualities in comparative terms, one might ask whether we can use JNDs between mental qualities themselves, and simply skip the step that involves JNDs among perceptible stimuli. Perhaps we can construct our QSs relying just on comparisons among the mental qualities and thereby type those qualities every bit as successfully as we can by extrapolating from JNDs among perceptible properties. One might hope thereby to combine taxonomy by appeal to QSs with the traditional view that subjective awareness is essential to mental qualities. One would simply start with JNDs among the conscious mental qualities themselves.

But seeking to save the traditional view in that way would come with a high price. As already noted, subjective awareness is subject to various confounds, such as attention and expectation, which we know can affect introspective judgments about qualitative states. And we can extract stable JND judgments when individuals take themselves merely to be guessing. In these cases the individuals have no confidence in their introspective judgments about their qualitative states; so their guesses about stimuli are more fine-grained than their judgments about conscious mental qualities. A reliance on JNDs among stimuli provides a more robust and reliable methodology than any reliance on introspective judgments can.

And we should not in any case seek to save the traditional view. The main support for that view has been that we cannot tell anything about the nature of mental qualities except by subjective awareness, and if that were so we could not even taxonomize mental qualities except by the way we are subjectively aware of them. But perceptual role, and in particular their role in perceptual discrimination, provides an alternative way to learn about their nature and taxonomize them, a way that is richer, more fine-grained, and more accurate than that provided by subjective awareness. Given the QST alternative, exclusive reliance on subjective awareness and the denial that mental qualities can occur without being conscious are stipulative and groundless.

The merits of the traditional view aside, the cost of a methodology that appeals to JND judgments about conscious mental qualities is even higher than already indicated. Subjective awareness can determine that two mental qualities are barely discriminable, but has no way to determine that the qualities would be indistinguishable were they even closer. And that is what it is to be JND. One can test for that only by manipulating the stimuli that result in those mental qualities.

In addition, one can replicate tests for JNDs between stimuli to confirm or disconfirm JND judgments. By contrast, if one elicits repeated discriminability judgments about token mental qualities there is no way to ensure that the tokens in subsequent tests are actually the same as those in earlier tests. This is not an idle concern, since there is some effect of top-down expectation on the earliest stages of visual processing (Kok et al. 2013). We cannot minimize the influence of such effects except by the manipulation of stimuli; direct subjective judgments about mental qualities cannot help.

There is yet another downside for the constructing of QSs by subjective discrimination among mental qualities. QSs do not extend indefinitely; there are stimuli beyond which no perceptual registration occurs, and so beyond which no perceptual discrimination is possible. We can readily test these limits by manipulation of stimuli, but subjective awareness is powerless to tell where those limits occur. One cannot determine by subjective awareness whether a mental quality could occur that lies just a bit farther along a particular qualitative dimension. For all these reasons, we cannot apply the QS-theoretic methodology directly to mental qualities, thereby combining that methodology with the traditional view that mental qualities cannot occur without being conscious.

Despite these considerations, one might seek to save the appeal to direct discrimination among mental qualities by appeal to some mental qualities that are privileged in reflecting perceptual primitives that provide fixed positions in the relevant QS. If such fixed positions are available, they might anchor relations among mental qualities, and thereby enable the construction of the QSs independent of JND judgments among corresponding stimuli.

In the case of mental qualities of color, there are two moves that might be tempting. One appeals to the so-called unique hues, which are said to contain subjectively no admixture of other hues.[12] Perhaps one can construct the color space by reference to a set of such unique hues. The other move appeals to color categories, which are said to be responsible for the cross-cultural and cross-linguistic prevalence of particular words for particular groups of hues (Berlin and Kay 1969), and are said to be operationalized by testing for rapid changes in color appearances near the boundaries between different color categories (e.g., Webster and Kay 2012; see also Hardin and Maffi 1997). Both unique hues and boundaries between categories might be thought to fix aspects of mental color qualities in ways that would enable the construction of QSs of mental color qualities independent of corresponding color stimuli.

[12] For discussion of the positing of such unique hues, see Gordon and Abramov (2005), esp. 109ff.

There is controversy about the objectivity of both unique hues and color categories.[13] But such controversies to one side, there is a methodological difficulty for purposes of constructing QSs for color. Both phenomena hinge on subjective judgments, one about whether a particular color experience involves any admixture of hues and the other about whether color experiences change more rapidly between two groups of subjective appearances. So the use of either to anchor objective locations or boundaries in the QS of mental color qualities is subject to the general difficulties noted above in relying on subjective judgments. We cannot responsibly factor out the appeal to JNDs among perceptible stimuli.

If there are unique hues and robust color-category boundaries, they would occur well within the outside limits of the color QS. So they could not do anything to establish those limits, that is, to determine mental color qualities beyond which no quality could occur along a particular qualitative dimension. But these limits are of substantial importance, since they determine the shape of the color QS. To establish those limits and the resulting shape requires appeal to JNDs of visible color stimuli.

And the shape of the color QS is important in connection with the conceivability of undetectably inverted qualities.[14] The shape of the color QS that JNDs of perceptible stimuli determine is asymmetric.[15] And that blocks undetectable inversion of mental color qualities, since an asymmetric shape guarantees that there will be no axis such that inversion around it would be undetectable. Even the one-dimension grayscale QS is asymmetric; the lightest shade in any local grayscale framework appears to be pure white, anchoring the grayscale shades by the lightest among them (Gilchrist 2006).

Indeed, there is no known QS constructed from JNDs among perceptible stimuli which is symmetric. Much experimental work remains to be done to map the QSs for perceptible properties other than color (see, e.g., Young et al. 2014). But one can see in advance of such work why no QS of JND stimuli could accommodate an axis around which inversion would be undetectable. If any QS did, the individual being tested would be unable to distinguish the areas that axis separates. So the overall QS would collapse to just one of those areas.[16] QST precludes undetectable inversion of mental qualities.

[13] On difficulties with unique hues, see, e.g., Logvinenko and Geithner (2013). For difficulties about color categories see Webster and Kay (2012) and more generally Hardin and Maffi (1997).

[14] Though it is not important, as we will see in section 1.3, for the individuation of the sensory modalities.

[15] See, e.g., *Commission Internationale de l'Eclairage Proceedings, 1931* (1932), Kuehni (2003), esp. ch. 6, and Ramanath et al. (2004).

[16] One could argue, as Sydney Shoemaker does, that though undetectable inversion is not possible, it is at least conceivable (e.g., Shoemaker 2003: 336). But even assuming with Shoemaker and many others that conceivability is weaker than possibility, if QST determines the nature of mental qualities, undetectable inversion is not even conceivable for mental qualities, just as it is not conceivable given the nature of water that water is not H_2O. Anybody who seemed to conceive of mental qualities as undetectably invertible would be conceiving of something other than mental qualities, just as anybody who seemed to conceive of

Mental qualities in subliminal perceiving occur without being conscious. But perception also occurs consciously, and a satisfactory theory must explain how conscious mental qualities differ from those that are not conscious. Qualitative states fail to be conscious when an individual is wholly unaware of being in the relevant states; so the natural move is to explain a qualitative state's being conscious by appeal to an individual's having some awareness of being in a qualitative state of the relevant type. Moreover, the typing of qualitative states is a matter of the relative location that their distinguishing mental qualities occupy in the relevant QS. So the awareness that results in a mental state's being conscious must itself be cast in terms of that relative location. That fits with the conclusion reached above that subjective awareness characterizes qualitative states solely in comparative terms.

I have argued elsewhere that the awareness that results in a qualitative state's being conscious can best be explained by appeal to a thought that one is in a state so characterized (e.g., Rosenthal 2005, ch. 1–4, and 2010, section IV). But this is not the place to rehearse those considerations. It is enough for present purposes to note just that since mental qualities occur both consciously and not, some explanation that goes beyond QST is needed to explain what it is for mental qualities to occur consciously. And whatever explanation one gives must be compatible with the typing of qualitative states in respect of the relative location of their distinguishing mental qualities in the relevant QS.

1.3 Individuating the Modalities

QST taxonomizes mental qualities by appeal to relative location in a QS constructed from JNDs among perceptible properties. So that methodology requires some way to determine which perceptible properties to compare in constructing a particular QS. Given a QS, we have a way to type mental qualities as well as the tools that allow us to give an informative theoretical account of what mental qualities are. But we won't get any QSs without first having a way to group some perceptible stimuli as relevant to the construction of a particular QS and others as not.

The natural move is to appeal to sensory modalities, and the foregoing account of QST took for granted the standard taxonomy of the modalities, using vision as the primary example. Vision is a modality we feel we understand well, because it has been so widely studied, because we feel we have an intuitive grasp of its nature, and because color stimuli and corresponding mental color qualities can be so readily captured in a QS with a small number of dimensions.

water as not being H_2O would not be conceiving of water, but just something superficially indistinguishable from water.

One could reject the analogy only by holding that we have access to mental qualities solely by way of subjective awareness; but without independent support that reply is question begging in evaluating the merits and implications of QST.

But there are other sensory modalities, and QST must apply to those modalities as well, accommodating QSs to taxonomize the mental qualities special to those other modalities. A QS for olfactory properties will likely require a far larger number of dimensions than the QS for color properties.[17] And QST will not in the end be satisfactory without some way of distinguishing among the sensory modalities. We must be able to distinguish the modalities to sort physical stimuli into groups to test for JNDs for the construction of QSs.

Each QS operates with properties that belong to a single modality, but the converse does not hold. A modality may well need more than one QS to exhaust the perceptible stimuli and mental qualities that occur in connection with that modality. Vision, for example, not only requires a QS for colors, but in addition QSs for the sizes, shapes, and locations that are accessible by vision.

Spatial properties require careful treatment. The physical spatial properties accessible to the various modalities are the same within the limits of what each sense can discriminate. But the corresponding mental qualities that pertain to these spatial stimuli differ from one modality to the next. Vision captures spatial location in respect of boundaries between distinguishable colors; audition captures spatial location by differences between a particular sound and its absence. Although the physical spatial locations are the same in the two cases, the mental qualities in virtue of which vision and audition capture those physical locations are distinct.

Aristotle famously noted that some perceptible properties are accessible to only one modality and others to more than one (Aristotle *de Anima* 1993: 425a–b); color is the perceptible property special to vision and sound to audition. But Aristotle confused things by identifying the mental qualities that occur in sensing things with the physical properties being sensed.[18] And since the sensed spatial properties are the same across modalities, he concluded that the corresponding spatial mental qualities must also be the same across modalities. But the connection between the way each modality senses spatial properties and the mental qualities that are special to that modality undermines that conclusion.[19] We need independent QSs to capture the spatial mental qualities for each modality that can discriminate location or other physical spatial properties.

Still, each modality will involve a single range of physical properties that are special to that modality and for which we can construct a single QS.[20] Distinct QSs of spatial

[17] Likely between 10 and 17; see Young et al. (2014).

[18] Aristotle does not speak of mental qualities as such, but it's clear that he has in mind the mental properties we speak of in that way: Perceiving on his view consists literally in the soul's taking on the perceptible properties of the object (Aristotle *de Anima* 1993: 418a4, 423b31, 424a18, 425b23).

[19] As Berkeley forcefully notes (1948/1710: I.10; 1948/1713: 194).

[20] Tactition is likely an exception. Even if we distinguish thermoception from tactition, we sense several distinct properties that are special to touch, such as pressure, texture, and hardness. And these are likely independently sensed by different mechanisms. For work that promises a basis for constructing a QS of sensed texture, see Weber et al. (2013).

and temporal properties[21] are needed for each modality because they are sensed as boundaries in respect of other physical properties that are special to the modality in question. I will return briefly in section 1.4 to mental qualities that pertain to the sensing of spatial physical properties, focusing in this section on mental qualities that figure in sensing stimuli that are uniquely accessible by a single modality.

We need a technique to individuate the modalities that allows us to tell which physical stimuli are distinctive of each modality and accommodates the construction of QSs for those stimuli. Two standard proposals for individuating the modalities plainly will not do. One appeals to the different sense organs that subserve the operation of each modality. Each modality does access a range of stimuli distinctive to it, and that requires a sense organ able to receive and suitably process those stimuli. But for the construction of a relevant QS, all that matters is the stimuli. Each sense organ is responsive only to particular ranges of stimuli, and so many provide a rough indicator of different modalities; but what matters to distinguishing the modalities is the range of stimuli, not the biological means of responding to stimuli in that range. If there were a single organ that somehow registered both auditory and visual stimuli, that by itself would tell us nothing about whether such registration involved one or two modalities.

A second popular proposal for individuating the modalities rests on differences in phenomenology, that is, on how the mental qualities distinctive of each modality appear to us subjectively. Nobody would confuse the subjective awareness we have of mental color qualities with that we have of mental sound qualities. But again, no matter how well one might think this proposal maps onto our commonsense taxonomy of the modalities,[22] it will not do. For one thing, this proposal by itself has no resources to classify mental qualities that occur without being conscious as falling within one or another modality. More important, it is less reliable for the construction of QSs even for conscious mental qualities than the use of JNDs among perceptible stimuli.

We want to individuate the modalities in a way that allows taxonomizing the mental qualities by appeal to QSs. That requires associating with each modality the right range of stimuli to use in constructing QSs from JNDs. It turns out that the methodology of QST itself allows us to do just this. I will first sketch how the resources of QST allow us to do this, and turn then to some problems about individuating modalities that this

[21] Even olfaction delivers information about location of stimuli, though it requires active exploration over time; see Young et al. (2014).

Physical temporal properties, like physical spatial properties, are sensed by different modalities in connection with properties unique to each modality. See, e.g., Klincewicz (2011) and (under submission).

[22] It is worth noting that in the cases of gustation and olfaction, the appeal to subjective awareness and our commonsense taxonomy both diverge from what we get by appeal to sensory mechanisms; there are conscious sensations we would introspectively classify as tastes that are processed by olfactory mechanisms. See, e.g., Stevenson et al. (1999). Here the QS-theoretic methodology developed in what follows sides with the sensory mechanisms.

QS methodology allows us to solve and to some challenges to this way of individuating the modalities.

We construct QSs by comparing stimuli in respect of discriminability relations, appealing in the first instance to JNDs and working out to more coarse-grained comparisons. To see how a QS-theoretic methodology can individuate the modalities, it will be convenient to start with the case of color and then generalize to other modalities.

We present an experimental participant with two color samples that are physically very close. If the participant can tell them apart, we successively present two samples that are closer until they appear indistinguishable to that participant. We label the last pair the participant could distinguish as JND, and proceed to test one of those samples paired against a new sample that is also physically close. We construct the color QS for that participant from the JNDs we collect.

Nothing matters except which sample stimuli the participant can discriminate under optimal conditions of perception. The physical properties of the samples serve only as a guide about which samples to test; those physical properties do not themselves figure in any way in the construction of the QS. We can expect that physical properties will often be good guides, leading to good hunches about which stimuli will be JND.

Physical properties will be especially good guides for modalities whose distinctive stimuli differ in respect of wavelength. Physical properties may not serve so well in guiding the testing for JNDs in modalities whose characteristic stimuli differ chemically; there we may well encounter some surprises, perhaps very many, about which stimuli are indistinguishable, which JND, and which more than barely distinguishable. In any case, it is only discriminability and not the physical properties themselves which matter in the construction of QSs. And the hunches for testing what the physical nature of stimuli suggest cannot stack the deck in any way, since they get factored out when we test for JNDs. Indeed, we need not rely on any hunches at all; we can apply the method to any perceptible stimuli whatsoever, that is, any physical properties or occurrences to which the individual responds perceptually.

For convenience, pick a color sample and test whether the participant can distinguish that sample from some randomly chosen auditory stimulus. Normal participants will always be able to distinguish them. But distinguishability is not what is basic here; what matters is near indiscriminability. And there we get the result that matters: There is no way to adjust the color and auditory stimuli or to choose such a pair so that a participant regards the two stimuli as barely distinguishable.

So there is no way to manipulate the stimuli so that the resulting stimuli are JND. Being JND requires that if the stimuli were any closer, they would no longer be discriminable at all. And there is no pair consisting of one color stimulus and one auditory stimulus that will be indistinguishable. If we have a pair of stimuli that cannot be adjusted so as to make them match or be JND, the stimuli belong to distinct sensory modalities. We have a reliable, experimentally testable mark of modalities' being distinct.

Let a bridge of JNDs consist of a succession of pairs of JND stimuli; each stimulus in the bridge will be JND from the next.[23] Constructing such a JND bridge will typically rely on the physical adjustment of stimuli, for example, changing a wavelength or increasing a concentration of some chemical. But the account of modality individuation does not itself depend on the physical manipulation of such stimuli. Two stimuli belong to distinct modalities if there is no bridge of JNDs that leads from one stimulus to the other. So we can establish that we have two modalities instead of just one by showing that there is a pair of stimuli such that no bridge of JNDs leads from one stimulus to the other. Whenever there is such a pair, the members of that pair belong to distinct modalities.

The absence of a JND bridge between any auditory stimulus and any visual stimulus shows we can never place a color stimulus in the same QS as any auditory stimulus. And that gives us reason to regard the two as belonging to distinct sensory modalities. We can use the failure to find JND stimuli, or equivalently matching stimuli that a participant cannot discriminate, to distinguish among the modalities. We have distinct modalities if we have two ranges of stimuli such that no stimulus from one range is JND from any stimulus in the other. The same appeal to JNDs that allows the construction of QSs in the first place also allows the formulation of a sufficient condition for sensory modalities to be distinct.

This appeal to JNDs satisfies the desiderata noted above. JNDs can be tested independent of subjective awareness of the stimuli; so the individuation of modalities does not rest on such subjective awareness. Moreover, the methodology appeals to nothing about sense organs or neural areas that subserve the discrimination of stimuli. Such sense organs and neural areas enable the relevant discrimination, but do not figure directly in testing for distinct modalities. Since discrimination depends on sense organs to serve as transducers for the relevant stimuli, we can expect a tight match between the modalities and the sense organs. And discriminability also reflects something about the physical nature of the stimuli. But the individuation of modalities appeals only to such discriminability, and not to the sense organs nor to the physical nature of the stimuli.

It is likely that this procedure will yield an individuation of modalities that largely conforms to our commonsense taxonomy of the modalities. We might need to revise our commonsense classification, as with the line between gustation and olfaction, and perhaps even larger revisions will be needed. But some such revising of commonsense categories is to be expected from any scientific treatment. It would be

[23] This requires an idealization, since JNDs are not in general transitive (see n. 3). But for the purposes of this test absolute JNDs are not needed; near indistinguishability of stimuli will suffice.

After this paper was completed, I came upon a passage in Goodman (1951) I had previously been unaware of which defines a notion of an M-path that resembles that of a JND bridge, though Goodman does not acknowledge the need for partial overlap described below and does not accommodate mental qualities that aren't conscious. There are significant similarities between Goodman's treatment of these topics and mine.

surprising if a traditional classification that has stood the test of time and served so well in everyday contexts did not survive at least in broad outline. But the JND-bridge technique provides a test that is independent of tradition, appealing only to the idea that modalities reflect continuity specifically in respect of discriminative response. So that test can tell us just how much revising is needed and where.

QST holds that the mental qualities are responsible for the discriminative abilities that generate the JNDs and matching of stimuli. The best explanation of the ability to make such discriminations is that we are in states that differ in a way that corresponds to discriminable differences among the stimuli. Mental qualities are simply the properties in virtue of which those states differ in suitable ways. This captures the role in perceptual discrimination that mental qualities evidently play, a role that is subjectively evident when the qualitative states are conscious and can be experimentally determined when those states occur without being conscious.

And with unusual exceptions to be discussed shortly, no JNDs occur across modalities. Any stimulus that is JND from another belongs to the same sensory modality. So it is natural to invoke the methodology used to fix the types that mental qualities fall under also to individuate the modalities. This has the theoretical benefit of providing a uniform, seamless treatment of mental qualities and the modalities. For stimuli and the corresponding mental qualities to belong to a particular modality requires that the stimuli and mental qualities be appropriately grouped together, in contrast with stimuli and mental qualities that lie outside that modality. The JND-bridge methodology provides a way to settle questions about that.

JND bridges allow the formulation of a sufficient condition for modalities to be distinct. If there are two ranges of stimuli such that no JND bridge stimulus from one range is JND from any in the other, we have distinct modalities. Is the absence of any JND bridge from one range of stimuli to another also a necessary condition for modalities to be distinct?

Here things arguably get more complicated, since there could be a bridge of JNDs from one range of stimuli to another even though we would want to regard the two ranges as belonging to distinct modalities. Imagine a creature that senses both colors and sounds, much as our vision and audition do, respectively. It is tempting to regard this creature as having two distinct modalities, one visual and the other auditory.

But imagine also that physical stimuli in a small range have JND bridges that connect them all, but also that some stimuli in that small range are also JND from at least one color stimulus that our creature can sense and also at least one sound stimulus our creature can sense. The physical nature of the stimuli in this small unexpected range is irrelevant; they could be a special range of physical colors or sounds and they could be stimuli with some altogether different physical nature.

The existence of this small range, however, results in an area in our creature's color QS that fully overlaps with an area in the sound QS, and is fully integrated by way of JNDs into the rest of the QS for each modality. Call this a partial overlap of QSs. Such partial overlap results in turn in JND bridges from any stimulus in the color QS to any in the sound QS, since there will be bridges from any such stimuli to stimuli in the area of partial overlap.

Such partial overlap may strike one as odd; we don't experience this with our modalities of vision and audition, though it is arguable that something like this may happen with gustation and olfaction, in connection with those olfactory stimuli that common sense classifies as gustatory. But odd though it may strike us, partial overlap is straightforwardly testable; we would have no difficulty in determining whether it held for any particular creature.[24]

We can expect that such partial overlap will be rare, and may for most creatures never occur. Still, its possibility presents a challenge for individuating modalities by appeal to JND bridges, since even a tiny partial overlap permits JND bridges between QSs we would otherwise have reason to regard as belonging to distinct modalities.

To deal with this challenge, we need a way to distinguish stimuli that occupy the area of partial overlap from stimuli outside that area, which are special to just one QS. The trouble is that an appeal to JND bridges cannot by itself do that, since such bridges by hypothesis connect the area of partial overlap to the rest of each QS. So we must instead appeal here to the physical nature of the stimuli themselves.

There are JND bridges that connect stimuli in the area of partial overlap with all the other stimuli in each of the two QSs. Nonetheless, stimuli in the area of partial overlap differ from those outside that area in each QS because the overlap stimuli cannot be manipulated or adjusted so as to be JND with other stimuli in both of the QSs in question. Consider the original example of an area of partial overlap between QSs that otherwise operate as our visual and auditory modalities do with color and sound, respectively. Whatever the physical nature of the partial-overlap stimuli, we cannot adjust them so that they are indistinguishable from stimuli in the areas of the two QSs that lie outside the partial overlap. The partial-overlap stimuli might themselves be physical sounds, colors, or stimuli of some altogether different type. But whatever the case about that, we will not be able to tweak them in small increments so they remain indistinguishable from both color and sound stimuli in the areas that surround the overlap.

This provides reason to regard the partial overlap as an oddity that we can dismiss, at least if the area of overlap is relatively small compared to that of the overall QSs. We can see the overlap stimuli as outliers, and comfortably take the two QSs to subserve distinct modalities. And we can save the spirit of the JND-bridge test for distinguishing modalities by noting that were we to disregard these overlap outliers, there would be no JND bridge leading from one QS to the other.

[24] Stimuli that are very different physically may be sometimes indistinguishable; this is likely the case for mentholated air and cool air. (I am indebted to Andreas Keller for this example, and for the challenge involving partial overlap.) Since these physically different stimuli can be indistinguishable by olfactory receptors, cool air will presumably be JND from some distinctively olfactory stimuli. This suggests that the imagined case of partially overlapping QSs is not so farfetched, even apart from cases involving olfaction and gustation, for which see below.

If the area of overlap were very large relative to that of the containing QSs, we might well conclude instead that we have only one modality, and not two. As often in dealing with natural phenomena, scientific judgment is needed here, and there may be no single strategy that will cover all cases. Individuating the modalities will in cases of some area of partial overlap need to follow whatever best serves our theoretical and explanatory purposes.

And though we must appeal to something about the physical nature of the relevant stimuli, individuation of modalities still rests firmly on JND bridges. Nothing matters about the physical nature of the stimuli except whether they can be manipulated in a way that is JND from other stimuli in a relevant QS. The JNDs that allow us to taxonomize mental qualities in the first place also underwrite individuation of the modalities.

One might seek to create areas of partial overlap artificially by presenting double stimuli, one from each of two modalities, say, each color stimulus accompanied by a distinctive auditory stimulus. If areas of partial overlap could be generated that way, large overlap areas would be available for any pair of modalities one might choose. But that maneuver will not work. No pair of stimuli would be JND from either of the single stimuli from that pair; double stimuli cannot generate areas of partial overlap.

Each QS of stimuli exhibits a geometrical shape determined by the JNDs used to construct the QS; similarly for the corresponding QS of mental qualities. But QSs with different geometrical properties might subserve the same modality; the QS a creature has for a particular modality might come in time to include a greater or lesser number of JND stimuli. If there are JND bridges from each stimulus in the smaller QS to every stimulus in the larger when the larger is operative, the two subserve the same modality. Sameness of geometrical properties of QSs is not necessary for two QSs to determine a single modality.

Sameness of geometrical properties is also not sufficient for two QSs to subserve a single modality. All that matters to the individuation of modalities is the possibility of JND bridges from any stimulus to any other. And one could have two QSs with isomorphic geometries but with no JND bridge from the stimuli in one to those in the other.[25] So distinct modalities can have QSs with identical geometrical properties.

An interesting illustration of this occurs with an imaginary variant of synaesthesia. Synaesthesia occurs when a stimulus from one modality evokes a mental quality distinctive of another, for example, when a sound stimulus evokes a sensation of color.[26] So one might imagine an extreme case in which every type of auditory

[25] One could imagine a creature whose one-dimensional thermoreceptive QS had the same geometrical properties as its one-dimensional temporal QS, but it would be clear that these subserve distinct modalities since no JND bridge would be possible from stimuli of the one to those of the other.

[26] Baron-Cohen and Harrison (1997) and Cytowic (2002). For a useful methodological review, see Mylopoulos and Ro (2013). Not all synaesthesia involves cross-modal associations; grapheme-color synaesthesia involves seeing letters and numbers as having consistent colors associated with each type of letter or number.

stimulus evokes a color sensation of a distinct type and every type of color stimulus evokes a distinct type of auditory sensation.[27]

This would not work for ordinary human perception, in which the QSs for color and auditory stimuli are not the same in respect of dimensionality, shape, and fineness of grain, and there are not enough color stimuli distinguishable by humans to cover all the distinguishable auditory stimuli. In addition, we have access to auditory stimuli that because of spatial location are visually inaccessible. But imagine a creature whose visual and auditory apparatus are adjusted so as to factor out these disparities, so that their visual and auditory QSs have the same geometrical properties.

Every color stimulus for such a creature would be JND from some auditory stimulus and conversely, since stimuli of each type would evoke mental qualities evoked by stimuli of the other. And since every stimulus of each physical type would produce mental qualities distinctive of both, every stimulus of each physical type would be indistinguishable from some stimulus of the other type.

Nonetheless, it may be tempting to imagine that despite the equivalent QSs and JND responses for physical visual and auditory stimuli, there would still be two sensory modalities in the imagined case, one auditory and the other visual. That temptation presumably stems partly from seeing the case simply as an extension of ordinary color–sound synaesthesia, in which it is plain that two modalities are operative. And it may strike us in any case that vision and audition are plainly distinct modalities. But if there were two distinct modalities in the imagined case despite the equivalence of QSs constructed from JNDs, we could not sustain a QS-theoretic taxonomy of both mental qualities and sensory modalities.

But seeing such a case as an extension of actual synaesthesia misleads. In actual synaesthesia, many stimuli lie outside the range of synaesthetic overlap. It is those stimuli that anchor distinct modalities, no matter how dramatic the area of overlap may be. But if the area of overlap were total, no basis would remain to see the case as involving two modalities. Having stimuli of distinct physical types is not enough to have distinct modalities, since the two types of stimulus would evoke identical discriminability responses and hence indistinguishable psychological responses generally.

One might hold that it would be obvious from a first-person point of view that mental qualities of two distinct modalities occur in the imagined case. But setting aside the issue about whether first-person impressions are relevant to individuating the modalities, it is far from clear that the first-person appearances would deliver that result in such total synaesthesia. If every distinct type of conscious color quality coincided with a distinctive type of conscious auditory quality, this would likely result in a first-person impression of a single range of conscious mental qualities, albeit one

[27] I owe this imagined case to Henry Shevlin (personal communication), who refers to it as perfect synaesthesia.

that we are unable to imagine subjectively. The temptation to think that first-person appearances would plainly point to two modalities again likely reflects our modeling the imaginary case on ordinary synaesthesia, in which first-person appearances of distinct modalities are anchored by the mental qualities for which there is no overlap.

The foregoing considerations fit comfortably with the appeal to JND bridges. For the imagined case of total synaesthesia, each color stimulus will be JND from at least one other very close color stimulus, and each auditory stimulus from at least one other close auditory stimulus. But each color stimulus results in the same mental qualities as some auditory stimulus. So any color stimulus will also be JND from auditory stimuli that evoke the same mental qualities as those that result from color stimuli JND from the target color stimulus. So total synaesthesia would permit a JND bridge from any color or auditory stimulus to every other color and auditory stimulus.

In actual synaesthesia, by contrast, there are color stimuli that evoke no auditory response and auditory stimuli that evoke no visual response. Consider two color stimuli that would be JND if they both evoked only visual responses, but one of which for some particular synaesthete evokes only a visual response and the other both a visual and an auditory response. For that synaesthete the two color stimuli are not JND. Being JND means that if the two stimuli were any closer they would be indistinguishable. But if these two color stimuli were closer for our actual synaesthete, either one would gain an auditory response or the other would lose it. So the two stimuli would be distinguishable even if they were to be closer, indeed, more readily distinguishable than before. For actual color–sound synaesthesia, there are stimuli in each modality from which there is no JND bridge to many stimuli in the other. Our test distinguishes two modalities for actual synaesthesia, and rules that there is only one in the imagined case of total synaesthesia.[28]

The taxonomy of mental qualities by appeal to relative location in a QS determined by JNDs proceeds in the first instance by testing one individual at a time, though we readily arrive at QSs for a species or other group by averaging those results. In determining which stimuli belong to a particular modality, we make no prior assumptions about the modalities, testing whatever stimuli we like for JNDs, though we follow hunches about which stimulus pairs are likely to be JND. But we construct QSs by testing for JNDs among stimuli that belong to a particular modality. And we must also test for JND bridges one individual at a time.

Again some averaging is needed. Different stimuli will be JND from one individual to another, and even for one individual at two times. And we can average over the JNDs themselves, building a set of JND bridges to assign to a species or to an individual across times. There is idealization in this procedure, as with averaging over individuals' QSs, but no more idealization than is inevitable in passing from

[28] It is also important that ordinary synaesthesia is asymmetric, so that shapes evoke sounds, e.g., but not conversely, adding to the anchoring of two distinct modalities.

individuals at specific times to the relevant species. We could even individuate modalities across species, relying on stimuli that overlap the modalities of the different species and disregarding areas that fail to overlap.

Mixtures of stimuli raise special challenges. Metamerism with colors results from distinct combinations of wavelengths that result in the same ratio of stimulation of the three types of daylight retinal receptors, and hence are indistinguishable as regards hue. As noted in section 1.2, the occurrence of such stimuli that differ dramatically in physical character poses no difficulty, since QST relies solely on JNDs.

But mixtures also raise questions about the individuation of the modalities, especially for the chemoreceptive modalities. Many experiences we count as taste result from olfactory input, rather than strictly gustatory stimulation. As a result, some speak of flavor as a combination of the olfactory and gustatory modalities.[29] However we may think of commonsense experiences of flavor, mixtures of olfactory and gustatory stimuli might seem to present a challenge to the JND-bridge method for individuating modalities.

Glucose is sensed by gustatory receptors and not by olfaction, whereas vanillin is the opposite, sensed by olfaction but not gustation. Suppose then one starts with pure glucose and then mixes in slight amounts of vanillin while decreasing slightly the amount of glucose, so that each successive mixture is JND from the one before, till one ends up with pure vanillin. One begins with a stimulus that is plainly a tastant and not an odorant, and ends up by JND steps with an odorant that is not a tastant. Other such examples of mixtures abound. And because we can construct a JND bridge from a tastant to an odorant, such mixtures may seem to challenge the JND-bridge method of distinguishing olfaction from gustation, yielding a single modality.[30]

But things are more complicated. The method for individuating modalities appeals not just to a single chain of JNDs, but to JND bridges among most of the stimuli distinctive of that modality. Otherwise the partial overlap noted above would have defeated the method. What matters is not that a single JND chain leads from pure glucose to pure vanillin, but rather which QS each stimulus in the glucose-vanillin chain is connected to by some JND chain. For each stimulus in that chain there will be a bridge of JNDs connecting that stimulus to others in the olfactory QS or to others in the gustatory QS. It is those JND bridges that determine whether a particular stimulus in the glucose-vanillin chain counts as gustatory or olfactory.

It may well be that some stimuli in the glucose-vanillin chain are JND from stimuli that occur solely in the olfactory QS and also from stimuli that occur solely in the

[29] Shepherd (2012) and Taylor and Roberts (2004). Commonsense classifications of flavor also are influenced by temperature and texture.

[30] I am indebted to Andreas Keller for pressing me about issues pertaining to such mixtures. For more, see Young et al. (2014).

gustatory QS. Indeed, this might well hold for many stimuli in that chain. We would then count those stimuli as belonging to both modalities. But as already argued, such partial overlap presents no difficulty. We have two modalities if there are many pairs of stimuli with no bridge of JNDs leading from one to the other. That is compatible with partial overlap between the modalities, in which JND bridges connect each stimulus inside the area of overlap to every other stimulus in each modality.

These considerations do not address questions about how best to conceptualize commonsense experiences of flavor. But they provide an independent test for whether particular stimuli and the corresponding mental qualities belong to a single sensory modality. And that in turn may shed light on useful ways to think about experiences that challenge our commonsense boundaries between the modalities.

Chemoreceptive modalities pose special challenges stemming from mixtures of stimuli, whereas modalities that sense wave phenomena seem not to. Differences among timbres of voice and musical instruments result in large measure, though not exclusively, from mixtures of auditory stimuli (Latinus and Belin 2011 and Handel 1995). But we can reasonably expect that JND bridges will reliably take one from any one auditory stimulus to any other. Similarly with the colors.

1.4 Some Applications

In a procedure known as tactile-visual sensory substitution, blind individuals are fitted with devices that receive visible information and produce tactile stimulation that provides the individual with strikingly accurate and detailed visual information (e.g., Bach-y-Rita 1972 and Bach-y-Rita and Kercel 2003). Subject to proper deployment, experience, and training, some blind participants have reported 'subjective experience... comparable (if not qualitatively identical) to vision.... Even the visual illusions that have been tested (e.g., waterfall effect) are the same as vision'. Congenitally blind participants have not yet reported such conscious visual experience, though they also have not yet had extensive training with these devices (Bach-y-Rita 2002: 497–8).

Individuals who are no longer sighted cannot compare stimuli that result from sensory substitution with those of ordinary vision in any fine-grained way, though their subjective memories evidently lead them to judge the stimuli to be different from those of their lost ordinary vision. It would be interesting to test sighted individuals for whether they can become sufficiently experienced with stimuli from a sensory-substitution device that such stimuli are ever JND from those of ordinary vision. One might anticipate a negative result, but that is not altogether obvious, especially if the stimuli presented to ordinary vision were degraded so as to match the coarse-grained character of stimuli presented by way of sensory substitution.

In any case, these considerations do not challenge the individuation of modalities by JND bridges. The modality of tactile-visual sensory substitution may well simply be distinct from any other; experienced participants also do not report the tactile stimulation as on a par with ordinary tactile stimuli. Or if testing of sighted participants' using sensory-substitution devices did yield JND bridges between ordinary vision and stimuli available by way of these devices,[31] that would encourage regarding the sensory-substitution modality as identical with, even if far more coarse grained than, the ordinary visual modality. In any case, the JND-bridge test provides a promising approach to settling questions about individuating the modalities that occur in sensory substitution.

Sensory substitution is intuitively striking because of a traditional reliance on the physical nature of the stimuli and sense organs, which makes it surprising, perhaps to the point of incredulity, that tactile stimuli applied to the organ of touch could result in visual experiences. The JND-bridge method serves as a corrective to that reliance. What matters for individuating the modalities is continuity in respect of discriminative responses, which is exactly what JND bridges reveal. Once we focus on such discriminative-response continuity as what is basic to individuating the modalities, it is no longer especially surprising that sensory substitution might result in distinctively visual experiences.

As noted at the outset of section 1.3, spatial properties, such as size, shape, and location, are discriminable only in virtue of perceptible boundaries that obtain among other properties accessible by the modality in question, colors in the case of vision, textures or resistances to pressures in the case of tactition, and so forth. So even though the physical stimuli of size, shape, and location are independent of whatever modality may sense them, the mental qualities that result from these spatial physical stimuli will differ from one modality to another. Because mental qualities of size and shape are tied to color boundaries in vision but not in tactition, for example, visual mental qualities of size and shape will differ from those of tactition. Similarly, sensing location is tied to color boundaries in vision but to differential sounds in audition, so that the mental qualities in virtue of which we discriminate locations by vision differ from those that figure in audition.

The observations recall the famous question William Molyneux posed to John Locke about whether a person born blind would on gaining sight immediately be able to recognize visually the shapes that person could discriminate by touch (Locke 1975/1700: 145–6, Molyneux 1978/1688: no. 1064, and Molyneux 1979/1693: no. 1069). If visual shape discrimination relies on visible boundaries among colors and tactile shape discrimination on boundaries among textures or pressures, it is difficult to see how such a person could calibrate the shapes perceived by sight with those perceived by touch without some learning. Similarly for early calibration in ordinary perceivers of spatial properties as those properties are accessed by the different modalities.[32]

[31] One possibility might be to let patients with congenital cataracts become highly proficient with sensory-substitution devices prior to surgery and test them for JNDs after cataract removal restores regular sight.

[32] Recent claims based on empirical findings that no such learning would be needed are not compelling; see, e.g., Schwenkler (2012 and 2013) and Rosenthal (2005: 221 and 222n). For a compelling empirical

That different mental qualities of size, shape, and location figure in the sensing of spatial stimuli by the different modalities again fits comfortably with the JND-bridge method of individuating the modalities. One cannot present a physical shape stimulus to vision except in connection with color boundaries, nor to tactition except in connection with boundaries of stimuli that touch can distinguish. The colors and tactile stimuli whose boundaries determine the shape in the two cases will ensure that any experimental participant could readily distinguish any shape stimulus presented to vision from the very same shape stimulus as presented to tactition. So there will be no way to manipulate a visible shape, for example, so that it becomes indistinguishable from a shape accessed by tactition. There will therefore be no JND bridges between shapes presented to vision and those presented to tactition. Visible shape belongs to a different modality from tactile shape, and similarly for stimuli of size and location as presented to the modalities that have access to those stimuli.[33]

JND bridges provide a precise, testable method for individuating the modalities, with exact factors that such individuation must take into account. And the method also explains the appeal of the traditional marks that have been used to individuate the modalities. It is inviting to think of individuating the modalities by way of organs, the physical nature of the stimuli, or the media used to transmit perceptible information from stimuli to organs because all these things tend to match the results that JND-bridges deliver. One would expect JND bridges to result from the use of particular sense organs in transducing physical stimuli, as well as from the similar physical nature of distal stimuli that affect those organs and the media used to transmit perceptible information to them.

The appeal to phenomenology to individuate the modalities also fits well with the JND-bridge technique. Each QS of stimuli that are JND fixes the mental qualities by means of which we discriminate among those stimuli. And though those mental qualities are not in themselves conscious, when they do occur consciously, we are subjectively aware of them in respect of their distinguishing characteristics, that is, their relative location in the relevant QS. And since that relative location is in turn fixed by JNDs, phenomenology will also reflect the considerations on which the JND-bridge method relies. The JND-bridge method arguably underlies and explains the appeal of all the traditional marks for individuating the modalities.

Still, the JND-bridge technique differs in an important way from those traditional approaches. The technique relies on discriminative responses to stimuli, as against

study that learning would be needed, see Held et al. (2011). Evidence from cataract-removal patients is unconvincing because such patients do have sight, albeit highly degraded, prior to surgery.

The Molyneux question relevant here and as usually discussed is what sensory discriminations a person born blind would have on gaining sight, not, as Evans (1985) casts it, what spatial concepts a person blind from birth would have.

[33] Location stimuli, e.g., belong to vision or audition depending on whether they are sensed by boundaries of color or sound. For issues about the spatial aspect of audition, see, e.g., Nudds (2009), Casati and Dokic (2009), and Grantham (1995).

reliance directly on the organs or the physical nature of stimuli or media. If a significant range of JND bridges exist between two sets of stimuli, they belong to the same modality; similarly for corresponding mental qualities. What matters to individuating modalities is how individuals perceive stimuli, and it is discriminative responses that reveal that. We can individuate the modalities in a way more robust and objective than any of the traditional methods.

It is also worth noting the ad hoc character of invoking, as Aristotle (1993 book II) did, combinations of the traditional distinguishing marks for the modalities. Inviting though it may be to correct the shortcomings of one by the strong points of another, we have no way to weigh and balance the various marks that is not wholly arbitrary. We cannot save the traditional marks by combining them.

Since the physical nature of stimuli and the functioning of sense organs and physical media all figure in determining which stimuli are JND, it is natural that traditional discussions, lacking appeal to techniques for measuring JNDs, should have focused instead on those other factors. Phenomenology too reflects JNDs, if somewhat imperfectly, since differences in phenomenology are due to differences in our subjective awareness of mental qualities, which in turn are taxonomized by way of JNDs. Appeal to JNDs both explains the appeal of the traditional methods and shows why relying on them can mislead. The traditional methods use factors that determine JNDs, but it is the JNDs themselves that matter, both for taxonomizing the mental qualities and individuating the modalities.

It might be thought that the JND-bridge technique has a shortcoming relative to traditional methods for individuating the modalities, because JND bridges allow for partial overlap of modalities. But allowing for the possibility of partial overlap is an advantage, not a failing. We know from gustation and olfaction that traditional methods of individuating modalities may lead us to assign stimuli and corresponding mental qualities to the wrong modality. And it is in any case an open question whether some stimuli and mental qualities might belong to more than one modality, a question we have no reason to decide in advance of empirical findings. The JND-bridge technique, unlike traditional methods, tells us how we might settle the question in an empirically sound way.

As with the appeal to relative location in a QS for taxonomizing the mental qualities, the JND-bridge method is at bottom a comparative matter. The individuation of modalities rests not on some absolute standard, such as the physical nature of the stimuli, the transductive powers of the organs, or the deliverances of consciousness about mental qualities. It rests solely on whether there is a suitable set of comparative responses to relevant stimuli.[34]

[34] The outline of a QST technique for individuating the modalities was developed while working on Young et al. (2014). I am grateful for the opportunity that working with Young and Keller afforded me to probe these issues and for the critical feedback I received from them. This material was presented at the December 2013 Conference on Olfaction at the University of Antwerp Centre for Philosophical Psychology; I am grateful for comments from those at the conference.

References

Aristotle (1993), *de Anima: Books II, III (with passages from Book I)*, tr. D. W. Hamlyn (Oxford: Clarendon Press, 1968); with a report on recent work and a revised bibliography by Christopher Shields (Oxford: Clarendon Press).

Avant, Lloyd L. (1965), 'Vision in the Ganzfeld', in *Psychological Bulletin*, 64/4 (October): 246–58.

Bach-y-Rita, Paul (1972), *Brain Mechanisms in Sensory Substitution* (New York: Academic Press).

Bach-y-Rita, Paul (2002), 'Sensory Substitution and Qualia', in Alva Noë and Evan Thompson, (eds), *Vision and Mind: Selected Readings in the Philosophy of Perception* (Cambridge, Mass.: MIT Press), 497–514.

Bach-y-Rita, Paul, and Kercel, Stephen W. (2003), 'Sensory Substitution and the Human-Machine Interface', in *Trends in Cognitive Sciences*, 7/12 (December): 541–6.

Balog, Katalin (2009), 'Phenomenal Concepts', in Brian P. McLaughlin, Ansgar Beckermann, and Sven Walter (eds), *The Oxford Handbook of Philosophy of Mind* (Oxford: Clarendon Press), 292–312.

Baron-Cohen, Simon, and Harrison, John E. (eds) (1997), *Synaesthesia: Classic and Contemporary Readings* (Oxford: Blackwell).

Berger, Jacob (under submission), 'A Holistic Theory of Perceptual Content'.

Berkeley, George (1948/1710), *A Treatise Concerning the Principles of Human Knowledge: The Works of George Berkeley*, edited by A. A. Luce and T. E. Jessop (London: Thomas Nelson and Sons), Vol. 2.

Berkeley, George (1948/1713), *Three Dialogues between Hylas and Philonous: The Works of George Berkeley*, edited by A. A. Luce and T. E. Jessop (London: Thomas Nelson and Sons), Vol. 2.

Berlin, Brent, and Kay, Paul (1969), *Basic Color Terms: Their Universality and Evolution* (Berkeley: University of California Press).

Block, Ned (1978), 'Troubles with Functionalism,' in C. Wade Savage (ed.), *Minnesota Studies in the Philosophy of Science*, IX (Minneapolis: University of Minnesota Press).

Breitmeyer, Bruno G., and Öğmen, Haluk (2006), *Visual Masking: Time Slices through Conscious and Unconscious Vision*, 2nd edn (New York: Oxford University Press).

Byrne, Alex (2001), 'Intentionalism Defended', in *The Philosophical Review* 110/2 (April): 199–240.

Casati, Roberto, and Dokic, Jérôme (2009), 'Some Varieties of Spatial Hearing', in Matthew Nudds and Casey O'Callaghan (eds), *Sounds and Perception: New Philosophical Essays* (Oxford: Oxford University Press), 97–110.

Chalmers, David J. (1996), *The Conscious Mind: In Search of a Fundamental Theory* (New York: Oxford University Press).

Chalmers, David J. (2007), 'Phenomenal Concepts and the Explanatory Gap', in Torin Alter and Sven Walter (eds), *Phenomenal Concepts and Phenomenal Knowledge: New Essays on Consciousness and Physicalism* (Oxford: Oxford University Press), 167–94.

Cheesman, Jim, and Merikle, Philip M. (1986), 'Distinguishing Conscious from Unconscious Perceptual Processes', in *Canadian Journal of Psychology* 40/4 (December): 343–67.

Clark, Austen (1993), *Sensory Qualities* (Oxford: Clarendon Press).

Commission Internationale de l'Eclairage Proceedings, 1931 (1932) (Cambridge: Cambridge University Press).

Cytowic, Richard E. (2002), *Synesthesia: A Union of The Senses*, 2nd edn (Cambridge, Mass.: MIT Press).

Dienes, Zoltán (2004), 'Assumptions of Subjective Measures of Unconscious Mental States: Higher-Order Thoughts and Bias', in *Journal of Consciousness Studies* 11/9: 25–45.

Dienes, Zoltán, and Seth, Anil (2010), 'Gambling on the Unconscious: A Comparison of Wagering and Confidence Ratings as Measures of Awareness in an Artificial Grammar Task', in *Consciousness and Cognition*, 19/2 (June): 674–81.

Ekroll, Vebjørn, and Faul, Franz (2012), 'Basic Characteristics of Simultaneous Color Contrast Revisited', in *Psychological Science* 23/10 (October): 1246–55.

Evans, Gareth (1985), 'Molyneux's Question', in Antonia Phillips (ed.), *Gareth Evans: Collected Papers* (Oxford: Clarendon Press), 364–99.

Gilchrist, Alan (2006), *Seeing Black and White* (Oxford: Oxford University Press).

Goodman, Nelson (1951), *The Structure of Appearance* (Cambridge, Mass.: Harvard University Press).

Gordon, James, and Abramov, Israel (2005), 'Color Vision', in E. Bruce Goldstein (ed.), *Blackwell Handbook of Sensation and Perception* (Malden, Mass.: Blackwell Publishing), 92–127.

Grantham, D. Wesley (1995), 'Spatial Hearing and Related Phenomena', in Brian C. J. Moore (ed.), *Hearing*, 2nd edn (San Diego, Calif.: Academic Press), 297–345.

Grice, Paul (1962), 'Some Remarks about the Senses', in R. J. Butler (ed.), *Analytical Philosophy, First Series* (Oxford: Basil Blackwell), 133–53.

Handel, Stephen (1995), 'Timbre Perception and Auditory Object Identification', in Brian C. J. Moore (ed.), *Hearing*, 2nd edn (San Diego, Calif.: Academic Press), 425–61.

Hardin, C. L. (1993), *Color for Philosophers*, 2nd edn (Indianapolis, Ind.: Hackett Publishing).

Hardin, C. L., and Maffi, Luisa (eds) (1997), *Color Categories in Thought and Language* (Cambridge: Cambridge University Press).

Harman, Gilbert (1990), 'The Intrinsic Quality of Experience', in *Philosophical Perspectives* IV: 31–52.

Held, R., Ostrovsky, Y., de Gelder, B., Gandhi, T., Ganesh, S., Mathur, U., and Sinha P. (2011), 'The Newly Sighted Fail to Match Seen with Felt', in *Nature Neuroscience* 14/5 (May): 551–3.

Jackson, Frank (1986), 'What Mary Didn't Know', in *Journal of Philosophy* 83/5 (May): 291–5.

Klincewicz, Michał (2011), 'Quality Space Model of Temporal Perception', in Argiro Vatakis (ed.), *Multidisciplinary Aspects of Time and Time Perception* (Berlin: Springer-Verlag), 230–45.

Klincewicz, Michał (under submission), 'Temporal Qualities and the Problem of Temporality'.

Kok, Peter, Brouwer, G. J., van Gerven, M. A. J., and de Lange, F. P. (2013), 'Prior Expectations Bias Sensory Representations in Visual Cortex', in *Journal of Neuroscience* 33/41 (October 9): 16275–84.

Kuehni, Rolf G. (2003), *Color Space and Its Divisions: Color Order from Antiquity to the Present* (Hoboken, N.J.: John Wiley).

Kuehni, Rolf G. (2010), 'Color Spaces and Color Order Systems', in Jonathan Cohen and Mohan Matthen (eds), *Color Ontology and Color Science* (Cambridge, Mass.: MIT Press), 3–36.

Latinus, Marianne, and Belin, Pascal (2011), 'Human Voice Perception', in *Current Biology* 21/4 (February 22): R143–5.

Lewis, David (1990), 'What Experience Teaches', in William G. Lycan (ed.), *Mind and Cognition: A Reader* (Oxford: Basil Blackwell), 499–519.

Locke, John (1975/1700), *An Essay Concerning Human Understanding*, 4th edn, edited by Peter H. Nidditch (Oxford: Clarendon Press), 145–6.

Logvinenko, Alexander D., and Geithner, Coryn (2013), 'Unique Hues as Revealed by Unique-Hue Selecting versus Partial Hue-Matching', in *Attention, Perception, & Psychophysics*, advance online publication March 8, doi: 10.3758/s13414-013-0432-2.

Macpherson, Fiona (2011), *The Senses: Classic and Contemporary Philosophical Perspectives* (Oxford: Oxford University Press).

Marcel, Anthony J. (1983), 'Conscious and Unconscious Perception: An Approach to the Relations between Phenomenal Experience and Perceptual Processes', in *Cognitive Psychology* 15/2 (April): 238–300.

Mealor, Andy David, and Dienes, Zoltán (2012), 'Conscious and Unconscious Thought in Artificial Grammar Learning', in *Consciousness and Cognition* 21/2 (June): 865–74.

Merikle, Philip M. (1992), 'Perception without Awareness: Critical Issues', in *American Psychologist* 47/6: 792–5.

Molyneux, William (1978/1688), 'Letter to John Locke, 7 July 1688', in E. S. de Beer (ed.), *The Clarendon Edition of the Works of John Locke*, 9 Vols (Oxford: Clarendon Press), Vol. 3, no. 1064.

Molyneux, William (1979/1693), 'Letter to John Locke, 2 March 1693', in E. S. de Beer (ed.), *The Clarendon Edition of the Works of John Locke*, 9 Vols (Oxford: Clarendon Press), Vol. 4, no. 1069.

Mylopoulos, Myrto, and Ro, Tony (2013), 'Synesthesia: A Colorful Word with a Touching Sound', in *Frontiers in Psychology*, October 22, doi: 10.3389/fpsyg.2013.00763, at <http://www.ncbi.nlm.nih.gov/pmc/articles/PMC3804765/pdf/fpsyg-04-00763.pdf>.

Nagel, Thomas (1974), 'What Is It Like to Be a Bat?', in *The Philosophical Review* 83/4 (October): 435–50.

Nemirow, Larry (1990), 'Physicalism and the Cognitive Role of Acquaintance', in William G. Lycan (ed.), *Mind and Cognition: A Reader* (Oxford: Basil Blackwell), 490–9.

Nudds, Matthew (2009), 'Sounds and Space', in Matthew Nudds and Casey O'Callaghan (eds), *Sounds and Perception: New Philosophical Essays* (Oxford: Oxford University Press), 69–96.

Öğmen, Haluk, and Breitmeyer, Bruno G. (eds) (2006), *The First Half Second: The Microgenesis and Temporal Dynamics of Unconscious and Conscious Visual Processes* (Cambridge, Mass.: MIT Press).

Ramanath, Rajeev, Kuehni, Rolf G., Snyder, Wesley E., and Hinks, David (2004), 'Spectral Spaces and Color Spaces', in *Color Research and Application* 29/1 (February): 29–37.

Rosenthal, David (1999), 'The Colors and Shapes of Visual Experiences', in Denis Fisette (ed.), *Consciousness and Intentionality: Models and Modalities of Attribution* (Dordrecht: Kluwer Academic Publishers), 95–118.

Rosenthal, David (2001), 'Color, Mental Location, and the Visual Field', in *Consciousness and Cognition* IX/4 (April): 85–93.

Rosenthal, David (2005), *Consciousness and Mind* (Oxford: Clarendon Press).

Rosenthal, David (2010), 'How to Think about Mental Qualities', in *Philosophical Issues: Philosophy of Mind* XX (October): 368–93.

Rosenthal, David (forthcoming), 'Quality Spaces, Relocation, and Grain', in James R. O'Shea (ed.), *Sellars and His Legacy* (Oxford: Oxford University Press).

Sasaki, Yuka, Náñez, José E., and Watanabe, Takeo (2010), 'Advances in Visual Perceptual Learning and Plasticity', in *Nature Reviews Neuroscience* 11/1 (January): 53–60.

Schwenkler, John (2012), 'On the Matching of Seen and Felt Shape by Newly Sighted Subjects', in *i-Perception* 3/3: 186–8.

Schwenkler, John (2013), 'Do Things Look the Way They Feel?', in *Analysis* 73/1 (January): 86–96.

Shankar, Maya U., Levitan, Carmel A., and Spence, Charles (2001), 'Grape Expectations: The Role of Cognitive Influences in Color–Flavor Interactions', in *Consciousness and Cognition*, 10/3 (September): 380–90.

Shepherd, Gordon M. (2012), *Neurogastronomy: How the Brain Creates Flavor and Why It Matters* (New York: Columbia University Press).

Shoemaker, Sydney (2003), 'The Inverted Spectrum', in Sydney Shoemaker (ed.), *Identity, Cause, and Mind: Philosophical Essays*, 2nd edn (Oxford: Clarendon Press), 327–57.

Stevenson, Richard J., Prescott, John, and Boakes, Robert A. (1999), 'Confusing Tastes and Smells: How Odours Can Influence the Perception of Sweet and Sour Tastes', in *Chemical Senses* 24/4 (December): 627–35.

Stoljar, Daniel (2005), 'Physicalism and Phenomenal Concepts', in *Mind and Language* 20/5 (November): 469–94.

Taylor, Andrew J., and Roberts, Deborah D. (eds) (2004), *Flavor Perception* (Oxford: Blackwell Publishing).

Watanabe, Takeo, Náñez, José E., and Sasaki, Yuka (2001), 'Perceptual Learning without Perception', in *Nature* 413 (October 25): 844–8.

Weber, Alison I., Saal, Hannes P., Lieber, Justin D., Cheng, Ju-Wen, Manfredi, Louise R., Dammann III, John F., and Bensmala, Sliman J. (2013), 'Spatial and Temporal Codes Mediate the Tactile Perception of Natural Textures', in *PNAS*, 110/42 (October 15): 17107–12.

Webster, Michael A., and Kay, Paul (2012), 'Color Categories and Color Appearance', in *Cognition*, 122/3 (March): 375–92.

Young, Benjamin D., Keller, Andreas, and Rosenthal, David (2014), 'Quality Space Theory in Olfaction', in *Frontiers in Consciousness Research*, at <http://www.frontiersin.org/Journal/10.3389/fpsyg.2014.00001/abstract>.

2

Neuro-Cosmology

Sam Coleman

Obviously there are volumes of pink. No inventory of what there is can meaningfully deny that fact. What is at stake is their status and function in the scheme of things.

Wilfrid Sellars, *Carus Lecture III*: 46

1. Consideration of a weakness in Nagel's argument for panpsychism, as highlighted by Rosenthal (§§2–11), points us in the direction of a modified argument for a nearby position (§§12–31). On *panqualityism* the basic building blocks of the physical world are qualitative without being yet phenomenally qualitative (i.e. intrinsically conscious). Panqualityism is developed and propounded as a promising form of physicalism (§§32–86). On this basis an objectivizing account is given of consciousness and subjectivity (§§87–99).

2. Distilled, the premises that carry Nagel to panpsychism are the following:

P1. *Material composition*: Any living organism is wholly composed of a huge number of particles.

P2. *Non-reductionism*: An organism's phenomenal properties are not implied by any physical properties alone.

P3. *Phenomenal realism*: Some organisms have phenomenal properties.

P4. *Non-emergence*: All high-level properties of a complex system intelligibly derive from properties of its constituents plus their arrangement.[1]

[1] See Nagel (1979: 181–2). I say 'distilled' because of two changes to Nagel's formulation: (i) Nagel talks not of phenomenal properties but of *mental* properties. Yet he defines mentality in terms of phenomenal consciousness (Nagel 1979: 188), and it is fair to say we home in on his main concern if we talk explicitly in terms of phenomenal properties from the outset. (ii) Nagel's *Non-reductionism* premise states additionally

Nagel gets from here to the conclusion that *all* micromatter has phenomenal properties via the following principle:

Fungibility: Any matter can compose an organism (including, notably, the sort mentioned in P3).[2]

The argument operates to inject an extra set of properties into micromatter, with the aim of supporting phenomenality[3] as we know it. Macrophenomenal properties are to be understood as complexes of microphenomenal properties, on this model.

3. The focus of Rosenthal's critique of Nagel's argument is Nagel's claim that 'A physical explanation . . . does not explain the mental because it does not explain its subjective features'.[4] This constitutes Nagel's support for *Non-reductionism*. Rosenthal's critique largely succeeds, we shall find, but leaves intact an important kernel of the Nagelian argument. Later we try to grow this kernel back into a worldview.

4. Why does Nagel hold that the subjective features of the mental prevent a physical explanation? To answer this we need to know what he means by 'subjective features'. One way to understand such talk involves Nagel's influential notion of a 'point of view'. A feature of experience is subjective, he says, when 'it can in principle be fully understood only from one *type* of point of view: that of a being like the one having the experience'.[5] So to fully understand the phenomenal properties corresponding to bat experiences, according to Nagel, one would need to be able to take up a point of view sufficiently close to a bat's. This might appear problematic for scientific treatments of phenomenal properties, since science aims to provide accounts from no particular point of view; i.e. objective ones, the grasp of which is not restricted in principle to certain kinds of experiencer.

5. Nagel does not claim that each *individual* creature occupies its own point of view, that no other individual can occupy, which would make phenomenal properties radically subjective, in effect private to their owners. Rather, he associates points of view with *species*: they get assigned to the bearers of different sets of sense organs. There is thus a bat point of view, a dolphin point of view, and a human point of view. But, as Rosenthal notes, this admits a certain relativity into the notion of a point of view, and the associated matter of subjectivity. We do not occupy the mouse point

that mental properties *are not* physical properties. But since if they were physical they would trivially be implied by certain physical properties, namely themselves, I omit this part of his formulation.

[2] Nagel (1979: 182). Again I've made slight and insignificant alteration to bring out the reasoning.

[3] By 'phenomenality' I will mean the determinable of which specific phenomenal properties, e.g. ostensibly seeing a blue sky, tasting chocolate, or feeling an orgasm, are determinates.

[4] Nagel (1979: 188). [5] Nagel (1979: 188).

of view, plausibly, yet we are doubtless closer to it than we are to the bat point of view, and likely closer to that than we are to the points of view of foot-inflating aliens and sentient robots. Thus the bar on comprehension of features belonging to other points of view would seem to be one only of degree. One may understand more and more features of a point of view depending upon how close one is to it. And perhaps, then (this goes beyond what Rosenthal explicitly says), there are no features of conscious experience *as such* inaccessible to investigating creatures as long as they too are conscious, and so share the 'point of view' of sentient life in its most general form. If 'objective' means 'accessible across all points of view', that would make the nature of phenomenality objectively comprehensible after all.

6. This leaves Nagelian subjectivity somewhat watered down. Rosenthal observes that Nagel's position seems to leave the door ajar for scientific methods. If features of experiences are available across points of view, who is to say that science cannot get some sort of purchase on them, or on phenomenality itself? So Nagel's notion of point of view, at least in the restricted form he employs, seems inadequate to support his claim that experiences cannot be physically explained *as a matter of principle.* Perhaps he could sustain on this basis the claim that certain features of conscious experiences, the most parochial ones, will remain physically mysterious; but not the much stronger, and correspondingly more interesting, thesis that phenomenality as such cannot be captured physically.[6] But it is this latter thesis which motivates panpsychism: panpsychism, in the first instance, is the view that the ultimate material constituents are required to be *conscious* in order to support macroconsciousness.

7. Elsewhere, Nagel's talk of the subjective features of experience seems best understood as referring simply to *qualia*: he says the relevant subjective features comprise 'what any conscious mental state is like for its possessor'.[7] What then is the difficulty for science in explaining qualia? Rosenthal suggests Nagel may believe that science simply cannot explain the fact of their *consciousness.* It is 'the passage from physical properties to *conscious states* with [qualia] which causes the difficulty',[8] as Rosenthal diagnoses Nagel's concern.

8. But, for Rosenthal, Nagel knits two things together here that ought to be kept separate, at least in our thinking. Entangling them can give the appearance of an impossible conceptual knot around phenomenality, yet when they are teased apart we gain explanatory purchase—or so Rosenthal believes. The two threads are one's

[6] This distinction is reminiscent of the point consistently pressed by Shoemaker (e.g. 1991), who holds that while inverted qualia cannot be physically ruled out, absent qualia can be. That is, *which* sensory quality an experience instantiates perhaps cannot be physically captured, but consciousness as such—what I called the point of view of sentient life in its most general form—is physically analysable.

[7] Nagel (1979: 188).

[8] Rosenthal (1983: 286, my emphasis).

consciousness, on one hand, and the *qualities* one is conscious of, on the other. The Rosenthalian divide-and-conquer strategy for phenomenality is familiar. Consciousness itself is explicated as a kind of awareness, supplied on Rosenthal's theory by one's having a higher-order thought (HOT) representing a certain sensorily qualitied state, e.g. a perceptual state.[9] As for the sensory qualities or qualia pertaining to the represented mental state, and which one experiences in phenomenal consciousness, Rosenthal believes these can exist in conscious and unconscious form. His understanding of blindsight cases seems to be that subjects have sensorily qualitied perceptual states, featuring (e.g.) fully-blown red qualia, but, lacking the requisite HO representation of these enqualitied states, the subjects do not consciously enjoy their qualitative features.

9. How does Rosenthal's two-component theory of consciousness bear on Nagel's position? As we've seen, Rosenthal dismisses the construal of subjectivity explicated via the notion of a point of view as useless to Nagel's argument. The other way of understanding subjectivity, for Rosenthal's Nagel, is as being bound up with consciousness.[10] Nagel's view seems to be that consciousness is physically inexplicable, and spreads this elusiveness over the sensory qualities inherent in it.[11] Now as regards consciousness itself, Rosenthal considers Nagel mistaken in holding that it is physically inexplicable (hence must be grafted onto lower-level matter, yielding panpsychism). If consciousness is a question of having a suitable HOT representing one's sensory state, as Rosenthal proposes, then it is indeed physically explicable in principle, since on the HOT account providing such an explanation would just seem to require identifying the neural architecture underlying HO representation; not a task without its complications, certainly, but not a project, either, that faces any obviously insuperable theoretical barrier.

10. Concerning the other component of phenomenal properties, sensory qualities, Rosenthal's Nagel considers these problematic for physicalists only because he is guilty of embroiling them with consciousness. Nagel is with the philosophical mainstream in holding that a red quale exists only in so far as someone is conscious of it. Sensory qualities are by nature phenomenally conscious on this view, which is why Nagel counts them as 'subjective'. Rosenthal's theory, however, separates qualia from what implements consciousness of them, and comprehends them as capable of

[9] This is a simplification. For full details of Rosenthal's HOT theory see e.g. Rosenthal (1986).

[10] Rosenthal (1983: 286). It's plausible that something has a point of view, in the relevant sense, if and only if it is conscious. Yet these do not seem to be exactly the same property. If the biconditional holds, the relationship looks to be something like as close as that between *having three sides* and *having three internal angles*, which are not the same property, albeit deeply connected. Though we, with Rosenthal, consider the ideas of *points of view* and *sheer consciousness* separately as possible Nagelian obstacles to scientific explanation, Nagel himself rather talks as though the two properties are more interpenetrating (e.g. Nagel 1979: 188–9).

[11] That would, overall, imply that conscious qualia—phenomenal properties—are physically irreducible, i.e. *Non-reductionism*.

existence outside of consciousness. Thus they are not, as properties, ineluctably subjective, where subjectivity is understood as having essentially to do with consciousness. Since qualia are no longer to be considered subjective features, they cannot constitute Nagel's sticking point for a physicalist account of mentality. Suitably distinguished from what goes into consciousness of them, Rosenthal takes sensory qualities to be perfectly capable of integration into the objective physical order.

11. Nagel's somewhat wispy notion of *subjective features* has failed to condense into any suitably solid impediment to physicalism, from Rosenthal's perspective. The notion of 'point of view' could not supply the needed substance. Meanwhile, Nagel's conception of phenomenal consciousness ignores the distinction between episodes of awareness and what those episodes supply awareness of, namely sensory qualities. This conflation lends phenomenality a deceptive aura of impenetrability: in accounting for sensory qualities one seems to have to include their conscious 'glow'; and in trying to capture conscious awareness one seems to have to analyse it so as to imply all the myriad forms of qualitativity. Indeed, as a general appraisal of his position, it seems that when Nagel considers consciousness as physically irreducible, this is because he thinks of it as consciousness *of sensory quality*, with the latter element deemed physically elusive.[12] Then, when he judges the qualities we find in consciousness to be physically irreducible, this is because he conceives of them as *conscious* qualities, and locates the difficulty in the former element.[13] In short, he does not quite settle on what is physically problematic about either element in itself. Yet once awareness is sanitized of the qualitative aspect, one starts to see that it might be given a merely relational treatment of some kind. And once sensory qualities are disassociated from consciousness they begin to look like rather more harmless properties, apt to be slotted into the physical world. So I read Rosenthal. Next we begin to rehabilitate Nagel's argument.

12. Without going so far as to endorse his HOT theory, the distinction Rosenthal draws between qualia (red patches in the visual field) and consciousness of them is valuable, in revealing texture in what otherwise appeared a forbiddingly smooth *explanandum*. Given this division between qualitative contents and conscious awareness, it seems likely the latter will prove relationally analysable. We plausibly have some species of intrinsic properties in play,[14] sensory qualities like visual redness, and what provides consciousness of them is putting their instances into some special

[12] See Nagel (1974), where the focus is on the physical elusiveness of *what it is like* to be a bat, i.e. bat-ish sensory qualities.

[13] This emphasis is evident in Nagel (1979), where we find the argument for panpsychism.

[14] This is plausible *prima facie*, but by no means obvious *ultima facie*. Whether qualia are intrinsic, and in what sense—not to mention why—is something to be explored and argued over. Exploration and argument come below.

relation with another thing, be it a Lycanian internal-scanner,[15] a Rosenthalian HOT, or something else.[16]

13. Pursuing this divide-and-conquer strategy does not yet make us reductionists about phenomenality, as normally understood. Reductionism seeks to naturalize phenomenality through explicating both the *conscious awareness* and the *sensorily qualitative* component in other terms.[17] But all we're contemplating is the division of phenomenality and analysis of the *conscious awareness* part. The story regarding qualities is more complicated. For anti-reductionists in spirit, it's worth noting that even a philosopher like James has a relational theory of conscious awareness.[18] In his neutral monist phase he takes the world to be constituted of 'pure experiences'—neutral data of some sort—with consciousness implemented by a relationship whereby one datum 'takes' another as its 'object'. It's hard to say exactly what James is getting at with this talk, but a relational view of conscious awareness it certainly is. In this much James and Rosenthal are peas in the same pod. I propose we enter their pod just that far.

14. Once we concede that awareness might be given some relational treatment or other,[19] it becomes little wonder that Rosenthal maintains a physical account could do the job. Physical science excels precisely in 'mechanistic' explanations of things in terms of their workings, relating parts x (lever-arm) and y (spring) to z (cheese-holder) to show how the whole realizes a given functional property (mousetrap-ness). To the extent we have scientifically pinned down the property of *life*, for example, it is because we were able to functionalize it to some degree, then mount an explanation in terms of how relationships between an organism's parts implement these functions. Perhaps something similar can be achieved for awareness, in the broad spirit of a HOT account.[20]

15. We've separated consciousness and earmarked it for relational analysis. This leaves us with qualia, like patches of visual redness: the *contents* of phenomenal consciousness. Rosenthal judges that, once disentangled from consciousness, sensory

[15] Lycan (1996).

[16] Perhaps the relevant relation is representation but borne by qualia to themselves. That would give us a self-representational theory like that defended by Kriegel (2009).

[17] I take this definition from Kriegel (2009: Ch. 1).

[18] See especially the first few essays of James (1912).

[19] Other than endorsing the distinction between consciousness and qualities as natural, and taking the relationality of awareness as a plausible consequence, I don't propose to argue for this move. The value is in where it leads us.

[20] I find the core reasoning of higher-order representationalists on this point attractive (see Rosenthal (2005) and Kriegel (2009) for examples): consciousness of sensory qualities amounts to one's being aware of (oneself as instantiating) sensory qualities, which awareness is naturally construed as one's representing to oneself mentally such quality instantiation. Depending as to the nature of the representation and the precise relation it bears to the represented qualities, one arrives at HOT theory or one of its kin.

qualities will slot relatively unproblematically into the physicalist worldview. But this is too quick. Qualia seem to be 'intrinsic properties', if any are. And if it's true that you cannot give an account of truly intrinsic properties in terms of relational goings-on, this will suffice to make qualia physically irreducible.

16. Talk of qualia as 'truly intrinsic' must be made more precise to be useful. Pereboom has something to say which may help: on his terminology qualia are 'absolutely intrinsic properties'.[21] These he contrasts with (merely) *comparatively* intrinsic properties. The circular shape of a hula-hoop is intrinsic to it, plausibly: anywhere you put the hoop—without subjecting it to undue forces, etc.—it's going to be circular: circularity belongs to *it*. Still, its circularity is only comparatively intrinsic, Pereboom explains, since this property is wholly accounted for by relations between the hoop's parts: roughly, the hoop's molecules are bonded into a solid, and they are arranged such that they form a circle. The intrinsic circularity of the hula-hoop is in fact explicable by mentioning only *extrinsic* properties of its parts: their organization. It doesn't much matter what the parts are like, only how they are interrelated. The same goes for individually non-liquid water molecules jointly composing liquid water: liquidity is just a matter of intermolecular relations, extrinsic properties (of molecules) again. Most macroscopic properties are like this, indeed. A property is comparatively intrinsic when it is *dissolvable* into extrinsic properties of the parts of the object to which it is intrinsic. Pereboom weighs seriously the hypothesis that qualia cannot be explained likewise, by mentioning only extrinsic properties of components of qualia-bearers (say, us), which would make them absolutely intrinsic properties.

17. Thus the standard physicalistically acceptable model of explanation of macro-features in terms of the configuration of parts would fail in this case: qualia, as absolutely intrinsic, would not be susceptible of capture within the conventionally conceived physical world.

18. The question would be: *What makes* qualia absolutely intrinsic properties? Absolute intrinsicness ensures a property goes all the way down to the lowest ontological level. If it cannot be accounted for by the arrangement of parts that lack it, then it—or something sufficiently like it—must be there in the mereological basement, if it is to be instantiated at all: thus in particles, or whatever is basic.[22] Explanation: Since mention only of relations between components of whole x cannot account for x's tokening property q, x's components must possess, intrinsically,

[21] Pereboom (2011: Ch. 5). I made a similar distinction in 2009, but not nearly so neatly or clearly. He takes the form of the distinction from Leibniz and the terminology from Kant.

[22] This is given the assumption that emergentism is ruled out. From here to §31 we're really just taking the long way around Leibniz's mill (Leibniz 1714/1991: §17). But the mill repays repeat visits.

something relevant to *q*'s generation—some property ontologically close enough to *q* (e.g. determinates of the same determinable). But if it is at non-basic mereological level *l* that *x*'s components first possess the *q*-relevant property, that would make the occurrence of that property at *l* emergent: since to be non-emergent it would have to be explicable in terms of the configuration of *x*'s components at still lower levels, yet by hypothesis none of *x*'s components at any sub-*l* level possesses anything like the relevant property, and we know this property to be inexplicable in terms of extrinsic properties, for it is not comparatively intrinsic. Therefore, if *x* possesses absolutely intrinsic property *q*, it is at the lowest level of *x*'s constituents that we must look for the *q*-relevant property. The model is charge: macroscopic items possess charge due, ultimately, to the charges of their fundamental constituents.

19. We would need good reason to rank qualia—qualities—alongside properties like mass and charge as ontologically fundamental. The deep reason, of which the intuition of their absolute intrinsicness is just the expression,[23] is that qualia are *qualitative*, and you cannot derive the qualitative from the non-qualitative.[24]

20. What do we mean by 'qualitative'? One is tempted to say, with Block's Louis Armstrong, that if you gotta ask you ain't never gonna get to know.[25] It's not 'non-relational' or 'non-dispositional', though the relational and the dispositional are often the relevant contrast classes. 'Not-merely-relational' is quite good, but one wants to know what the *something more* then is. We mean *positively* qualitative. We could approach by way of examples, but these are all likely to involve qualia, which doesn't carry us very far.[26] We can certainly say that its quality is what makes each type of

[23] Note that, as concerns mass and charge, there is plausibly no similar *intuition* that they are absolutely intrinsic.

[24] Rosenthal (see especially his 1999) considers that it is construing them as essentially conscious which makes sensory qualities appear physically irreducible. But his analysis of this apparent irreducibility is questionable. He maintains that sensory qualities come in and out of consciousness unchanged (so an unexperienced red quale is every bit as *red* as when conscious). He then notes that we find a difficulty in accepting the physical reducibility of sensory qualities when they are experienced. But he subsequently suggests that we find no such difficulty when we think of qualities as unexperienced, despite the fact that they are (by his lights) unaltered by consciousness. One might have thought that if we find a problem with qualities as experienced, and they are unaltered by going into the non-experiential darkness, then there would be a problem with reducing them *qua* unexperienced, too. At least, Rosenthal provides no reason why we should reason from the (alleged, by him) lack of difficulty associated with naturalizing unexperienced qualia to the reducibility of conscious qualia, as he recommends, rather than from the (admitted, by him) difficulty with naturalizing conscious qualia to an equal difficulty (in light of the 'no-change' doctrine he advances) concerning unexperienced qualia.

[25] From Block (1978). Michelle Montague reminds me that Block uses Armstrong to evoke *conscious* qualities, whereas we concentrate on qualities alone here, even taking it that qualities can exist without consciousness. But this is no problem: the only way we know what these qualities are like is by being conscious of them, and the Block/Armstrong point still applies.

[26] Armstrong, discussing much the same point, gives this list of qualities (1961: 188): 'Colours, sounds, tastes, smells, heat and cold'. It's probably no accident that the list has the same members and order as Hume's in 'Of the Modern Philosophy' (1738/1975: Treatise, Bk I part IV sect. 4).

conscious experience the type it is, as distinct from experiences featuring other kinds of quality. But this is really only to say that different qualities are different, and it still only comes at the nature of qualities from a relational angle. It seems we simply have to rely on an inherited intuitive sense of the qualitative,[27] and plough on. That's so, at least, as far as the *general* class of qualities is concerned: but to confine ourselves to an amenable example, on which everyone can easily enough fix their mind, a colour will do, like *occurrent pinkness.*

21. Concerning the alleged impossibility of deriving qualitative properties from the non-qualitative, we can perhaps do little better than Sellars, who bluntly greets the suggestion as 'absurd... How, we would surely expostulate, can an object's having occurrent pinkness consist in facts about its parts, none of which facts involves occurrent color?!'[28]

22. The following thought experiment captures the Sellarsian sentiment. We can imagine God shuffling around colourless tiles, combining them hither and thither in ever more complex forms and relationships. Maybe the tiles possess basic dispositional properties like pushing and pulling one another at a distance, and depending on their shapes they attract or repel similarly or differently shaped other tiles—let the tile-world be rich in such properties. Can any amount of divine shuffling of these colourless tiles *by itself* generate colour in the scenario? It doesn't seem that it can. For how could we obtain items for which there is an answer to the question 'What is it like?' (Answer, for instance, 'pink') *just* by re-arranging items for which the answer to this question is: 'Qualitatively? Nothing at all'. How could *all there is* to the quality of the sum be but the relationships holding between qualityless items?[29] To be sure, we can easily imagine God simply 'pushing the colour button' at a certain point, and the whole scene flooding with colour. But that would be not at all on the model of a reductive explanation. To be naturalistically respectable, higher-level properties demand to be understood as *configurational*: they are the mere product of the arrangement of lower-level bits and pieces *given the properties already in play.*[30] If God, or Mother Nature, has to press the quality button at a certain level of material organization—say, the level of enbrained creatures—then qualities (qualia) emerge, and emergentism is true. That is not the way to capture qualia within the physicalist

[27] E.g. Armstrong (1961) seems to use the term as I do, and he follows Hume, and others, closely.

[28] Sellars (1981: III 25).

[29] This difficulty seems in no measure subdued by taking into account the history or 'teleology' of assemblies of tiles, attributing some sets 'response-dependent' properties with respect to other sets, inserting 'tracking' relations, etc. All the standard physicalist manoeuvres consist in *arranging the essentially qualityless.*

[30] Here we reassert Nagel's *Non-emergence* premise, kith of Sellars's principle of the *strong reducibility of properties* (e.g. Sellars 1963: 27).

worldview. Even most Type B physicalists don't hold that qualia emerge—they only think that for contingent reasons we can't see how it is that they *don't* emerge.[31]

23. Further support for qualitative irreducibility can be drawn from Mary's familiar story. The knowledge argument is usually deployed to show at least a conceptual gap between phenomenality and the physical.[32] But it's important to see that whatever force the argument has derives not from the epistemic elusiveness of consciousness as such. Mary knows about consciousness, after all, since Mary is a normal conscious person. So if there's something it is like simply *to be conscious*, that's not something which eludes Mary. The slippery quarry for Mary is what it's like to be conscious of *red*. Plausibly what escapes her is just what redness is like, its quality. Mary doesn't know this, since she's never come across any redness, in the only manner we are able to come across such qualities—by being conscious of them. The qualitative character of red cannot be gleaned from Mary's Galilean scientific textbooks, which make no use of qualities in their explanations of phenomena. What Mary's story indicates is just the gulf between orthodox physical goings-on and qualities. This is not to say that consciousness isn't something important and difficult to explain. But the real power of the knowledge argument flows from the difficulty of accommodating qualities within the conventionally conceived—i.e. qualityless—physical world.

24. The divine tiles thought experiment and Mary together supply good evidence that qualities are metaphysically irreducible, which explains why they are absolutely intrinsic in Pereboom's sense. Pereboom, for his part, turns to a non-qualia-like, i.e. non-qualitative, class of absolutely intrinsic properties to try to account for macro-phenomenal properties.[33] These more physicalistically respectable fundamental properties are stipulated to produce phenomenal properties in configuration, despite being non-qualitative (and non-conscious). In fact, their defined role in generating phenomenal properties aside, the character of Pereboom's absolute intrinsics remains unspecified—they are categorical *blanks*. But adding a mysterious absolutely intrinsic *non-quality* to the divine tiles improves matters not a jot, so we should reject Pereboom's proposal. His stipulation is a metaphysical cheque doomed to bounce. This is just another variation on a hopeless theme—to analyse qualities as mere complexes of the qualityless. The Galilean physicalist's ambition to conjure a painting from a pencil sketch is impossible.

[31] I take it that those who posit brute necessary *a posteriori* connections between qualia and the physical—in effect psychophysical laws—qualify as emergentists in the relevant sense. I won't directly tackle epistemic Type B physicalists—those who think we are (e.g.) conceptually barred from understanding the non-emergent production of qualia. My instinct is to do all we can to mount a positive theory of consciousness, and I'm not convinced this will entail any violation of physicalism. One way to counter a position is to offer a more warm-blooded alternative.

[32] For this version of the knowledge argument see Jackson (1982). Jackson draws a stronger metaphysical conclusion than we do, the truth of dualism.

[33] Other advocates of this sort of view are Tom McClelland and Daniel Stoljar.

25. The naturalist's arsenal is all but exhausted: it needs supplementing. Life was problematic, appearing at one time an irreducible property, because consciousness was implicitly mixed in with it. Then it seemed that consciousness was the last bastion against science—but if we make the move of dividing conscious awareness from quality, and attack consciousness relationally, this outpost too will fall. Quality is the truly insurmountable rampart. At notable points in its history, science has seen fit to admit a new class of basic properties, out of explanatory necessity. Given its extant repertoire of things and properties, it could not make sense of some salient phenomenon, and progress was blocked. We are at such a moment: a Maxwell moment. Basic matter will have to be qualitative, since we experience qualities.

26. Accommodating this fact constitutes not an abandonment of physicalism, as much as a step towards its completion as a theory of all that is. This undercuts the motivation for adopting some of the unsustainable protective contortions into which physicalists press themselves, such as insisting that qualities simply *must* be derivable from the non-qualitative, *somehow*; or that qualities are an outright illusion; or else that we are actually designed—as if by Descartes's demon—to be unable to comprehend their generation; or, that this happens to be the *very spot* in nature for the uniquely brute production of a significant macroproperty. It would likely be but plain distaste for qualities which prevented physicalists from even exploring the line to be traced below, and there is nothing essentially scientific about *that* sentiment.[34]

27. Here, then, is our revised Nagelian argument:

P1. *Material Composition*: Any living organism is wholly composed of a huge number of particles.

P2. *Non-reductionism*^{Q}: Qualitative properties are not implied by any non-qualitative properties alone.

P3. *Quality Realism*: Some organisms instantiate qualities. (Evidence: we consciously experience qualities.)

P4. *Non-emergence*: All high-level properties of a complex system intelligibly derive from properties of its constituents plus their arrangement.

Therefore: Basic matter has qualities.

Assuming it holds as before that:

Fungibility: Any matter can compose an organism (including, notably, the sort mentioned in P3).

[34] Though scientists do routinely express such distaste. See Heisenberg (1937: 119).

We derive:

Conclusion: All basic matter has qualities.

This is not panpsychism, but *panqualityism*.

28. Compared with the argument attributed to Nagel, this incarnation lacks reference to *phenomenal properties*, and to *physical properties*. It makes no mention of phenomenal properties because these are now taken to be composite: being conscious of a quale is a bipartite state of affairs consisting of a *conscious awareness* on one hand of the *quale* on the other. Our main concern is the elusiveness of qualities.

29. Nagel assumed that phenomenal properties are intrinsic to an experiencing creature. This argument takes experienced qualities to be intrinsic to the experiencer. Nagel's internalist assumption is understandable given his strong association of qualia with consciousness, added to the plausible doctrine that consciousness is an intrinsic property of experiencers. But since our topic is qualities ontologically independent of consciousness, it is less obvious why the argument focuses on those qualities instantiated by experiencers, instead of the putative qualities of external perceptual objects. The argument's conclusion is that there are qualities *everywhere*, but it departs from those of which we can be most certain: these are the qualities we experience, and which belong to us. This is not a paper directly about perception, but rather ontology, therefore we are within rights simply to assume *quality internalism*—the view that the qualities of which we are immediately aware belong to our organism. This line will be partly justified by epistemological rewards we receive later on.[35]

30. Regarding the conscious awareness of qualities: we should allow that, as a relational affair, it might well be capable of conventional physical explanation. Hence Rosenthal's criticism of Nagel's argument—effectively, that Nagel takes for

[35] P3 signals a rejection of the treatment of qualities, as *merely* represented—i.e. wholly uninstantiated—properties (see e.g. the first half of Pereboom 2011). Someone might reasonably think that not all our encounters with qualities are encounters with instantiated qualities (see e.g. Johnston 2004), but the idea that qualities are *nowhere* instantiated is hard to take seriously. Eliminativist representationalists must answer two tough questions, which come at the representational mechanism from either end: (i) What could provide the representations in question with their contents, in the sense of intentional objects, if there are not, and have never been, qualities, nor anything like them, instanced anywhere? (ii) What could enable the sensory states in question to represent—i.e. stand for, portray—qualities if they are precluded from the use of qualities in the representations? (When we want to represent qualities *outside* the head we routinely use other quality instances to do this: as in holding up a swatch for a suit; and non-qualitative representations, e.g. text, are clearly parasitic on acquaintance with such exemplars.) These questions correspond to asking just *what* these representationalists hold to be ascribed to the environs in consciousness, and *how* it would be ascribed. Sellars is again highly sensible on this topic; on such a view, he says: 'we have taken [qualities] out of our world picture altogether. We will have made it unintelligible how things could even *appear* to be coloured.' (Sellars 1963: 30).

granted something called 'subjectivity' which will elude the objective point of view—does not apply. Our argument makes no use, implicit or otherwise, of the notion of the subjective. That is the fat trimmed from Nagel's argument. Distinguishing qualities from episodes of conscious awareness of them, we need not take qualities to be restricted to phenomenal consciousness; *a fortiori* their existence is not exhausted by figuring in consciousness. They are not subjective in this, the second, Nagelian sense. We needn't take them to be subjective in the first sense either, i.e. restricted to particular points of view, though this will require some explaining.[36] Nagel rhetorically asks 'what would be left of what it was like to be a bat if one removed the viewpoint of the bat?'[37] The ready answer is: whichever qualities the bat was experiencing—much as, for common sense, a perceived object is left with its qualities when we look away from it.

31. This brings us to the omission of 'physical properties'. Since the argument gives no reason for holding that qualities are non-objective in any significant sense, there is no in-principle motivation, at least for all the argument says, for discounting them as physical properties. Thus Nagel's *Non-reductionism* premise, as he frames it, is ultimately false.[38] Given contemporary mores, the conclusion that basic matter is qualitative in something like the way qualia are qualitative amounts to Russell-style neutral monism. But this will turn out to be compatible with physicalism; or at least, all of physicalism one could reasonably want—indeed, physicalism is well served by this move. These are murky ideas at first sight; one aim of the remainder is to make them clearer. What follows is a fairly detailed sketch of a certain picture of how qualities and the physical integrate. For reasons of space, many of the details are exhibited rather than defended—although most are defensible. However, assuming physicalism, *something like* this picture in its broad outlines must be true, by the argument just given.

32. Basic matter is qualitative. How to understand this claim? As physicalists we defer to physics when it comes to characterizing ultimate ontology. So what's called for is integration of the thesis that quality is a fundamental property with what physics tells us about the attributes of the tiniest entities. Sellars initially dismisses the possibility of this marriage: 'whatever other difficulties such a view would involve, it doesn't make sense to say of the particles of physical theory that they are coloured'.[39]

[36] Strictly, I should say qualities are not restricted to points of view *except* in so far as this is an objectively explicable matter. But that is a wrinkle we will smooth out below (§§93–5).

[37] Nagel (1979: 173).

[38] Assuming, that is, the physical reducibility of (relationally construed) awareness. The premise would be true were the sense of 'physical' restricted to the non-qualitative. One rhetorical question running through this paper is: *Whyever would we want so to restrict it?*

[39] Sellars (1963: 35). The 'other difficulties' would include the grain problem—how do discrete particles realize the homogenous colour-fields we experience? (Note that this is not a problem with the sheer idea of particles being coloured: in fact Sellars (1963) broaches coloured particles directly as a response to the grain

33. *Colours* will do as a conceptual hook for this issue, since they are qualities we can easily latch onto and imagine as filling spatial volumes. But their usefulness is probably limited to providing an analogy. Though Unger conceives of quarks and electrons literally being blue and red,[40] it seems problematic to commit ourselves as to the primitive qualities of particles existing outside of brains. It appears we do know *some* of the qualities particles carry, at least in massive conglomerations, because those are qualities we encounter in consciousness when such conglomerations constitute the relevant portions of our brains. But given that we only experience the qualities of these particles *en masse*, and in a special (cerebral) context, there seems little reason to hold that the qualities of extra-cranial particles will be qualities of our acquaintance. They are just required to be qualities that, in the right (exceedingly complex) combinations, yield the qualities we know. This doesn't seem to place much restriction on their nature, at least that can be obvious to us at this stage of theorizing. The fundamental qualities will certainly be *of a kind* with the qualia we know, a kinship best explicated via the connection to *what-it-is-like-ness*. Were you to be directly consciously aware of an isolated particle, its quality (plus your awareness of it) would go into what it was like to be you at that moment. What it—the particle—was like qualitatively would help to constitute what it—consciousness—was like for you. However, seeing that nothing appears lost by the move, we will for now use colours as convenient placeholders for the fundamental qualities.[41]

34. Why does Sellars dismiss coloured fundamental physical particles?[42] Re-treading this territory later, he 'take[s] it to be a conceptual truth about molecules that they do not have color in the occurrent sense'.[43] He would presumably extend this remark to physical particles, and now we have our clue: the trouble with coloured particles is *conceptual.* In Sellars's framework, an analysis of the interactions of our various conceptual schemes, physical particles are introduced under the *scientific image*, a conceptual network embodying a Galilean worldview of qualityless matter in motion, whose quantities and interrelations science charts.

problem.) A field conception of matter would seem to promise an answer: when considered in highly localized form, the fundamental physical field is helpfully conceived of as particulate. This is only the start of an answer to the grain problem; see Coleman (2015a) for more on this, and related issues. Sellars (1963) airs, without quite endorsing, the solution to the grain problem that ultimate reality is 'non-particulate' (Sellars 1963: 37). By 1981 he embraces it, in the form of an 'absolute process' conception of basic ontology, discussed below.

[40] See Unger (1998). Unger holds the qualities of basic particles to be epiphenomenal: they can be changed without altering the powers of an enqualitied entity. It's unclear why he holds this. I take it a more satisfying view will tie qualities to the causal roles of physical entities, thus providing qualities with a respectable home in the physical world. More on this below.

[41] The obliging reader will keep this placeholder status for colours in mind.

[42] Certain commentators consider the claim not in need of support, thus Richardson and Muhlenberg (1982: §9) aver that '[Sellars' claim] that... particles are not colored surely needs no argument'. But it would be helpful at least to know what makes the claim so obvious.

[43] Sellars (1981: III 20).

35. This amounts to noting that our inherited conception of physical particles doesn't ascribe them anything like occurrent colour (colour in Sellars's 'aesthetically interesting'[44] sense). Hence we cannot *within* the extant frameworks of neuroscience or physics define entities with the qualitative properties of sensations.[45] However, we are effectively in the business of *revising* the scientific image to accommodate qualities, so that science can explain phenomenality; or, should a Sellarsian maintain that science is not thus revisable, of building a framework to succeed it, which achieves a synoptic view of material conscious creatures and their world.

36. In fact Sellars is only a false foe, for he knows more or less exactly what to do towards a synoptic view. It is only that, we will see, he does not go far enough in certain respects. Sellars's favoured position will serve as a stalking horse behind which to reach another theory.

37. Elsewhere he argues:

> a theory which is to explain the properties of core persons will involve a family of families of predicates which would be a *categorial transformation*, but not substantive reduction, of raw feel predicates, and which would apply only to systems of scientific objects . . . at the most fundamental level.[46]

By this 'categorial transformation' Sellars means that colours, unreduced—which is to say, taken just as they are qualitatively—are to be shifted in ontological category and rehoused in basic physical ontology. In his mature philosophy he abandons the ultimate reality of fundamental physical *objects*, in favour of a conception of 'absolute processes'[47] (this for two main reasons, one of which will concern us shortly[48]).

38. Processes are ongoing, and causally charged. *Absolute* processes differ in two main respects, while inheriting these valuable characteristics. Where processes are object-bound, so that a buzzing belongs to a bee, absolute processes are self-standing—there is (simply) a buzzing, or: buzzing.[49] Processes are spread out over time—the bee's

[44] Sellars (1971a: 408).

[45] A slightly stronger formulation might claim that the very meaning of particle terms excludes such properties as colours from being predicated of their referents. But it's not clear that terms like 'atom' or 'fundamental particle' have their meaning fixed exclusively by their role in our physics. Doesn't it make sense to say that Plato in *Timaeus* (360BCE/1997) was effectively talking about fundamental particles, and if so, don't we have to say that he attributed qualities like 'brightness' to them? In any case—as against Grossmann (1975: 131)—does physics positively exclude, as opposed simply to omitting mention of, coloured particles?

[46] Sellars (1965: 448).

[47] Sellars credits C. D. Broad with the terminology.

[48] This ontology is non-particulate, which helps Sellars to finesse his grain problem: particles, and other objects, are to be seen as logical constructions out of the absolute processes. The reason that will soon occupy us has to do with meeting a threat of epiphenomenalism.

[49] They can take 'dummy' logical subjects, as in 'It buzzes'.

buzzing has a beginning, a middle, and an end, and these are not compresent. An absolute process is all here in one go—like Mozart hearing one of his symphonies all at once.[50] Nonetheless, an absolute process is an essentially active, fluxy kind of existent, but fundamentally *non-particulate*—it *is*:

the actualization of an 'intrinsic character' or 'dynamic quality'.[51]

39. Sellars demands this categorial transformation because the manifest image (naïvely) views colours as macroscopic 'stuffs' composing objects,[52] or (maturely)[53] as mere states of perceivers. Their ultimate rehousing in the realm of fundamental processes requires us to transport the same 'content' from the manifest to the synoptic conception, i.e. the colourfulness of colours. Nowadays philosophers, perhaps non-philosophers too, are apt to construe colours in terms of surface properties of perceptible objects—textures, or propensities to reflect light in varying keys, corresponding to different colours. This sort of view has plausibly become part of our manifest image.[54] We cannot carry colours over into fundamental ontology while retaining this aspect of our way of framing them, since basic particles lack surface textures, and electrons alone among them are candidates for light emitters.[55]

40. To isolate the content to be transposed intact, we need to extricate colours from these associations and behold them in pure form. Here are two methods. The first is simply to consider all the ways of understanding colours mentioned above, and subtract everything except what they have in common. The second route is positive: consider colours as they figure in dreams, where light reflectance properties play no role, there are no relevant perceptible objects, etc.[56] Now *hold it*: that is, try to avoid immediately leaping to (e.g.) contemplating the neural 'basis' of such colours. For a brief period the philosopher must stand still and consider something *just as it is*.

[50] This ability is probably, sadly, only apocryphally ascribed.

[51] Seibt (2000: 279), punctuation as in original.

[52] So an apple is a slab of red with a slab of white 'inside'.

[53] Because, in deVries's paraphrase, even in the manifest image 'the notion that colours, tastes, smells, sounds and feels are the very substance of the objects that confront us in the world cannot hold up' (deVries 2005: 204). Our ultimate recommendation is roughly 'back to basics', marrying the naïve conception with modern microphysics.

[54] I also frequently encounter the view among non-philosopher friends that colours are (belong to?) different wavelengths of light. All such proposals call for the same treatment.

[55] Noren (1977: 78): 'the color a thing has is explained by reference to the electromagnetic radiation given off by the atoms said to constitute the thing, i.e. given off by the atom's electrons as they "move" from a higher to a lower energy state, etc. It follows, then, that neither the atoms nor the electrons *can* be colored.' Despite an easy first appearance, it's hard to say exactly why what is alleged to follow is taken by Noren so to do.

[56] I'm unreceptive to philosophers who deny dreaming colour experience, and claim we only misremember such experiences. Why not say that I confabulate *all* my waking memories of having seen colour?

Clasp colour in its role as *explanandum*, for a moment, suspend it there, and go no further.

41. What we now want to say, with Sellars, is that colour, taken just as such, *constitutes* the fundamental physical world. For Sellars colours are 'a dimension of natural [absolute] process'.[57] Among the world's fundamental furniture are such items as 'reddings', the 'transposition of [colours] into the framework of absolute process'.[58]

42. Processes are dynamic and causally charged. This is to the good, because a major preoccupation Sellars shares with us is that qualities should be understood as causally efficacious—they make things happen in the physical world. His way of overcoming historical tendencies to quality epiphenomenalism is to place the conventionally physical *alongside* the qualitative as equally kinds of absolute processes, basic layers of a world which is a 'tissue of goings-on'. There are thus 'quarkings' as well as 'reddings'. With this *categorial* monism established, Sellars reckons, reasons to see the qualitative as causally isolated evaporate; qualitative absolute processes can be seen to interact perfectly sensibly with physical absolute processes.

43. Sellars maintains that qualitative processes arise uniquely in the context of those physical processes constitutive of what (at a higher level) we call brains. The world surrounding sentient creatures features only recognizably conventional, non-qualitative, physical processes, obediently following the established laws of physics. Once a central nervous system is built—according to these extant laws—a new sort of absolute process comes into being, the qualitative 'dimension'. Qualitative absolute processes and conventional physical processes thence *combine* in the construction of our familiar qualia.[59]

44. Sellars has therefore two radically different sorts of absolute process in play—one qualitative, the other utterly not. But the starting point of all these enquiries was the apparent gap between the *qualitative-as-experienced* and the *physical-as-understood-through-science*. Sellars might be accused of replicating this dichotomy at the fundamental level. Perhaps these two sorts of process interact. *Perhaps*, even, there's no

[57] Sellars (1963: 37) and (1981: III 128). The addition of 'absolute' is more appropriate to the latter context. Sellars seems here very close to his father's proposal that consciousness is 'a qualitative dimension of integral activities of an emergent order'. (R. W. Sellars 1938: 475). More on the emergence element momentarily.

[58] Sellars (1981: III 115).

[59] Sellars (1981: III 121, 123, 124). Seibt (2000: 281): 'sensory processes, we are told, can function as "ingredients" of those process-bundles which constitute neurons in the ideal successor theory of present-day science'. A Sellarsian 'sense-impression' of a pink ice-cube is therefore a double-sided entity—a winding together of conventionally physical with qualitative absolute processes. It is in part coloured, in part not. Clearly we are unaware of the non-coloured element...

problem around seeing how that might be so.[60] But there's no escaping the fact that our world is left with a deep chasm down its middle. Wasn't it this chasm we were trying to close up? What we are offered is at best an unstable bridge.

45. Since the qualitative processes are of a fundamentally different sort to the conventionally physical ones ('quarkings' etc.), and since they are said to be causally efficacious, it follows that, in the context of sentient creatures—their phenomenal states and consequent actions—the laws of physics are broken. Sellars is sanguine about this: in such situations a new set of laws begins operation.[61] We should not be: Sellars is making an empirical bet that physical laws won't suffice to explain the behaviour of conscious creatures. Should they prove to suffice, Sellarsian absolute qualitative processes will be left epiphenomenal after all.[62]

46. Sellars's qualitative processes *emerge.* Purely physical laws do not account for their coming into being, rather there must be *physical-to-qualitative* laws governing their systematic production.[63]

47. The interest of physicalism as a doctrine, and the reason for the controversy as to its truth, lie in the idea that *whatever rules govern the operation of matter in non-sentient contexts, just those laws account both for the arising of sentience and, on its having arisen, the subsequent operations of the sentient system.*[64] This is surely the sense in which we are physical creatures, if such we are. So it is in vain that Sellars defines an extended sense of physical, physical_1 (meaning roughly: figures in the spatiotemporal causal network), under which the activities comprising the constitution and operations of the conscious mind may be classified. It remains the case that: (i) qualitative physical_1 absolute processes and conventional physical ('physical_2') processes are of radically different sorts of being and (ii) their interaction is governed by a novel and fundamental set of laws. Despite Sellars's delicate dialectical dance, we seem to have retained most of the bad points of Cartesian dualism, only transported now to microcosm.

[60] Though it seems there is such a problem: all there is to one sort of process is qualities, while the other kind lacks qualities altogether. This marks them out as fundamentally different kinds. Categorial monism didn't save Descartes from interaction worries, so it's hard to see why it will save Sellars, or why shifting from substances to processes constitutes a *decisive* advance.

[61] Sellars (1981: III 102/4, 113, 122). He had defended the coherence of this possibility with Meehl (1956).

[62] See the appendix of Papineau (2002) for persuasive argument that there exists a good inductive case for physical completeness.

[63] Sellars calls these 'psycho-physical laws'.

[64] As implied, it seems part of physicalism that there *are* non-sentient contexts—in this regard (at least) it is opposed to panpsychism.

48. For proper physicalism we must go further. In saying that all matter *everywhere* is qualitative (though not intrinsically conscious) and governed by the familiar laws of physics, we avoid the Sellarsian schism, and emergentism. We will encounter further reason to say this later, connected with the basis of physical causation. There is only one kind of absolute processes, the qualitative—to stick with our placeholder, ours is a world of *absolute colour processes.*

49. 'Colour-process' is a term we balk at, because colour instances don't appear active in the way processes do. Sellars's original preoccupation was with coloured *expanses* and *volumes*, and indeed this is what we encounter in perceptual consciousness. There was a good reason why the naïve manifest image could construe perceptible physical objects as made of colour *stuff.* To retain the activity and causal efficacy of process, while giving qualities just that bit more solidity, we should prefer an absolute process-*stuff*; or perhaps *stuff-process*, even a 'stuff-ing',[65] to plain absolute process. If one squeezes out a tube of red paint into a curly pile, it's possible to come close to thinking of it as a heap of *redness*, of redness *stuff*, through and through. This is to approach the recommended conception of matter. But this is still rather static: can *stuff* and *process* marry? Think of the material inside a lava lamp—it is stuff, but it moves, changes, and *does*—it is process-stuff. It is also—appears—coloured throughout. This is our prototype image for the stuff-ing of the material universe.[66]

50. This conception requires that we relinquish, as far as possible, the picture of colours as 'coating' (or 'painted' onto) macroscopic objects. Colour is not a mere attribute. We must think of a particle—a logical parcelling of absolute stuff-ing—literally *as* colour, a volume (or field) of colour-stuff-ing. Colour is what particles (hence material volumes) simply are made of. Their being colour*ed* thus derives from their being *colour*. Most strictly, a 'particle' is just what the colour stuff-ing *does* at a particular (more or less precise) co-ordinate.

51. We should resist the temptation to say colours are mere (even essential) *attributes* of absolute stuff-ings. That would be to enshrine some non-qualitative nature as the deeper reality, with the resurfacing threat of inexplicable and epiphenomenal qualities.[67] To go as far as saying that absolute stuff-ings have the sole core characteristic of colour (*redding*, *pinking*) equates to admitting colour stuff-ings in our sense.

[65] This term is in part homage to Armstrong's discussion of these issues. Though he talks initially of a need for physical objects merely to 'have' qualities, he revealingly lapses into talking of these as providing the 'stuffing for physical objects' (Armstrong 1961: 189).

[66] Thanks to Paul Coates for this image.

[67] This will likely be why Sellars of the Carus lectures does not embrace Hooker's suggestion (Hooker 1977: 348 n.5), to posit *one* set of physical *and* qualitative basic entities.

52. Sellars's qualitative absolute processes are 'physical' in the meagre sense of lacking intentionality, and 'playing a genuine causal role in the behaviour of sentient organisms'.[68] Our colourful absolute stuff-ings mount a much stronger claim to physicality: beyond the Sellarsian properties, they are, first, intrinsically non-conscious—and independent of consciousness. Second, they express the standard laws of physics. Third, as earlier indicated, but not yet explicated, the qualities of such processes are understood to be intersubjectively accessible in principle.

53. Does our *matter-as-colour-stuff-ing* conflict with what physics tells us about ontology? There are two possible points of conflict, relating to the *content* and the *structure* of the physical representation of the world.

54. As is familiar from the work, most notably, of Russell,[69] the physical description is completely silent as to the world's content, what it is like 'in itself' or 'categorically'. What we know of basic physical entities is limited to relational characterizations, which effectively encode expectations about their behaviours in varying contexts.[70] What is an electron? An item with a certain mass, spin, and charge. To say it has these properties is to capture the sorts of effect it *would have* in proximity to other items similarly specified—e.g. repelling a fellow electron, resisting acceleration—to package its anticipated behaviour into the ascription of characteristics. Even spin is construed relationally, being a sort of internal angular momentum. Physics, overall, knits a *pattern* of items and their properties, defined in terms of their interactions. These interactions themselves heap relation upon relation: charge is a tendency to alter the *distance between* charged things.

55. We are bound to a structural characterization of the external world, since our encounter with it comes via its impact on our sensorium of experienced qualities. We gain some idea of its architecture through taking the array of sensory events as isomorphic with their causes. Hence we know a patterned world of *somethings*.[71] This is also why scientific—structural—knowledge is objective, not dependent on its anchoring in any particular set of sensory qualities, or modality.[72]

[68] Sellars (1981: III 126). The former characteristic may not be all that desirable—see §70 and note 86.

[69] Russell (1921) and (1927b). This theme is also prominent in the work of R. W. Sellars and Eddington. See also Hartshorne (1934) and (1977). The core point, that we are ignorant of the 'nature' of matter, is of course a much older one.

[70] See also Hume (1738/1975: Treatise, Bk I part IV sect. 4) for stylish expression of the same essential idea. An item's behaviours are of course only *evident* in so far as they affect another item (albeit the contents of a cloud chamber), so 'behaviour' in physics is a deeply relational concept.

[71] R. W. Sellars (1922: 58): 'the knowledge gained by physical science is inevitably *external to its object* in this sense that it can grasp only those characteristics which are reproducible in another medium (order or form)'. See also Russell (1927b).

[72] Compare Feigl (1956: 143–4).

56. What are these things *like* whose interrelations we understand to ever finer degrees of precision? We have no idea, based on their physical characterization. What is the nature of the properties that confer these propensities? Ditto. We say two particles are of differing mass and charge, thereby abbreviating their potential interactions. What *about* these particles that makes it the case that they behave like this? We do not know. All we are able to record relies on their twitching: what makes them twitch thus-and-so is a mystery. So, were we to conceive of an electron as a (more or less discrete) volume of greenness (say),[73] this couldn't conflict with what we know about electrons' non-relational character, since we just don't know about that character.[74]

57. Taking physics' structural characterization at face value, and coupling a strong allegiance to science as ontological arbiter, yield *ontic structuralism*—the view that structure is all there is. But we know ontic structuralism is false as a *global* thesis, since we know of at least one physical system possessing content as well as structure: that conscious qualitative portion of brains. The idea of quality as the mere structuring of the qualityless is one we have already rejected. Ontic structuralism could be true *outside* brains only at the cost of throwing us back to emergentism. Brute laws would forcibly extract content from assemblies of contentless structure.

58. On the structure side, there is nothing *in principle* to prevent colour filling in physics, since 'we do not know of any intrinsic character which could be incompatible with the logical properties that physics assigns to physical events.'[75] There is room, then, for qualities to supply the music to the physical score.

59. How this is implemented depends on one's preferred interpretation of physics. We might envisage, for example, the fundamental physical world as a continuous but variegated quality field, or several intersecting quality fields, like enormous sheets of different colours.[76] As with a board in the game Othello, the colour instanced at any co-ordinate is determined by the surrounding colours. What results is a massive relational quality-web.[77] Crucially, however, relations are not *all there is to it*—this is

[73] Really, it would be a logical construction from *greenings*, but I will talk loosely for ease.

[74] Armstrong (1961: 190): 'Might not physics be able to produce a theory which correlated real secondary qualities of the true "fundamental particles" with their real primary qualities *in a simple way*?... what objection would there be to admitting these qualities into an account of physical reality?' We of course go far beyond *correlation*.

[75] Russell (1927b: 384). See also Feigl (1956: 87, final paragraph).

[76] Or perhaps a single field of stuff-ing of every possible quality in blended superposition. My liking for Bohm's non-collapse interpretation shows in the following discussion, but the core idea, that quality underpins the physical structure, can be adapted to suit.

[77] Notwithstanding the time it takes for human players to move the pieces, colour changes in an Othello game could be construed as the almost instantaneous products of the rules of quality-determination across

not the *bare* relational web of structuralism. Rather, the universe is like one of Mozart's instantaneous symphonies—with every qualitative value in the series deeply informed by the character of its fellows.[78] *Space* might be grounded in the extent of, and qualitative differences among, sectors of the colour field—*something* must extend, after all, for space. *Time* might be grounded in the changes effected according to the rules of qualitative interplay, with the colour at a co-ordinate giving way to a new quality as determined by interaction with its environs. The symphony would thus evolve.[79]

60. Physics describes the evolution of this field(s) of quality stuff-ing. Particles can be thought of as relatively stable nodes in the web. Given its suite of dispositions, it is perhaps inaccurate to view an electron as a genuine unit. We could expect the basic colour stuff-ings to be wholly *actual* and *simple*, hence without hidden tendencies, which bespeak complexity.[80] Instead, we might envisage electrons as certain intersections between a mass quality-field, a negative charge quality-field, etc., visualized most easily as meeting points between differently coloured, angled sheets in space-time. The specific *electron values* for these properties would then be a function of the point of field intersection—their quantized character perhaps explicable by deeper facts about the interface possibilities between the underlying quality fields. There may well be natural 'notches' where quality fields readily, and relatively stably, interlock—just as some colours and flavours fit naturally together, forming *gestalts*.

61. What is evident in experience? A continuous, four-dimensional field of (*inter alia*) colours. The panqualityist proposal is that in consciousness we have intimate contact with (a small portion of) the universal fabric. The posit of a unified, active field as the underlying physical reality finds empirical confirmation in experience.[81]

62. Colours and physical causal/relational profiles cannot be merely correlated. Colour is the stuff-ing of the physical world, hence what a given 'particle' is literally

the grid. One plausible general lesson from quantum physics is that our universe behaves as if strongly unified and non-local, with even distant parts deeply interrelated (see e.g. Smolin 2001, Bohm 1980). As Whitehead (1925) emphasized, some such features would be needed to ground induction, since if one part of the universe made no intrinsic reference to what was outside it, it's hard to see how empirical generalizations would ever be justifiable.

[78] For a familiar piece, a musical note is strongly conditioned by (i) one's knowledge of the note(s) just gone and (ii) one's expectation of the note(s) to come.

[79] Or we might say, with Sellars, that it is continuously *becoming*.

[80] Sellars envisages absolute processes as lacking 'iffyness' (conditionality). Bohm (1980: 62) similarly suggests that the dispositional complexity of our current basic particles hints at a deeper, simpler fundament.

[81] Though some account would have to be taken of the extra (perhaps 'curled up') dimensions posited by modern physics.

of. To construe its quality as immaterial, mere accompaniment, to its behaviour is then more absurd than imagining the sphericity of a ball as irrelevant to its disposition to roll. And having different qualities confer identical dispositions—if electrons came in various colours—would be more absurd than allowing different shapes to confer identical dispositions. Its quality is all there is to a particle: this would be to make the very being of a physical entity epiphenomenal. Perhaps we can conceive an *attribute* to be epiphenomenal with respect to its possessor's powers, but we cannot possibly conceive the bearer of those powers' *very stuff* to be so epiphenomenal. We can ascribe some of the ease of conceivability of *epiphenomenal qualia* to the miscategorization of qualities as mere attributes.[82] On our view each particle-type corresponds to a quality-type, the product of the values at the intersection point of the underlying quality-fields corresponding to basic physical properties.

63. Nature demands to know why an electron has its particular mass and charge. Why does it behave in *these* ways, as opposed to *those* ways? Had it different dispositions, that fact would correspond to differences *in* the disposed—but what kinds of difference?

64. Where an ageing vase becomes fragile we can point to changes in its intrinsic molecular structure. But the evolving features of this structure resolve into relations among its parts, down to ingredients like the electron just considered. The same moral applies to a story explaining a person's movement in terms of her brain-state, itself comprised of interactive neuron-structures, comprised of molecules, etc. We reach at bottom, again, mystery—*mere* regularities. Even if physical science attains perfect predictive ability, it will still omit the basis of these patterned occurrences.

65. Qualities, however, are *ultimate explainers*. Certain pains demand movement, or attempts to move. If we are *given* that a person suffers such a screaming kind of pain, no further explanation is really called for of her jerk away from the stimulus. The question is settled, macroscopically. Say that two already irritable-feeling people encounter each other in a crowded café, both keenly desirous of seating. The meeting of these qualitative states accounts for their ensuing shouting match with an explanatory richness no neuroscientific theory could match, restricted as it is to describing the outsides of the events involved.

66. Qualities needn't be conscious to play this explanatory role, as Freudian psychology illustrates. It is their quality that counts, *felt* or not.

[82] This echoes Sellars's diagnosis, on which qualities were left to 'dangle' from neurophysiological objects and their interactions.

67. It could hardly be more false, then, that 'there is *nothing dispositional*, to the subject, in the onset of a pain or a flash in the visual field'.[83]

68. Causal power varies with macroquality. Consider the diverse propensities conferred upon one by a tickle and the pain of stepping on a pin. Within a qualitative type, distinct determinates key different propensities: severe pain tends more to avoidance behaviour than mild pain. It is hard to envisage a psychological situation where, all else being equal, two different qualities subsequently added to the mental mix would have the same result, i.e. confer exactly the same propensity. It seems plausible, conversely, that qualitatively identical phenomenal fields, as instantiated by two experiencers, confer on those subjects just the same dispositions to activity.[84]

69. It would be unbelievable if nature worked utterly differently lower down—after all, we are just the top of the pyramid, a high-level congregation of natural processes. The *grounds* of particle dispositions, then, are their qualities. Likely these are quality kinds not directly known to us, though ultimately the ingredients of our own qualia. Causal/relational profiles *supervene* on quality. Moreover, they *logically* supervene. Analogously to the way two instances of irritable quality repel one another, or produce an explosion, in everyday senses of these terms, and do so *intelligibly*, there are qualities of particles that account with the same perspicuity for their behavioural tendencies.[85]

70. It has frequently been felt that the mental is the exclusive realm of final causes. Injection of qualities into physics endows our efficient causes with the potential for finality.[86]

71. While we think—conveniently—of *colours* as the fundamental properties it is challenging to understand them as conferring causal power on their microphysical bearers thanks only to their quality. But we can edge our way towards this understanding.

[83] Blackburn (1990: 65, my emphasis). Blackburn is right to stress that a quality instance can't be *reduced to* bare dispositionality/relationality.

[84] Which isn't to say the subjects *do* the same things, once other facts about their constitution and environment are included: the same disposition expresses differently across circumstances.

[85] The present view would make a natural fit with the 'powerful qualities' theory of Heil (e.g. 2005), Martin (e.g. 1997), and Strawson (2008). Of these only the last would likely entertain fundamental powerful *qualities* in our exact sense (*qualia*-tative).

[86] Martin (1997) sees a form of proto-intentionality in the way a disposition is directed towards its manifestation. Kriegel (2011) and other members of the 'Phenomenal Intentionality Research Program' see intentionality as grounded in phenomenal quality. Panqualityism can integrate these ideas in a productive direction (to the taste of neither party).

72. Qualities, far from being inert and isolated, stand *essentially* in relations to one another—hence they are not intrinsic in one use of that term. It is impossible to put two (or more) colours, flavours, musical notes, etc. in series but they seem mutually to affect and condition, existing now as a unit distinct in kind from each element taken individually. These relationships are quite *objective*, independent of our experience of them. It is not because we *experience them as* harmonious that we arrange roast beef qualia to be accompanied by red wine qualia. It is due to their harmony that we so arrange their accompaniment that we can experience it.[87]

73. Such qualitative relations often supply change and constraint. Notoriously, a colour is altered by varying its coloured background. Pain qualia displace itch qualia, but not conversely. Bitter qualia will exclude other flavours. Etc.

74. Some qualia we also understand as causal, even if we don't perhaps think of them *as* qualia. There are qualia of effort, as in pushing against a heavy obstacle, qualia of pedalling hard. We *expect* the upshot of such qualities to be movement.[88] There must be something similar in the qualia of magnetic attraction.[89]

75. We incline to viewing qualities as epiphenomenal because they supply the paint with which perception represents the world. It will never, therefore, seem that something happens *in the world* because of an object's sensed quality, which is just its mode of representation to us. Correlations abound—like the silver surface of a kettle radiating little heat—but these turn out to be due to *mechanical* effects intrinsically unconnected with perceived quality.[90] This is how science initially undermines common sense.[91] It's when we turn to our own causal doings, contemplate the mental determinants of action, and the relations between qualities in themselves, that we escape the powerlessness of mere paint. The evident interactions of mental qualities are plain physical happenings, because the mind is a plain chunk of the physical world. There's little reason to take such activity, in its essentials, as of anything other than commonplace physical character.

[87] That you might not *like* this harmony doesn't mean there is no harmony.

[88] To see this imagine (a) the effort without the qualities, (b) the qualities without the effort.

[89] So in experiencing our qualia of causation we plausibly gain insight into the nature of causation itself—we escape Hume's problem. Hassel (2014) develops this idea in a panpsychist direction.

[90] It's because of the kettle's radiative properties that it appears silver to us, so the colour is a mere signal for a physical property; one can easily imagine that property being signalled by a different colour (response in us). This point concerns *tertiary qualities*, i.e. the effects we observe objects having on one another, with us out of the equation except as percipients. The colours, etc., with which perception paints the world of course have effects *on us*, as when we buy baby blue t-shirts. Conventional science, and physicalism, have been—impossibly—trying to rid qualities from such transactions as well.

[91] E.g. the felt warmth we associate with it is discovered in science classes to have nothing to do with heat's power to melt things. This is hard to swallow, and keep down, even in adulthood.

76. The rules of physics, charting the evolution of absolute quality stuff-ings, are, on their inside, qualitative rules—rules relating qualities to one another on the basis of qualitative relations of mutual constraint. Ratios are qualitative ratios. Causation is qualitative constraint: the world is an Othello board, massively expanded in colours and dimensions.[92]

77. A traditional thought is that the physical world, relationally understood by science, offers such a deep contrast to qualities, allegedly *non-relational*, that the latter cannot be fitted into the former, but must slip away to another metaphysical realm. This provides the basis of Sellars senior's emergentism, among many others.[93] Commenting on this transition, his son inquires: 'But . . . Why could not . . . sensible redness, etc., be . . . qualitative features of neurophysiological events *which play specific roles* in the functioning of the visual system centers, and in the discriminative behavior of the . . . organism as a whole?',[94] proceeding to accuse his father of elsewhere *implicitly* accepting that 'the qualitative dimension of the brain state can be determinately characterized in terms of its explanatory role in the theory of the functioning sensory cortex'. Sellars junior is exactly right. The contrast we've emphasized as crucial is between *the qualitative* and *the non-qualitative*, not between *the relational* and *the non-relational*. Qualities are relational, intrinsically so—they wear their relationality on their sleeve; they helplessly reach out to one another. They are not however *mere* relations; they are what ground all relations. Trying to capture them just in terms of the relations they ground would give us something like the empty coats and hats Descartes sees passing in the street. Bare relations couldn't capture qualities because this would be one *instance* of the unfeasible qualityless analysis of quality. Relations do not support quality; but quality supports relations, so it is obvious which has to ground which, and what we must say about the ultimate content of the physical world. Science may see the world purely relationally, but this isn't the same as, nor implies, seeing the world as purely relational. Pure relationality is an *epistemological* predicament (see §55).

78. The relations among qualities are *qualitative relations*—'brighter than' or 'reddish' are evidently stained through by the character of the relata to either side. So the point about the conventionally conceived physical world is not that qualities are something ontologically *beyond* the relations they sit in; it is that we, through science, know these relations in only a bare, *see-through* fashion. Except for in the mental case, we are ignorant of the qualities of the relata. What we know of the relations between physical items is also relational—it concerns ultimately their effects on us in

92 Since relations of qualitative constraint stretch across the universe's entire quality-web, this might help to account for apparent faster-than-light causal effects, as with entangled particles.

93 R. W. Sellars (1922).

94 Sellars (1971b: 287) my emphasis—I have also put the quotation into the 'material mode'.

perception. In the end, once we see that relations are qualitative relations, we glimpse a deep *identity* of the 'relational' with the 'non-relational', in the form of a field of qualities. Neither aspect eludes the other. This is the final analysis of the physical world.

79. As particles of different qualities combine, their composites will be fixed by their components equally in quality and causal/relational profile. Each atom-type will be a unique overall quality, matching its unique set of constituents and correspondingly unique propensities.[95] The interactions, as determined by the qualities in play, are what physics traces, in outline form.[96] Molecules are larger quality-complexes (the models of coloured plastic balls shown to schoolchildren being then oddly close to the truth). Chemical powers vary with, deriving from, molecular quality. A molecule's powers have much to do with its shape—but this shape is fixed by the powers of its atoms, and these powers, on the present account, flow from the qualities of the deeper atomic constituents. Naturally there are shapes (if only of field configurations) at the lowest level too—but shapes *of what*? Of colour (quality). As in the visual field, there are shapes *because* there are colours. Quality is basic.

80. In this way physical matter, qualitative through and through, develops up the ascending mereological levels just as science, skeletally, understands. What we now have is the possibility of rendering our familiar macroqualia smoothly as mere configurational properties of matter, qualitative physical ingredients structured neurally. Varied material constitution across different species' brains, and intrabrain areas, accounts for their distinctive associated qualia, thanks to the differential assembly and interaction of qualities. Our macroqualia are comprehensible as having their causal powers by their compositional provenance, in the way macroscopic objects are understood to inherit their powers from the interplay of their physical constituents.[97]

81. The brain's conscious areas offer a unique cosmological laboratory. In those regions we discover not only the physical structure, but access directly the underlying

[95] At the current quantum level there are fixed units and levels for quantities, which would suggest leaps from one quality across interlinking shades to another one, with some never featuring at all. But we might anticipate a deeper level of being of which quantum mechanics is just the aggregative description, taking in effect statistical averages of the finer-grained behaviour (Bohm's (1980) analogy is with Brownian motion). On that deeper level we would perhaps see all possible 'shades' expressed. This would be confirmed in the discovery of ever greater quantities of particles, occupying more and more determinate qualitative nodes. The fit between fundamental quality intersections constrains the combinations and their stability.

[96] The idea of the universe as qualitative stuff-ing seems formally similar to Bohm's (1980) concept of the universal 'holomovement'; one notable difference is that Bohm does not try to build quality directly into the physical system.

[97] We already employ this synoptic model when cooking. One essentially thinks of a dish under construction—say a lasagne—as an *assembly of qualities*, with the flavour of the whole the intelligible combination of the qualities of the ingredients. And one understands the causal powers of the dish as directly deriving from the overall quality. We should think of brains after the model of lasagne.

qualities. This is the spot, nature's lens, where we might grasp the exact manner of the connection between physical causal/relational profiles and quality.[98] *We must start from the qualities, which ground the physical structure*. Holding a quale fixed, its quality ought to give us some clue—beyond our current crude, correlative techniques—to the neural structure it supports. The relationality of the quale will match the relationality of the neural state. At present we attempt to build backwards from the relational profile to its ground—but we inevitably fall down. Knowing *nothing else* but that two people acted thus-and-so in a crowded café, it is hopeless to try to analyse the mental qualities they each instantiated *just in those terms*: that is the failure of behaviourism, and the relational physicalisms descended from it constitute no improvement in this respect (they only drive the bare relational construal inside the skull). Knowing, though, that both *felt irritable*, and *desirous of seating*, explains—even perhaps implies (given their other mental states and qualities)—how they subsequently interrelated.

82. The physical structure of things, being but a web of relations between qualitative instances, would be intelligible given knowledge of the qualities involved. Carnap's *Aufbau* failed to reconstruct the colour spectrum in terms merely of similarity relations, yet once we know the colours these relations immediately fall out. In other words, we would need to extrapolate the qualitative content of the world to understand why the physical laws hold. The methodological recommendation is that we (i) cease attempting to analyse qualities away relationally, instead (ii) take them as our starting point, aiming to (iii) understand their qualitative structure and (iv) how they support their relations.

83. Neuroscience is an indispensable enrichment of our direct qualitative knowledge. Inhabiting a certain pain quality, one doesn't feel its interconnections with non-conscious states. One feels how the pain pushes one *towards* avoidance, but not how it locks teeth with other unfelt neural cogs to *effect* movement. In this way conscious states are, in R. W. Sellars's phrase, 'insulated' from their neural surround. Obviously, we feel only what we feel.[99] Introspection gives us depth, but without breadth of vision. To know how states lock together we need the relational science. Where relating states are both conscious, though, we ought to be able to map felt connections to neurological structure.[100] Good neuroscience already begins its

[98] Hartshorne (1977) writes in this spirit when he says that '[conventional physicalists] are in effect telling us that from animals we can learn only about animals, but not about gases, fluids, or minerals . . . if it is conceivable that these thinkers are wrong, they are barring the path of inquiry'. Instead: 'we can learn from animals something important about inanimate nature'.

[99] He puts the point by saying that a felt quale 'can *be* only itself and therefore cannot draw its context into itself and open it up to inspection' (R. W. Sellars 1938: 475).

[100] R. W. Sellars (1938: 481) expects that in this way neuroscience may get 'cues' from consciousness. Feigl (1956: 149) is more forthright: 'by doing introspective-phenomenological description of immediate experience, we are in effect . . . doing also a bit of (very crude, vague and preliminary) brain physiology.' Must it remain crude, vague, and preliminary?

individuation of neural states from their felt properties—the craving to dissolve felt states into bare structures appears to be a disease of *philosophical* etiology.

84. More ambitiously: As we develop ever finer understanding of the physical structure of the brain and its matter, we should aspire to a compositional understanding of macroqualia to match. This is the route to a completed—qualitative—physics. A first step is to isolate the ingredients of our macroqualitative states: we would aim to draw up a periodic table of *qualitative elements*, from which we might start to infer the qualities of the deepest physical processes. This would require us to model the constitution of macroqualia by the underlying qualitative ingredients, down to the ultimate physical elements of the absolute quality stuff-ings (or as far as we can go). We must begin with qualitative chemistry to advance to qualitative physics.[101] We require, in this enterprise, a conservation law. The conservation of energy framed physics' ontology, for chemistry the conservation of mass. With qualia the rule is conservation of *total experienced volume of quality*. Considering one's overall experience at a time, including all perceptual, sensory, and cognitive phenomenology, there is evidently a finite 'sphere' of quality instances of which one can be simultaneously aware. If something new becomes consciousness's object, or an existing element claims a more prominent place (as attention switches) other elements fade, or disappear. Likewise, there is only *so much* you can see in the visual field; and when some new colour-patch enters, it is at the expense of a previous occupant. Knowing that *quantum of experienced quality* is conserved should help us to get a theoretical grip on qualitative reactions (after: chemical reactions), like the combination of sweet and bitter in the taste of lemonade, and identify their components.[102] Among many other things, it remains unclear how to determine where a quality is irreducible, or whether we directly experience any such.

85. Knowing the qualitative chemistry, we would see from the constitution of a pain quale why it was the seat of just those causal powers. Its functional profile in the mental economy would follow transparently. We could then banish those physicalist bogies, colour inverts, and zombies: for it would neither be the case that a quality could conceivably have a different causal profile, nor that that causal profile, at the limit of

[101] I'm inspired in this proposal about theoretical procedure by Ch. 6 of McGinn (2004) ('Consciousness, Atomism, and the Ancient Greeks').

[102] We would know that the upshot of a qualitative reaction, like the addition of sweet qualia to those of bitter lemon, contained only the qualities inputted at the start. Similar knowledge allowed chemists to find the elements; by permutation they were able to identify stable ingredients across different reactions. It would be immensely helpful if we could be sure that the qualities of the visual field at a time were just the product of the qualities a moment before, but the visual field is also interacting with other brain (quality) systems of which we're not conscious. Hence we are restricted to purely conscious cases like the addition of taste qualia in lemonade flavour, or white and red giving pink—these are marked by perspicuity.

precision,[103] could be underpinned by a different quality, *let alone* by no quality at all.[104] Making qualia fundamental, strangely enough, gifts us the opportunity to drain hoary dualist intuition-pumps. The different neuronal-activity configurations corresponding to our experiences of colours, tastes, smells, etc. can then simply *be* those qualitative instantiations. We will have established the mind/brain identity thesis, though more after the style of Feigl than that of Smart and Place.[105]

86. We have been propelled to this position by the pressures involved in taking equally seriously the qualitative and the physical: it is an attempt to integrate their respective logical spaces into one.

87. What of the realm Nagel marks out as *subjective*—of the experiencer and her consciousness of qualities? Qualia are not intrinsically conscious. What then makes them conscious? What makes a quality, though it is there in the brain, there also *for you*?[106] The natural answer is that what makes you conscious of the quality is bearing a certain relation to it, if it is non-conscious in itself. James insisted that 'consciousness' picks out no entity, but a *function*, a relationship qualities bear to the mind. Rosenthal's Jamesian relation is *representing a quality in higher-order thought*. Some judge Rosenthal's theory phenomenologically inadequate. Might it seem more adequate in our setting, where qualia are already imported wholesale—so that HOT theory need not *produce* qualia, only analyse our awareness of them?

88. Sheer consciousness comprises surprisingly little of the famous *what-it-is-like-ness*. Instead, in detailing what an experience is like, we refer exclusively to *qualities* of which we're aware. The conventional equation of phenomenality with what-it-is-like-ness conceals two independent quantities. Consciousness is only the fact that certain qualities are *there for you*, whereas others are not. This property, which we might label 'that-it-is-for-ness', seems suited to relational analysis. What-it-is-like-ness properly so-called just involves the particular qualities that are for you. The phenomenological challenge to representational theories of *consciousness* (i.e. that-it-is-for-ness) is then unexpectedly slight: for the phenomenology lies with the qualities.

[103] Nearby qualities might support broadly the same set of causal powers, the functional difference being undetectable except at the finest grain. Thus functionally similar creatures will have *something like* our pains.

[104] To conceive a full zombie, on this model, is to entertain the idea of a set of causal/relational profiles being in place, but absent their actual and necessary (since quality fixes causal power) qualitative categorical grounds. This relational house of cards could not conceivably stand up. And the idea of having *different* qualities standing in the same relations is like imagining that green could bear red's precise closeness to orange.

[105] (Early) Feigl (1956) is clear that qualia *as such* are picked out by neurological predicates, whereas Smart (1959) and Place (1956) more or less explicitly aim to eliminate qualia before seeing physical identifications underway. See also the position advocated in Sellars (1965).

[106] Another way to ask the same question: *What's the difference between those qualitative brain-areas of which you're aware and those of which you are unaware?*

Panqualityism helps itself to any promising physical mechanism for the awareness relation.

89. We must now develop our relational models of awareness. The naturalistic project is due no progress while we insist that for qualities *being* equates to *being felt by someone*. Seventeenth-century Cartesian sensibility confined qualities to the mind so the world might be mathematically traced. But this confinement, predictably, saw *qualities* fall in conceptually with *consciousness*, with both flying free of the physical world as a result. To shrug off Cartesianism, to put qualities back into the world—to reclaim *one* world—we must understand how qualities are physical. A first step in this reconception is to distill them from consciousness.

90. For panqualityists the brain is attributed two principal roles. First, it is the site where lower-level physical qualitative ingredients are assembled, to build the qualia-complexes of our familiarity, which aid perception.[107] Second, it enables awareness of these qualia for the system they belong to, by the implementation of consciousness. Brains are a unique species of self-directed viewing instrument. As with a periscope: by viewing directly, first, an interior area which mirrors the outside, we are able, indirectly, to perceive.

91. Our merely *indirect* perceptual access to external physical reality is more than offset by the intimacy of our *direct* interior access in awareness to the physical region of the brain. Given the deep relatedness of the physical universe, and our perception-based grasp of its structure, this is a powerful inductive springboard.

92. We might propose a *relational higher-order representational* (HOR) mechanism as implementing awareness. The difference between relational and non-relational HOR accounts concerns the need for the sensory first-order target. On Rosenthal's theory, it suffices for a red London bus-ish visual experience that a HOT representing such a percept obtains.[108] That is to say, there need *be* no such percept. This feature identifies the theory as non-relational: the HOT wholly determines phenomenality. On a relational HOR theory the conscious episode is *essentially* a transaction between the HOR component and an existent sensory target. For instance, a simple self-representationalism has a quale represent itself using itself—the represented therefore cannot go missing without consciousness elapsing. Identity is a little too tight a relationship for our purposes, however.

[107] A non-reductive intentionalism would be the most appropriate perceptual theory—see Chalmers (2004).

[108] This characterization does some violence to the details of Rosenthal's theory for the sake of brevity. For him the relevant representations are subject-involving, so that a HOT represents to the subject that she is in a state involving such a percept.

93. Imagine a bridge with 'under construction' painted on it. Crossing, you think 'This bridge is under construction'. Plausibly you have the very sentence *beneath* you, with the bridge itself playing the noun role. In this sort of unusual quotational structure—a 'display sentence'—the referent is deployed, framed within the construction, to represent—really, *present*—itself.[109]

94. Say that a red London bus-ish visual quale exists in a subject's brain. Without the HO representer this percept is unconscious—as in blindsight. On the *quotational higher-order thought theory* the quale is made conscious by being embedded in a 'quotational' HO thought (its structure: 'This quality is present "—"') which enlists the quale to present itself, like the bridge.[110] The qualitative state serves as sense and referent within the context of this demonstrating frame. This special operation of mentally displaying a quale is, perhaps, that in which consciousness consists.[111]

95. Mental quotation likely demands considerable neural integration between HO state and quoted quale. This would make the fact that you can be conscious of your qualia, but not of mine, a simple product of the reach of your neural quotational system: you cannot quotationally embed the qualia currently composing the relevant portions of my brain, so as to display them. No more can you digest last night's dinner for me. Some entities we can only see using microscopes. The qualitative nature of matter is analogous: it requires specialist, rather short-sighted, machinery to access.[112] The fact that I cannot experience your qualia is therefore no more interesting or mysterious than the fact that I cannot observe the specimen currently under your microscope using my own. It implies nothing subjective about the *target*.

96. We could *move* the specimen from your microscope to mine—can we also move your qualia into such a position that I can be conscious of them? This is an in-principle possibility. If the material portion currently constituting your visual percept of the sunset could be somehow transposed intact to my cortex, and there

[109] The bridge example is from Kriegel (2009), the idea of a display sentence from Zemach (1985). Kriegel (2009: 164) feels, and I agree, that the display sentence structure may possess that 'special' something to allow us to make an explanatory 'quantum leap' to consciousness.

[110] The structure is reminiscent of Papineau's (2002) proposal for *quotational phenomenal concepts*, which use the experiences they refer to as sense and referent, by embedding them in a demonstrative concept. The central difference is that we propose the quotation of a *non-experience*—a quality—turning it *into* an experience—providing that-it-is-for-ness. See Coleman 2015b for a clearer picture of QHOT theory—it is blurred here for ease.

[111] A pleasing feature of this account is that given such a mechanism the qualitative target can neither be misrepresented, nor can qualitative consciousness occur in its absence. These possibilities are frequently raised as objections to Rosenthal's non-relational theory (see e.g. Neander 1998).

[112] Perhaps the machinery is pre-frontal monitoring of sensory cortex activity, as some now believe. See e.g. Kriegel (2009: Ch. 7) for a sketch of this idea, and further references.

quotationally displayed, then I will 'see' what you saw.[113] Perhaps more constitutionally robust aliens have cerebrums able to reach out beyond their skulls and 'grab' (quotationally embed) the qualities in each other's brains—this is the irresistibly intelligible possibility of telepathy. Our ignorance of bat qualia is, consequently, a purely contingent circumstance, akin—as some physicalists say, for the wrong reasons—to our not being able to fly. Qualia—qualities—being intrinsically non-conscious, and awareness being only a relation to them, there is nothing, metaphysically, to stop us passing their tokens around.[114]

97. Since *all* matter is qualitative, there is even the opportunity for these aliens to know what a rock is like, in the '*what-it-is-like-ness*' sense—rocks are not *conscious* of their qualities.[115]

98. *Qualia turn out not to be subjective in any important sense.* Intrinsically non-conscious, they are also perfectly *public* properties—in principle—only requiring dedicated equipment to access. Objectivity, the key criterion of physicality, demands *intersubjective accessibility.*[116] Notably: (i) This means access *by subjects.*[117] (ii) It is *potential* access at issue. Our relational theory of consciousness has permitted us to complete the picture of qualities as physical, when added to their integration into—grounding of—the structure of physics, and intrinsic non-consciousness. This, despite their irreducibility. We can now agree wholeheartedly with Rosenthal that 'the subjective is simply a particular form of the objective'.[118] And we bemoan the prevailing doctrine that qualia are subjective properties as conceptual contamination of an item by our particular mode of accessing it—like cats expecting milk to appear only in bowls.[119]

[113] Since qualia are likely neurally highly complex, implicating multiple brain areas, this may block more than an in-principle possibility, for human experiencers anyhow—see below.

[114] Note how much stronger this result is than the counterfactual (which will still strike many as impossible) *that you could have been the one to have this very token quale of mine*—on our theory you could still have it. Jackson's Fred (1982), who sees an extra colour where we see plain red, has his visual system transplanted after death so other people can finally know what red$_2$ is like. This is good intersubjective knowledge of qualia—something Jackson underplays—but plausibly restricted to types. Cf. Feigl (1956: 30–1).

[115] So it may not be impossible, against R. W. Sellars, for us to 'peer into' the being of physical systems other than the brain. This also counters Armstrong's (1961: 34) objection to indirect realism—understood by him as entailing that direct awareness of physical objects is logically impossible. Armstrong argues that any indirect relationship must have at least the possibility of being direct. The quasi-acquaintance relationship of mental quotation permits direct awareness of physical objects, in principle—at least if they are brought within range!

[116] See e.g. Pereboom's (2011: 118) account of Carnap's *Aufbau* project (Carnap 1928).

[117] Armstrong on length (1961: 182): 'in the case of the ruler, it is necessary to *see* that the thing to be measured coincides with points on the ruler ... this reliance on perception does nothing to cast doubt on the objectivity of lengths'.

[118] Rosenthal (1983: 292).

[119] *Still, the episode or property of* you experiencing this token quale *is subjective, because even if I can have the* quale *I cannot have* your experience *of it.* But this 'your experience of it' only invokes the fact that

99. If the qualities in another's mind are (contingently, given human constitution) beyond your quotational reach, then you cannot access them from the 'inside'. The only access you have to that mind is indirect. You could open the other person's skull and take a literal look at the relevant portions of her brain. Why don't you 'see' her qualia then? The answer is Russell's.[120] All that can happen is the causal impact of her brain on your own: her consciousness can modify yours by bouncing light rays into it through your eyes, provoking the relevant neural reactions. But that gets you only an extrinsic peek into what's occurring. That's why looking at other brains doesn't reveal their qualia.[121] The question 'How do you get technicolour qualia from soggy grey brain-matter?' is thus ill-posed: the green/grey appearance to you of another's brain is a matter of *your* qualia modified so as to represent an external state of affairs. This aspect of the explanatory gap rests on a mistaken view of perception: that in perceiving another's brain we get at that brain as it is, naked. In fact we directly experience only our own brains, which are evidently rife with qualities.

100. The first scientific revolution began when qualities were stripped from the world scientists were to describe. Science can only be completed, which entails comprehending conscious beings as just another part of the material world, when qualities are put back into matter, in a realist and non-dualistic way. Since every moment of waking experience confirms that there are qualities, and since we are material creatures, we must reconcile the qualities with the material, without making them an extraneous aspect. As irreducible, they have therefore to be in the core of our conception of the stuff of the world. Nagel is wrong that there are irreducibly subjective facts involved in or implied by conscious experiences. Rosenthal, along with conventional materialists, is wrong to insist that qualia, to be something physical, really have to be something else.[122]

References

Armstrong, D. (1961), *Perception and the Physical World* (London: Routledge and Kegan Paul).

Blackburn, S. (1990), 'Filling in Space', in *Analysis* 50 (2): 62–5.

my token HO quoting *of*—consciously entertaining—the quale is a different token to yours. I cannot occupy your conscious perspective, it's true—but that is just to assert the numerical distinctness of distinct events. Neither can I occupy your physical body, which is not subjective in any relevant sense. Plain old video cameras also have 'subjective perspectives' in this sense, which is frankly undeserving of the aura of mystery that has descended upon it.

[120] See his (Russell 1927a: Ch. 13). See also Mach (1906/1914: e.g. Ch. 4, section 3).

[121] Equally, in tasting the brain of someone eating chocolate, the neuroscientist would not experience the foreign chocolate qualia (Nagel 1987: 30). Rather, after Russell, he tastes his own brain.

[122] Thanks to Philip Goff, Galen Strawson, John Heil, Frederik Willemarck, Dan Cain, and especially Paul Coates for comments on an earlier version of this article, as well as to David Chalmers, Hedda Hassel Mørch, and Michelle Montague for helpful discussion.

Block, N. (1978), 'Troubles with Functionalism', in *Minnesota Studies in the Philosophy of Science* 9: 261–325.

Bohm, D. (1980), *Wholeness and the Implicate Order* (London: Routledge and Kegan Paul). References are to the 2002 imprint by Routledge Classics.

Carnap, R. (1928), *Der logische Aufbau der Welt* (Berlin: Weltkreis). English translation: (1967) *The Logical Structure of the World*, translated by R. George. (Berkeley and Los Angeles: University of California Press).

Chalmers, D. J. (2004), 'The Representational Character of Experience', in B. Leiter (ed.), *The Future for Philosophy* (Oxford: Oxford University Press).

Coleman, S. (2009), 'Mind under Matter', in D. Skrbina and G. Globus (eds), *Mind that Abides* (Amsterdam: Benjamins).

Coleman, S. (2015a), 'Panpsychism and Neutral Monism: How to Make up One's Mind', in G. Brüntrup and L. Jaskolla (eds), *Panpsychism* (New York: Oxford University Press).

Coleman, S. (2015b), 'Quotational Higher-Order Thought Theory', in *Philosophical Studies.*

deVries, W. A. (2005), *Wilfrid Sellars* (Chesham: Acumen).

Feigl, H. (1956), 'The "Mental" and the "Physical"', in *Minnesota Studies in the Philosophy of Science*, 2: 370–497. References to the reprint as an essay and postscript: H. Feigl (1967) (Minneapolis: University of Minnesota Press).

Grossmann, R. (1975), 'Perceptual Objects, Elementary Particles, and Emergent Properties', in H. Castaneda (ed.), *Action, Knowledge and Reality* (Indianapolis, IN: Bobbs-Merrill), 129–46.

Hartshorne, C. (1934), *The Philosophy and Psychology of Sensation* (Chicago, IL: University of Chicago Press).

Hartshorne, C. (1977), 'Physics and Psychics', in J. B. Cobb and D. R. Griffin (eds), *Mind in Nature: The Interface of Science and Philosophy* (Lanham, MD: University Press of America), 90–122.

Hassel Mørch, H. (2014), *Panpsychism and Causation: A New Argument and a Solution to the Combination Problem* (PhD thesis: University of Oslo).

Heil, J. (2005), 'Dispositions', in *Synthese* 144: 343–56.

Heisenberg, W. (1937), 'Gedanken der Naturphilosophie in der modernen Physik', in *Die Antike*, XIII.

Hooker, C. A. (1977), 'Sellars' Argument for the Inevitability of the Secondary Qualities', in *Philosophical Studies* 32 (4): 335–48.

Hume, D. (1738/1975), *A Treatise of Human Nature*, edited by L. A. Selby-Bigge, 2nd edition revised by P. H. Nidditch (Oxford: Clarendon Press).

Jackson, F. (1982), 'Epiphenomenal Qualia', in *Philosophical Quarterly* 32: 127–36.

James, W. (1912), *Essays in Radical Empiricism* (London: Longmans, Green and Co.).

Johnston, M. (2004), 'The Obscure Object of Hallucination', in *Philosophical Studies* 120 (1–3): 113–83.

Kriegel, U. (2009), *Subjective Consciousness: A Self-Representational Theory* (New York: Oxford University Press).

Kriegel, U. (2011), *The Sources of Intentionality* (New York: Oxford University Press).

Leibniz, G. W. (1714/1991), *The Monadology*, in *Discourse on Metaphysics and Other Essays*, edited and translated by D. Garber and R. Ariew (Indianapolis, IN: Hackett Publishing).

Lycan, W. (1996), *Consciousness and Experience* (Cambridge, MA: MIT Press).

Mach, E. (1906/1914), *The Analysis of Sensations, and the Relation of the Physical to the Psychical*, 5th edition (London: Open Court Publishing Company).

Martin, C. B. (1997), 'On the Need for Properties: The Road to Pythagoreanism and Back', in *Synthese* 112: 193–231. Updated version in C. B. Martin (2008), *The Mind in Nature* (New York: Oxford University Press).

McGinn, C. (2004), *Consciousness and Its Objects* (Oxford: Clarendon Press).

Nagel, T. (1974), 'What Is It Like to Be a Bat?', in *Philosophical Review* 83: 435–50.

Nagel, T. (1979), 'Panpsychism', in T. Nagel, *Mortal Questions* (Cambridge: Cambridge University Press).

Nagel, T. (1987), *What Does It All Mean? A Very Short Introduction to Philosophy* (New York: Oxford University Press).

Neander, K. (1998), 'The Division of Phenomenal Labour: A Problem for Representational Theories of Consciousness', in *Philosophical Perspectives* 12: 411–34.

Noren, S. J. (1977), 'Micro-Reduction, Scientific Realism and the Mind-Body Problem', in *Critica* 9 (25): 73–88.

Papineau, D. (2002), *Thinking about Consciousness* (Oxford: Oxford University Press).

Pereboom, D. (2011), *Consciousness and the Prospects of Physicalism* (New York: Oxford University Press).

Place, U. T. (1956), 'Is Consciousness a Brain Process?', in *British Journal of Psychology* 47 (1): 44–50.

Plato (360 BCE/1997), *Timaeus*, in J. M. Cooper (ed.), *Plato: Complete Works* (Indianapolis, IN: Hackett Publishing Company).

Richardson, R. C., and Muhlenberg, G. (1982), 'Sellars and Sense Impressions', in *Erkenntnis* 17: 171–211.

Rosenthal, D. (1983), 'Reductionism and Knowledge', in L. S. Cauman, I. Levi, C. D. Parsons, and R. Schwartz (eds), *How Many Questions?* (Indianapolis, IN: Hackett Publishing).

Rosenthal, D. (1986), 'Two Concepts of Consciousness', in *Philosophical Studies* 49: 329–59.

Rosenthal, D. (1999), 'Sensory Quality and the Relocation Story', in *Philosophical Topics* 26: 321–50.

Rosenthal, D. (2005), *Consciousness and Mind* (Oxford: Clarendon Press).

Russell, B. (1921), *The Analysis of Mind* (London: Kegan Paul).

Russell, B. (1927a), *Outline of Philosophy* (London: George Allen and Unwin).

Russell, B. (1927b), *The Analysis of Matter* (London: Kegan Paul).

Seibt, J. (2000), 'Pure Processes and Projective Metaphysics', in *Philosophical Studies* 101: 253–89.

Sellars, R. W. (1922), 'The Double-Knowledge Approach to the Mind-Body Problem', in *Proceedings of the Aristotelian Society* 23: 55–70.

Sellars, R. W. (1938), 'An Analytic Approach to the Mind-Body Problem', in *The Philosophical Review* 47 (5): 461–87.

Sellars, W. (1963), 'Philosophy and the Scientific Image of Man', in his *Empiricism and the Philosophy of Mind* (London: Routledge and Kegan Paul).

Sellars, W. (1965), 'The Identity Approach to the Mind-Body Problem', in *Review of Metaphysics* 18 (3): 430–51.

Sellars, W. (1971a), 'Science, Sense Impressions and Sensa: A Reply to Cornman', in *Review of Metaphysics* 24: 391–447.

Sellars, W. (1971b), 'The Double-Knowledge Approach to the Mind-Body Problem', *New Scholasticism* 45: 269–89.

Sellars, W. (1981), 'Foundations for a Metaphysics of Pure Process: Carus Lectures', in *The Monist* 64 (1) 3: 90.

Sellars, W. and Meehl, P. E. (1956), 'The Concept of Emergence', in H. Feigl and M. Scriven (eds), *Minnesota Studies in the Philosophy of Science* (Minneapolis: University of Minnesota Press), 239–52.

Shoemaker, S. (1991), 'Qualia and Consciousness', in *Mind* 100 (4): 507–24.

Smart, J. C. C. (1959), 'Sensations and Brain Processes', in *The Philosophical Review* 68: 141–56.

Smolin, L. (2001), *Three Roads to Quantum Gravity* (New York: Basic Books).

Strawson, G. (2008), 'The Identity of the Categorical and the Dispositional', in *Analysis* 68 (300): 271–82.

Unger, P. (1998), 'The Mystery of the Physical and the Matter of Qualities', in *Midwest Studies in Philosophy* 22 (1): 75–99.

Whitehead, A. N. (1925), *Science and the Modern World* (New York: Free Press).

Zemach, E. M. (1985), 'De Se and Descartes: A New Semantics for Indexicals', in *Noûs* 19 (2): 181–204.

3

Phenomenal Qualities
What They Must Be, and What They Cannot Be

Howard Robinson

3.1 Phenomenal Qualities, Transparency, and Our Conception of the Physical World

The following doctrine of weak transparency should be, and probably is, uncontroversial.

The principal phenomenal qualities that characterize experience in our major sense modalities are the qualities that we prima facie and naïvely take to be the qualities/properties that characterize the physical world at the macroscopic level. These are such qualities as colour, shape as presented in vision and touch, hardness/solidity as presented in touch.

This is transparency because it takes central features of experience—the features that characterize the What it is Like (WIL) of experience—to be essentially the same or similar to the features we attribute to the common sense or manifest image world. It is a weak version of this doctrine because it does not claim (or deny) that all the features of experience or qualia can be treated in this way, both because it does not try to apply this idea to sensations, such as pains or itches, nor does it claim that every feature of perceptual states such as visual experience can be so dealt with. It only claims that it is true for certain central features. It is also weak because it does not claim that even these features actually are features of the external world, only that they purport to be and are features of our naïve or manifest image conception of the world. It is because of the minimalness of my claim that I take it to be uncontroversial. Though uncontroversial, it is not, however, inconsequential.

It follows from this limited transparency that what it is like to see red, for example, and what red, as naïvely conceived, is like are two sides of the same coin. This applies not only to secondary qualities, for what it is like to see square, and what square, as naïvely understood by the sighted, is are similarly linked by the transparency relation.[1] This has serious consequences for any attempt to give a physicalist reduction of the WIL of experience. If the WIL of experience is a reflection of what the qualities of our manifest world are like, then no account of WIL that deprives them of this world-constituting nature will be plausible. For example, if one were to claim that different WILs were really just different spiking frequencies of neuronal electrical activities, one would be at a loss to see how our picture of the world could be merely a transparent projection of such frequencies: I do not experience the world as an externalized set of electronic firings, nor as a set of my own behavioural dispositions or functional states. This is not, of course, to say that the experience does not causally depend on such physical states, but it does mean that, if anything like identity is asserted to exist between the qualitative states of experience and their neural grounds, then an explanation must be given of how such a thing can be that out of which our manifest world is (to a significant extent) constructed.[2]

This point is salient because the discussion about WIL and qualia is conducted as if it simply concerned certain intra-mental phenomena—things that leave one's conception of the external, physical world untouched. These qualia are embarrassments to be somehow accommodated into one's independent conception of the world. If they were all like itches and pains—sensations that do not form part of our construction of external reality—this would be fine. But this is not so. Qualia must be construed in a way that makes sense of their world-constructing role. Given transparency, qualia must be construed in a way that enables them to retain such a quality of 'mental paint' that they paint not only avowedly subjective experience, but our manifest world as well.[3]

3.2 Transparency, Direct Realism, and the Status of Qualia/WIL

I suspect that what I have said above will cause a confused reaction. On the one hand, it looks as if it should be uncontroversial, resting, as it does, on a very weak doctrine of transparency; on the other, the world-constructing role that transparency gives to

[1] I argue for this in Robinson (2013)

[2] I attempted to show how behavioural/functional accounts of experiential states lose our grasp on the world in Robinson (1994: 128–36).

[3] Lycan (1996) distinguishes between the qualitative content of experience—the qualia—and WIL, on the grounds that the latter is higher order: our experience can have qualitative content without our noticing this, and in such a case there will be nothing it is like for us, according to Lycan. Even if this is correct, it would not follow that the quality is not the object/content of WIL, just as it is the object/content of the experience, noticed or not. When you are in the higher order state of noticing what your experience is like, it is still the lower order content—the quality—that you are coming to notice—perhaps plus the fact that you are noticing it. So even if Lycan is correct about the difference between qualia and WIL, this does not affect my point that phenomenal red and what it is like to see phenomenal red are two sides of the same coin.

the qualitative content of WIL seems to guarantee that WIL cannot be treated reductively, whereas transparency is often nowadays cited by physicalists as helping them to disembarrass themselves of phenomenal qualities as properties of the mental or inner realm and so becomes a part of a reductionist strategy. From Ryle's Concept of Mind, through U. T. Place's 'phenomenological fallacy', to Harman and Tye's deployment of the term 'transparency', the hope is to plant all phenomenal contents firmly in the external world.[4] There are two versions of this approach. One is naïve realist, the other representationalist. The former faces all the problems of naïve realism, which include how to deal with the relativity of perception (the 'argument from illusion'); the need for a simple realism about secondary qualities; and being saddled with disjunctivism to cope with hallucinations. I shall say no more about this here. Representationalism does not export phenomenal content into the external world, but hopes to render it harmless by making it into an intentional object. But, unless it is given some further reductive treatment, the subjective states 'of-redness', 'of-squareness', etc. remain the bearers of the content that characterizes our lived world.

There is, of course, much more to be said here about the philosophy of perception, some of which I have said in Robinson (1994) and (2012), but nothing plausible can be said to make WIL non-subjective, nor to cut its connection with the world as we experience it. What it is like with us subjectively and what the world seems like to us, are two ways of describing the same thing. If this were not so, experience could not even seem to be revealing to us how the world is.

3.3 The Phenomenal Concept Strategy: What Is It a Strategy for?

I suggested at the end of section 3.1 that the role of phenomenal qualities in constituting our lived world, together with the interdependence of such qualities, via transparency, with WIL makes it difficult to see how any reductive account of WIL or qualia could work. I want in this section to look at one prevalent physicalist attempt to deal with phenomenal qualities, namely the Phenomenal Concept Strategy (PCS). Of the philosophers I shall discuss, only Block, I think, with his 'mental paint' theory, could explain how these qualities contribute to constituting our world.

Almost everyone believes in phenomenal concepts—most especially dualists. Phenomenal concepts are those concepts that can only be fully understood by a process of ostension, because they designate features of the world as they are revealed only in experience. Paradigmatically, these concepts include secondary quality concepts, concepts designating sensations, such as pain, moods, feelings, and the like. It used to be the case that dualists were the only people who believed in these concepts,

[4] See G. Ryle (1949), U. T. Place (1956), Harman (1990), and Tye (1992).

because accepting them seemed to commit one to accepting special referents of a 'logically private' or 'privileged access' kind, that fall outside the range of the public, physical world. The qualities which can only be ostensively defined, it was thought, belong to an inner, Cartesian world.

But then a strange thing happened. Physicalists discovered phenomenal concepts, and, in the context of 'the phenomenal concept strategy', began to talk as if they had discovered some previously ignored conceptual phenomenon, recognition of which enabled one to understand why physicalists appeared to have problems accommodating the apparent privacy of experience. The strategy, as most generally expounded, consists in some way of claiming that phenomenal concepts contain the experience within themselves, on the model of quotation within a sentence. The result is meant to be that the 'explanatory gap' (EG) and all that goes with it, cease to be challenges to physicalism once one realizes that these things are merely the by-product of the difference between physical and phenomenal concepts, and not a difference between public and private properties or qualities.

This is very strange in at least two ways. First, it is strange because, as traditionally understood, phenomenal concepts have their content because of the experiential qualities that they designate, and it is precisely these qualities—what Mary did not initially know about and what she learned about when leaving her room—that seem to fall outside the physicalists' remit. One challenge, therefore, facing PCS as a physicalist strategy is to explain how these concepts work and why they are needed if they do not designate special 'private' qualities. Second, it is strange because the quotational model mimics dualism in a further way. Katilin Balog (2012) describes this theory as 'speculative', by which, I think, she means to include 'innovative', but the quotational model is simply a version of Russell's semantics of logically proper names, according to which that with which one is acquainted (restricted, for him, to sense-data and the self) itself figures as part of the content of the thought which is the recognition of its presence. So in a proposition such as 'that is red', indicating a sense-datum, the datum itself figures as part of the proposition. So PCS is not presenting a new kind of concept or strategy, it is boldly claiming that semantic features originally regarded as specifically designed to cope with the peculiar features of dualistic inner life can be transferred wholesale to a physicalist account. But, as I shall argue below, this semantic transfer is not the only or main challenge facing PCS, for it is also necessary to explain how PCS solves 'the hard problem' of the nature of qualia or sensations. Or if it does not solve this problem, at least to say how it relates to this problem, and how it could still be interesting as a physicalist strategy if it leaves the 'hard problem' untouched. For, after all, the hard problem is the problem for the physicalist.

3.4 Why I Have Difficulty Understanding the PCS

There is a sense in which PCS is not dealing with 'the hard problem', as are other physicalist theories of consciousness.

Why do I say this? First, what is 'the hard problem'? No doubt it can be expressed in various ways, but it is roughly as follows:

> How can a physical state—presumably neural—taken as being just the way that physical science understands it, be the same thing as the 'what it is like'—the phenomenal, subjective, qualitative nature—of experience?

Chalmers states the problem in similar terms:

> we can say that a mental state is conscious if it has a qualitative feel—an associated quality of experience. These qualitative feels are also known as phenomenal qualities, or qualia for short. The problem of explaining these phenomenal qualities is just the problem of explaining consciousness. This is the really hard part of the mind-body problem. (Chalmers 1996: 4)

Why does this seem to be a problem? As physicalists like J. J. C. Smart and others acknowledged from early on in the contemporary discussion, it is because the properties ascribed to neural states by science and the qualitative properties revealed in the 'what it is like' of experience seem entirely different, and, by Leibniz's Law, things with different properties cannot be identical.

So the problem can be put as follows. The physicalist claim that phenomenally conscious states are identical to, or in some other way 'nothing over and above', physical states or processes, seems to run up against Leibniz's Law. The challenge for the physicalist is to say what, if anything, it could be about a physical state or process that constituted it as, or made it count as, or made it to be, an experience with phenomenal character without imputing to it the kind of non-physical property that leads to the Leibniz Law problem (LLP).[5]

Traditional physicalist theories, such as behaviourism, functionalism, and the topic neutral analysis, are clearly attempts at direct answers to this problem, and they do so by arguing that the phenomenal data are not what they seem to be (or have seemed to certain philosophers to be), namely the transparent presentation of phenomenal qualities. Thus a behaviourist says that the 'what it is like' of experience is just some sort of behavioural readiness to respond, grounded, no doubt, in neural structures. The functionalist says more or less the same thing, namely that 'what it is like' is just being in a functional state, realized in the brain and characterized in terms of the discriminatory responses appropriate to the stimulus in question. The topic neutralist (who is normally simply trying to improve on one of the above two) says that there is no problem because 'what it is like' states don't reveal their nature, only their similarity/dissimilarity relations to other internal states that occur when

[5] Kati Balog in her (Balog 2012) gives eight versions of 'the traditional puzzles about consciousness', but none of them are put in this explicit LL form, and so, in my opinion, none does justice to the hard problem, neat, so to speak.

prompted by certain stimuli. Thus there is no Leibniz Law clash because the 'what it is like' states do not make manifest properties of a kind different from those ascribed to physical objects.

These answers may be judged radically inadequate, but it is intuitively clear how, if they were correct, they would constitute a solution to the problem they are intended to address: their relevance is not in doubt, only their adequacy to the apparent data of experience. My main difficulty with PCS is that it is not clear how it is meant to address the traditional problem in the first place. In other words, how does the fact that phenomenal concepts are in some sense discontinuous with physical concepts show how a physical state can manifest itself (or seem to do so?) as a phenomenal quality?

In fact, supporters of PCS are divided on how to express the theory themselves. The disagreements are not about details but about how to state the core of the theory. PCS is not so much a particular general theory—as even behaviourism or functionalism might be thought to be—but a framework for a theory: somehow the special ostensive nature of phenomenal concepts should explain the Explanatory Gap and, with it, the 'hard problem'.

3.5 The Problem Facing PCS

One cannot deny that prima facie at least, there are three things in the game. (i)There is the neural state, as represented in science. (ii)There is the WIL/the phenomenal quality, which is how it seems to the subject. (iii)There is the phenomenal concept.

The core of what is obscure and problematic in PCS, I think, turns on how it handles (ii). The fundamental issue is what it is for a neural state to be experienced as a phenomenal quality, and how one explains the fact of its being so experienced. The physicalist and PCS-ist say this is just the neural state as it is present (or presented) in experience, but the whole problem is to explain this latter notion. This is the root of the LLP: how can the standard neural properties and what appears to be a quite distinct phenomenal quality be identical?

Loar, who inspired the PCS, says nothing which is both plausible and illuminating on this point. He says that

> What [Mary] lacked and then acquired...was knowledge of certain [physical] properties *couched in experiential terms.* (Loar 1997: 599, italics added)

What can this latter expression mean? Something is usually 'couched' in words. Here it obviously contains the idea of something expressing itself experientially but what—if anything—it could be for a physical state to do this is what is at stake. Given that it is not verbal, the 'terms' in which it is 'couched' can, in this context, only be concepts. Loar is similarly unilluminating in the following passage:

odd though it may sound, the properties these conceptions *phenomenologically reveal* are physical-functional properties—but not of course under physical-functional descriptions.
(Loar 1997: 602, italics in original)

The implication would appear to be that the physicalist can help himself to some such notion as phenomenal mode of presentation and treat it as primitive, in the sense that it is only by appealing to this notion that one can express the idea that some brain state is an experience, whilst, at the same time, claiming that ontologically one need only admit the physical-functional properties that science ascribes to the brain. This leaves completely untouched the question of how we are to explain how certain brain states manifest themselves phenomenally, unlike the rest of the physical world.

There seem to me to be four ways of tackling this. (a) The first is to say that certain physical states manifest themselves phenomenally simply by being conceptualized in the way that PCS suggests: stated bluntly, a brain state is 'turned into' an experience simply by our thinking of it in a certain way. (b) The second is to accept that it is just a brute fact that some neural states are experiences, and that is that! (c) The third is to say that some neural states are experiences and this is a brute fact, but why this seems so mysterious is somehow connected with the fact that experiences are conceptualized by phenomenal concepts. In other words, if [*per impossibile*?] they were not conceptualized in this way, there would be no Explanatory Gap. (d) The fourth is to explain how a neural state is presented as an experience by saying it is presented topic neutrally, so that the way it comes across in experience reveals nothing about its real nature.

My impression is that both (a) and (d) are positions most PCS theorists want to avoid, though they cannot avoid saying things that seem to suggest them. (b) is often adopted but usually with some gesture to (c). I shall discuss these positions in turn.

3.6 Taking Option (a): Phenomenal Concepts Are What Present Brain States as Experiences

Option (a) has the advantage that it is clear how it makes PCS relevant to the hard problem: it makes the phenomenality of experience simply into a way of conceptualizing certain brain states. But it purchases this relevance at a great price. The idea that, for example, a neural spiking frequency is rendered as an experience by being conceptualized in a certain way seems to hover between the radically implausible and the barely intelligible. It at least seems to put into the notion of conceptualization a very special kind of content. It seems to put on the physicalist the obligation to provide an account of conceptualization, which is both consistent with physicalism and able to perform this trick. Without something like this, it would just be the suggestion that one 'turns a brain state into' an experience by conceptualizing it—thinking of it—in a certain way and this makes even behaviourism look intuitively plausible: think of your brain in a certain way and it will seem to you like an experience! I do not see how this is improved by saying (as supporters of PCS usually do) that the relevant brain state is actually part of or quoted in the phenomenal concept. It is wholly opaque how including a spiking frequency within a concept could bring it to phenomenal life. I do not believe that supporters of PCS want to say anything as bizarre—or as straightforward—as this; but, on the other hand they often seem to be falling back on a move of this sort. If one says, for example, that there is only one property present, namely the spiking frequency, but two ways of conceiving of it, one as a spiking frequency and one as a phenomenal quality (and I have often come across this formula in discussion, at least) then I think one is falling back on (a).

The idea that the Hard Problem can be thought of as essentially a conceptual problem has, I think, the following source.

The 'hard problem' can be broken down into two parts. One is the apparent Leibniz Law problem, namely, how the experiential state and the neural state can be the same, given the apparent manifest difference in their properties. But there is a second problem waiting in the wings, namely, given the answer (whatever it is) that one gives to the first problem, why should it seem so intuitively obvious that these states instantiate different properties? Suppose, for example, that one thought that What It Is Likes (WILs) were neuro-functional states; why should it seem that they were something completely different—for example, the presentation of simple qualities? The PCS approaches the 'hard problem' through this second problem—it attempts to explain why any physicalist solution to the Leibniz Law problem is so counterintuitive. It does this by claiming that there is a discontinuity between the concepts of science and those involved in recognition of our own phenomenal states and that this makes impossible an intuitive grasp on the ontological affinity of what they are conceptualizing. So PCS is trying to answer the question 'if physicalism is true, why is it so counterintuitive?' It is not trying directly to answer the question, 'given the apparent facts, how can physicalism be true: how can a physical state be, or constitute, a phenomenal state?' The thought behind PCS, then, seems to be that if PCS can explain away physicalism's counterintuitiveness, then rational resistance to physicalism will have been overcome. Accepting for the moment this strategy, the question then becomes 'does explaining the misfit of the two kinds of concepts actually explain why physicalism seems so counterintuitive?' This is, I think, the point at which the failure of PCS to address the fundamental Leibniz Law problem comes in. If you think that the correct focus for the problem facing physicalism is the explanatory gap, then conceptual misfit could plausibly seem to be the answer. But if you think that the problem is to explain how a physical state can do the job of being a phenomenal state without invoking non-material properties, then explanatory relations between concepts do not seem to get to the heart of the question.

Some protagonists of PCS argue that it is not concerned with the hard problem, but with the Knowledge Argument, the Explanatory Gap, and the Conceivability of

Zombies.[6] This presupposes that there is a serious difference between the Hard Problem, as exposed by Leibniz's Law, and the Knowledge Argument. The Explanatory Gap is, it can plausibly be said, about the relation between two sets of concepts, the physical and the phenomenal, not about how a brain state can also be an experience. Similarly, the Conceivability of Zombies is also about the conceptual separability of these groups. But which of these two issues—conceptual distinctness or the Hard Problem—does the Knowledge Argument concern? It seems to me that the problem facing Mary when she has her first chromatic colour experiences is not best expressed (let alone only expressed) as 'why could I not previously derive this conceptual characterization of this situation from the conceptual characterization of it I received from science?' Rather her puzzlement would be in the form 'how can that quality/property I am now experiencing be the same property as those that were exhaustively characterized by the science I already knew?' The problem is a *de re* not a *de dicto* one. It is to explain how the phenomenal quality figures in the experience, not just the role of the concept that characterizes it.

The Explanatory Gap and the Conceivability of Zombies are consequences of the Hard Problem, whereas the Knowledge Argument is a way of focusing on the Hard Problem itself. The transferring of discussion from the Hard Problem and the Knowledge Argument to the Explanatory Gap and the Conceivability of Zombies seems to me not to be helpful when trying to evaluate the adequacy of physicalism as an account of phenomenal consciousness.[7]

In fact, this way of misconstruing the Knowledge Argument (KA) dates back to Brian Loar's initial statement of PCS (1997). He reports it as follows:

> The knowledge argument is straightforward on the face of it. Consider any phenomenal quality and any physical property however complex. We can know that a person has the physical property without knowing that she experiences the phenomenal quality. And no amount of a priori reasoning or construction can bridge this conceptual gap. That is the intuitive premise. The conclusion is drawn that the phenomenal quality cannot be identical with the physical property. The argument is equivalent to this: since physical and phenomenal conceptions can be connected only a posteriori, physical properties must be distinct from phenomenal properties. (Loar 1997: 598, italics added)

The idea is that the separateness of the concepts misleads us into believing in a separateness of properties. Notice that there is nothing here about Mary's first personal perspective. We are presented with something rather like the other minds problem, because Loar sets the issue up in terms of our not being able to infer a priori from someone's physical properties that they are phenomenally conscious. This

[6] This point was made in discussion to me by David Papineau.

[7] This is certainly the way I intended and understood my version of the knowledge argument when I used it as a way of setting out the challenge facing physicalism, at the opening of my (Robinson 1982).

approach is closely connected to the conceivability of zombies: if zombies were not conceivable, we could not doubt whether other people had minds—at least if we were allowed to examine their brains as well as their outer behaviour. This approach says nothing about how the content of her experience strikes Mary when she sees chromatic colour, and how different that quality seems from the properties about which science had told her: the approach is entirely third-personal and this enables it to bypass the real issue.

Barry Loewer has suggested to me that my way of describing the situation in terms of properties and Loar's in terms of concepts are just two ways of characterizing the situation and that Loar's has the advantage of not leading directly to dualism. It is important to my position that Loar's way is actually defective, and does not constitute another empirically adequate theoretical framework. It is important that Loar actually misses something out. That there is experience and what experiences are like are not just artefacts created by a peculiar mode of conceptualizing something which is essentially different from how experience presents it.

Also, I think that the argument in section 3.1 above shows this to be the case, because it showed that the qualitative content of experience—the generalized version of what Mary came to know when she left her room—has to be the kind of thing out of which our lived world can be (to a great extent) built. The world as it presents itself to us is not a mere conceptual construct but rich with vivid qualities and properties. This is so whether or not these are actual properties of the world itself or only the way that it seems.

3.7 Options (b) and (c): Identity Is Given but PCS Explains away the Mystery

Options (b) and (c) are normally taken together. Consider first the idea that one can assume that phenomenal states and brain states are identical. This, after all, is the physicalist hypothesis, so how can it be wrong to take it *ex hypothesi* in the present discussion?

There are in fact two different positions in this vicinity. One is exemplified by Block and Stalnaker (1999) and by Searle (1992). According to this view, all identities in science suffer from an 'explanatory gap' which is bridged simply by the fact that the best theory requires one to posit the identity: the properties belonging to the two 'levels' always seem to be different. In this respect, the identity between a brain state and an experience is no different from that between liquidity or heat, on the one side, and various kinds of molecular motion on the other. It is not clear why someone who took this line should need PCS, any more than such an account is needed to justify or explain the other identities posited in science.

The other view, exemplified by Papineau, Balog, and most supporters of PCS, accepts that there is no explanatory gap in cases other than that of the mind-body relation, and that PCS is needed to explain it in that case. Nevertheless, they hold, it is not question-begging to take the identity *ex hypothesi.* The issue for this theory is to make clear how PCS relates to the hard problem and the Leibniz Law problem; whether it somehow dissolves them, if so, how, and, if not, whether PCS is much help to the physicalist in facing the major challenge which they constitute. Unless it makes a significant contribution to these issues, assuming identity will simply be question-begging.

An example of someone who seems simply to assume identity is David Papineau. Reporting his 2002 views, he says the following

> To have a phenomenal concept of some experience, you must be able introspectively to focus on it when you have it, and to re-create it imaginatively at other times; given these abilities, you can form a term with the structure the experience: –, in which the gap is filled either by a current experience or by an imaginative re-creation of an experience. (Papineau 2007: 112)

Here the idea that certain brain states are experiences is simply taken as primitive. Of course, as I have conceded, physicalists believe that certain brain events are experiences, but the challenge they face is to explain what it is about a brain process that makes it an experience, not to take their theory as needless of an explanation. This potentially question-begging position remains in his later theory:

> [The new] model of phenomenal concepts as a species of perceptual concept retains one crucial feature from my earlier quotational-indexical model, namely that phenomenal references to an experience will deploy an instance of that experience, and in that sense will use that experience to mention it. (Papineau 2007: 123)

Once again, the fact that certain brain states are experiences is taken as a given and unproblematic, and phenomenal concepts are explained in terms of how these experiences are deployed in concepts. This transfers the answer to the 'hard problem' away from the nature of phenomenal concepts to certain accounts about the constraints on property identity. If the idea that certain brain states are experiences is essentially unproblematic, then it might seem that there was no 'hard problem' in the first place.

The supporter of PCS can try to bring together the ideas behind (a) and (b)—namely, the idea that phenomenal concepts create experience and the idea that the experiential status of certain brain states is essentially unproblematic—by uniting them in (c). They might argue that identity between phenomenal states and physical states only seems bizarre because of EG, and it is the discontinuity between the different kinds of concepts that causes EG: so, if there were no EG, which is caused by the conceptual structure, one would not find the identity strange. This just seems completely false. The identity is strange because of the apparently manifest difference between the phenomenal quality as it is presented in experience and neural states as they are characterized by science or external observation. It is the fact that the quality as presented in experience can only be accessed by the subject that gives phenomenal concepts their different and discontinuous status.

The suggestion that this radical discontinuity can be explained simply from the conceptual features of phenomenal concepts can be seen to be inadequate by considering those features and the other places in which they occur.

Phenomenal concepts are what pick out phenomenal qualities, whether primary or secondary. In fact most of our initial empirical concepts are given content for us wholly or largely by ostension—that is, by experiencing their instances. I think that this generates a problem for PCS. Consider the concept of liquidity, or the concept of flowing, as it applies to liquids. It would be very difficult to get these notions without experience of liquids and their typical behaviour. 'A liquid is that sort of thing'—'flowing is behaving like that—get it—you see what I mean?' But if ostension, which involves quoting, or reactivating, or some such, the WIL of the experience itself, is what creates the explanatory gap between the physical account and experience, why do we not feel any problem in understanding the behaviour of liquids as being adequately explained by the behaviour of molecules? If the manifest world is, as I argued in section 3.1, just (or largely) WIL plus transparency, why is there not an explanatory gap between physical science and the world of common experience, in its primary as well as its secondary qualities? The only reasonable conclusion is that the conceptual features picked on by PCS are irrelevant to the real hard problem, which is founded on the Leibniz Law problem.

Ned Block appears to accept that there is some genuine feature in experience which is only accessible to the subject and which is not an artefact of conceptualization, but claims that this is no threat to the physicalist because such properties are 'thick' and the neural structure is their hidden nature, just as H_2O is the hidden nature of water. So the subjectively available feature can be identified with the 'deeper' physical structure, as water can be with H_2O. Kripke has argued, seemingly convincingly, that this model cannot be applied to experiential states. How does Block respond to this?

I agree that the two terms of the identity 'Q = cortico-thalamic oscillation' pick out the referents via different aspects of that referent, different MMoPs [Metaphysical Modes of Presentation]. And I also agree that the aspect used by the mental term of the identity is available to the first person whereas the aspect used by the physical term is not. But it does not follow that the aspect used by the mental term is thin. It is true that no neurological property is explicitly part of the first-person route, but that does not show that it is not part of the first-person route, albeit ontologically rather than explicitly. The MMoP of Q is stipulated to be phenomenal, and may be taken to be the property of *being* Q. But being identical to Q, on the physicalist view, is both a thick property and available to the first person... Being identical to Q is a physical property (being identical to cortico-thalamic oscillation) but is nonetheless distinct from the MMoP I have been supposing for 'cortico-thalamic oscillation', which has to do with the oxygen uptake that functional magnetic resonance scanners use to identify it. On the physicalist view, the feel and the neurological state are not different aspects of one thing:

they are literally identical. If they are aspects, they are identical aspects. But the MMoP of the right-hand term of the identity is still different from the MMoP of the left-hand term.

(Block 2007: 292–3)

This will work if we accept Block and Stalnaker (1999) on what is involved in scientific claims that two seemingly different properties are really the same.

Block and Stalnaker maintain that there are explanatory gaps between every explanatory level.[8] The properties associated with liquidity, for example, do not follow from those of the molecules making up the liquid. The identification is made simply on grounds of theoretical neatness and unity. In this case, a resilient prima facie difference and actual identity are both preserved, giving a 'thick' property, so property identities can then follow the model of 'stuff'—e.g. water = H_2O—identities. But the claim that there is an EG in cases such as liquidity is hard to maintain [as Searle, at least, now concedes]. So it seems to be generally accepted that the case of phenomenal qualities presents an EG in a unique way. It would undermine the plausibility of Block's claim that property identities can be thick if the phenomenal quality-brain state cases were the only ones to which it applied. So if thickness is general but the EG is unique, thickness must be independent of whether there is an EG. It would have to be the case that all cross-level property identities were thick, but EGs existed only when there was the kind of conceptual breach created by phenomenal concepts.

Now it might seem that liquidity is a 'thick' property, because there might be different mechanisms in different possible worlds—or even in the actual world—by which it is realized. But they will still all manifest liquidity, because that is a behavioural property. In other words, there is no way that that very ostensively identifiable feature could be essentially dependent on a certain realization. If you allow this same fact for, e.g. red qualia, namely that they could be multiply realized, and add the fact that, unlike liquidity, this is not a behavioural property, then you reach the real problem, which is that one cannot see how this property—phenomenal red, as opposed to liquidity (the latter being a behavioural property)—can be wholly implemented—sufficiently explained—by the mechanism that underlies it. Moreover this difference cannot be explained by the unique nature of PCs, as I argued above against Papineau: PCs are not unique to the intra-mental case, but apply also in the case of liquidity and others similar, where there is no EG. Given that the Block and Stalnaker theory, in so far as it depends on taking liquidity and the like as thick properties, does not explain why there is an Explanatory Gap in the phenomenal

[8] It might come as something of a surprise to note that Block and Stalnaker's position on this is not significantly different from Searle's (1992). In both cases it is maintained that throughout the sciences (i) the lower level remains closed, (ii) there are explanatory gaps between the levels, and (iii) these together do not entail epiphenomenalism for the higher level or over determination. Searle does not talk of identity between the levels, but given (i) to (iii), this is a verbal difference.

case, and that PCS cannot assist it, it seems that the Block and Stalnaker theory is no help to a physicalist who wants to appropriate phenomenal qualities.

So taking the identity of experiential and neural states as primitive begs, rather than answers, the question.

3.8 Option (d): The Topic Neutral Approach

The fourth, topic neutralist, option seems to be how Janet Levin interprets PCS when she says that phenomenal concepts 'aren't supposed to characterize phenomenal properties at all' (Levin 2007: 105). She is also against the 'quotational' approach and the idea that phenomenal concepts are partially constituted by the experience or that one can speak of 'acquaintance'. Her conception of the concepts, therefore, seems very neutral. But resort to topic neutrality takes the whole issue back to Jack Smart's theory of 1959—which is to admit that no serious progress has been made by physicalism in the last fifty years!

This, though correct, is not the most serious objection to the topic neutral approach. If normal experience gives us topic neutral knowledge of our inner workings, and Mary already has topic specific knowledge, then she already knew more before she had colour experience than can be acquired by having it.

3.9 A More General Objection to PCS as a Whole

All the above versions of PCS take for granted the idea that a physicalist can contrast the physical system with the way it is conceptualized, in such a manner that Mary might know all about the former whilst being in some kind of ignorance about certain important features in the latter. This itself can be disputed.

PCS is essentially a version of Churchland's early response to the Knowledge Argument (KA). Churchland argued that what KA showed was not that Mary learned something new on leaving her room but that she gained a new way of knowing something she had already known. PCS is just an attempt to fill out how this 'new way' works. I argued in (Robinson 1993: 165–6) that if this 'new way of knowing' was itself a physical process then it had to be included in what Mary already knew.

> The idea behind the 'mode' theory is, presumably, that if the phenomenal is merely another mode of access to respectable physical facts, then it does not itself constitute an extra fact: it is not an addition to ontology, but an extra mode of access to part of the previously accepted ontology. A moment's reflexion will, however, show this to be sophistical. Call the set of physical facts P and the scientific modes of access which [Mary] has to these facts S, and the experiential mode of access [she] lacks H. If we regard S and H as external to P, then the addition of a new mode of access will not alter P. But the physicalist hypothesis is that everything relevant is included in P: modes of access to physical facts are themselves simply

physical processes and are included in physical facts. Therefore, if [Mary] knows all the relevant members of P, [she] should know all the facts about H, including the fact of what that mode of access is phenomenally like.[9]

The same applies to the PCS, which is just a version of the 'different mode' theory. Chalmers uses a similar, but fuller, argument. Papineau summarizes it as follows.

> Let C be the thesis that humans possess phenomenal concepts. As Chalmers sees it, type-B physicalists require both (a) that C explains our epistemic situation with respect to consciousness and (b) that C is explicable in physical terms. However, Chalmers argues that there is no version of C that satisfies both these desiderata—either C can be explained in a way that makes it physically explicable or in a way that allows us to explain our epistemic situation, but not both. (Papineau 2007: 136)

Papineau claims that one can do both, as a full physical account still leaves an epistemic gap. Mary works out how phenomenal concepts work physically, but she is still mentioning them, not using them, so she still does not know them in the phenomenal concept way.

This response is sound if we are allowed to take the fact of identity as a primitive that overcomes the EG by force, so to speak. No amount of physical conceptual knowledge entails phenomenal conceptual knowledge, just as (if the primitive identity theory is correct across the board, as Block, Stalnaker, and Searle claim) no amount of description of molecules entails that there is a liquid present. But all the weight is now on defending that theory of property identity: PCS alone cannot explain how it is true of consciousness and not—against Block and Stalnaker, and Searle—of other cases.

Katalin Balog (2012) puts herself into a similar position to Papineau. She gives as one of the puzzles facing physicalism:

> Only subjects who have undergone or who are currently undergoing the relevant phenomenal states can token the corresponding phenomenal concepts. This underlies Jackson's 1982 Knowledge Argument and is widely accepted.

The verb 'token' here is somewhat evasive. The question is whether Mary in her room should, if physicalism were true, have been able to understand what colour was like, not whether she was in a position to deploy colour concepts recognitionally. Now the response might be that one cannot understand these concepts unless one can apply them recognitionally, but on what grounds could a physicalist say this?

[9] When I first discussed what is now known as 'the knowledge argument', in Robinson (1982), I introduced a deaf scientist (presumed male) whom I dubbed DS and who played the counterpart to Jackson's Mary. I was still keeping to this practice in 1993, so I have modified the quotation to substitute Mary for DS.

Mary can observe exactly how these concepts work in others and can recognize that experiential neural states (of a kind she has never had) constitute part of them. If she can understand other things that people are thinking, not by empathy—i.e. by having had the same thoughts herself—but by studying their brains, why cannot the same obtain in this case? No orthodox physicalist can retreat to the position that there is any state of which you cannot have complete knowledge unless you are, or have been, in it yourself, or can imaginatively recreate what being in it is like: the third-person perspective must command everything. There will be certain things you cannot do unless you are in the state yourself, but that will be strictly knowledge how.

Perhaps one might claim that someone cannot understand a concept unless they can deploy it, but this is not necessarily true. It may often be the case that someone cannot deploy a concept *because* they cannot understand it, but it is possible to understand a concept and not be able to deploy it because you are not in a situation that makes deployment possible. I cannot myself deploy the concept 'solemnizing a marriage' in a first-person way because I am not a legal registrar of marriages, but I understand it perfectly well. Mary cannot deploy the concept 'recognizing red' in a first-person way because she never has the experience that licenses its use. I can, of course, deploy the concept 'solemnizing a marriage' in a third-personal sort of way, but so can Mary deploy 'recognizing red' in such a way, for she can know when others are doing so. So appeal to 'deploying the concept' is irrelevant against Chalmers's objection.

3.10 Papineau and the Leibniz Law Problem

David Papineau in effect challenges the Leibniz Law problem by characterizing it as 'the intuition of distinctness' (Papineau 2007: 139). In other words, the sense that there are clearly different properties involved is deemed to be an 'intuition'. I think that the use of the word 'intuition' here is likely to be misleading. In fact the word as used in natural language and in philosophy has, if not two senses, at least two poles. On the one hand it means something close to intellectual hunch or putative insight. On the other it means something that seems plainly and obviously true; a blatant fact that cannot be ignored because it is a datum of experience. Philosophers who denigrate something as an intuition are assimilating both kinds to the former. The former is the sense behind Dennett's powerful metaphor of the intuition pump, and also behind his citing as a case of an 'intuition', in a relevant sense, the belief that if you fart, burp, and cough at the same time you will die. I have the intuition that the world could not be infinitely old and that Cantor and Hilbert were right in thinking that their logico-mathematical treatment of infinity cannot be empirically interpreted, only formally. This is an intuition in the first sense and I may very well be completely wrong in this belief. One person's insight is another's prejudice. But if you show me a red patch, a blue patch, and play middle C on the piano, it is intuitively obvious to me that these are qualitatively different phenomena. This is not a speculative hunch or a putative insight. If there is such a thing as experience at all, I am plainly right. The claim that phenomenal red is the same property as electrical activity between neurons, as these are characterized in physical science, is intuitively obviously false in pretty much the same way as it is intuitively obviously false that phenomenal red is the same quality or property as phenomenal blue, or as the sound of middle C. This is why Smart and Armstrong desperately tried to magic away the positive content from the phenomenal side with their topic neutral analysis.

3.11 Conclusion

Phenomenal qualities are amongst the fundamental building blocks of our, lived, manifest or common-sense world. As such all attempts to conceive of them physicalistically seem to be self-destructive. In particular, the purportedly non-reductive phenomenal concept strategy can give no account of how a neural state can manifest itself as an experience, nor even explain why its so manifesting itself seems so inexplicable to us. As far as the existence and status of phenomenal qualities are concerned, a primitive empiricism is much nearer the truth than physicalist realism.

References

Balog, K. (2012), 'Acquaintance and the Mind-Body Problem', in Christopher Hill and Simone Gozzano (eds), *New Perspectives on Type Identity: The Mental and the Physical* (Cambridge: Cambridge University Press), 15–45.

Block, N. (2007), 'Max Black's Objection to Mind-Body Identity', in T. Alter and S. Walter (eds), *Phenomenal Concepts and Phenomenal Knowledge* (Oxford: Oxford University Press), 249–306.

Block, N., and Stalnaker, R. (1999), 'Conceivability, Possibility and the Mind-Body Problem', in *Philosophical Review* 108: 497–528.

Chalmers, D. J. (1996), *The Conscious Mind* (Oxford: Oxford University Press).

Harman, G. (1990), 'The Intrinsic Qualities of Experience', in *Philosophical Perspectives* 4: 31–52.

Levin, J. (2007), 'What Is a Phenomenal Concept?', in T. Alter and S. Walter (eds), *Phenomenal Concepts and Phenomenal Knowledge* (Oxford: Oxford University Press), 87–110.

Loar, B. (1997), 'Phenomenal States', in N. Block, O. Flanagan, and G. Guzeldere (eds), *The Nature of Consciousness* (Cambridge, MA: MIT Press), 597–616.

Lycan, W. (1996), *Consciousness and Experience* (Cambridge, MA: Bradford Books).

Papineau, D. (2007), 'Phenomenal and Perceptual Concepts' in T. Alter and S. Walter (eds), *Phenomenal Concepts and Phenomenal Knowledge* (Oxford: Oxford University Press), 111–44.

Place, U. T. (1956), 'Is Consciousness a Brain Process?', in *British Journal of Psychology* 47: 44–50.

Robinson, H. (1982), *Matter and Sense* (Cambridge: Cambridge University Press).

Robinson, H. (1993), 'The Anti-Materialist Strategy and the "Knowledge Argument"', in H. Robinson (ed.), *Objections to Physicalism* (Oxford: Clarendon Press), 159–83.

Robinson, H. (1994), *Perception* (London: Routledge).

Robinson, H. (2012), 'Qualia, Qualities and our Conception of the Physical World', in A. Göcke (ed.), *The Case for Dualism* (Notre Dame: University of Notre Dame Press), 231–63.

Robinson, H. (2013), 'The failure of disjunctivism to deal with "philosophers' hallucinations"', in F. Macpherson and D. Platchias (eds), *Hallucination: Philosophy and Psychology* (Cambridge, MA: MIT Press), 313–30.

Ryle, G. (1949), *The Concept of Mind* (London: Hutchinson).

Searle, J. (1992), *The Rediscovery of the Mind* (Cambridge, MA: MIT Press).

Tye, M. (1992), 'Visual Qualia and Visual Content', in T. Crane (ed.), *The Contents of Experience* (Cambridge: Cambridge University Press), 158–76.

4

Real Acquaintance and Physicalism

Philip Goff

4.1 Real Acquaintance versus Acquaintance Physicalism

In the old days physicalists refused to compromise. They not only denied the existence of mental *properties* over and above physical properties, but also of mental *concepts* over and above physical/functional concepts. For the old school physicalist mental properties are just physical properties we pick out in virtue of their functional role: the concept 'pain' picks out c-fibres firing as the state that plays 'the pain role' in humans. On such a view, zombies are inconceivable and Mary learns no new propositional knowledge when she sees red for the first time.[1]

Physicalists these days tend to be more conciliatory. Those physicalists who adopt the 'phenomenal concepts strategy' concede to the anti-physicalist that there is a special class of *phenomenal concepts*, formed when conscious states are conceived of in terms of what it's like to have them, which bear no a priori association to physical or causal concepts. The existence of phenomenal concepts entails that zombies are conceivable, and that Mary gains new propositional knowledge.

Despite this concession regarding mental *concepts*, the phenomenal concepts strategist gives no ground on *ontology*. Although we have two very different kinds of concept—physical/functional concepts on the one hand, phenomenal concepts on the other—each phenomenal concept co-refers with some physical/functional concept: the concept 'what it's like to feel pain' picks out the very same state of the world as the concept 'c-fibres firing'. Because phenomenal concepts refer to physical states, zombies are impossible. And Mary's new knowledge is just a matter of her gaining a new way of thinking about a property she already knew about under a physical description. Mary used to know that seeing red involves 'physical property P', now she knows that seeing red involves 'phenomenal quality Q', but 'physical property P' and 'phenomenal property Q' are just two ways of thinking about the same thing. In general, to adopt the phenomenal concepts strategy is to accept that there is an

[1] Armstrong (1968), Dretske (1995), Harman (1990), Lewis (1966, 1970, 1994), and Rey (1995).

epistemic gap between the mental and the physical, but to account for it in terms of a dualism of concepts rather than of properties.[2]

All versions of the phenomenal concepts strategy agree with the anti-physicalist that there is no a priori association between phenomenal concepts and physical/functional concepts, and hence that the phenomenal facts are not a priori entailed by the physical facts. But a subclass of phenomenal concepts strategists want to go further, to have a view of the working of phenomenal concepts which more closely resembles that of the dualist. Specifically, these physicalists want to agree with the standard dualist position that we are 'acquainted' with our phenomenal qualities, that is, that we refer to the qualities of our experience in virtue of standing in some special, epistemically intimate relationship to those qualities. Call this kind of view 'acquaintance physicalism'.

There is a natural sense of the word 'acquaintance', according to which acquaintance affords the acquainted an understanding of the real nature of the thing with which she is acquainted. Call acquaintance so understood 'real acquaintance'. Something like real acquaintance was taken by the British empiricists to hold between a mind and its ideas, and by the sense-data theorists to hold between the self and its sense-data. It is a familiar and intuitive idea in the history of philosophy that the mind is somehow 'so close' to the qualities of experience that their nature is 'laid bare' to the thinker.

On the face of it physicalism—at least the kind of physicalism adopted by proponents of the phenomenal concepts strategy—from now on 'PCS physicalism'—cannot consistently believe that we bear the *real* acquaintance to our phenomenal qualities. For physicalists take the real nature of phenomenal qualities to be physical or functional. If this were the case, then a real acquaintance with our phenomenal qualities would allow us to discern their real physical nature. Attending to pain would reveal it to consist of c-fibre stimulation. There would not be, contrary to what the PCS physicalist supposes, an epistemic gap between the physical and the phenomenal.

This much seems to be conceded by the acquaintance physicalists. Katalin Balog, who gives a detailed exposition and defence of a form of acquaintance physicalism, says that with respect to phenomenal qualities we have a 'direct, unmediated, substantial insight into their nature' (Balog 2012: 17). However, she also says that 'this kind of direct insight... does not reveal anything about the metaphysical nature of phenomenality' (Balog 2012: 18). So whatever Balog means by 'substantial', it does not involve knowing the real nature of the object of thought. David Papineau, one of the original proponents of acquaintance physicalism (although he never actually used the word 'acquaintance' in expounding his view), makes it clear that there is no basic

[2] Block and Stalnaker (1999), Hill (1997), Hill and McLaughlin (1999), Levine (1983), Loar (1990 and 2003), Papineau (1993 and 2002), and Perry (2001).

mode of thought which affords us an understanding of the real nature of the thing thought about:

> No doubt there are ways of thinking of things that make certain essential properties *a priori* knowable. But I take such a priori knowledge to derive from (possibly implicit) compositionality in the relevant modes of thinking, and so not to be associated with the most basic ways in which thought makes contact with reality... When it comes to these basic points of contact, I find it hard to take seriously any alternative to the assumption that our atomic concepts are related to reality by facts external to our *a priori* grasp, such as causal or historical facts.
> (Papineau 2006: 102)

In place of real acquaintance, acquaintance physicalists give a *constitutional account* of a certain subclass of phenomenal concepts, according to which those phenomenal concepts refer to phenomenal qualities in virtue of being partly constituted by those qualities. When I am in agony, and I deploy a phenomenal concept to think about my agony, that concept, and the thought it is involved in, are literally constituted by the feeling of agony itself.[3]

We can understand this view by analogy with quotation marks. When we put quotation marks around a word, we create something that refers to a word by containing that word as a part. For example, the term 'dog' refers to a certain three-letter word of the English language, and it does so by containing that word within itself. We can think of phenomenal concept as 'quoting' the phenomenal qualities they refer to, on the constitutional account. This model is not—at least not obviously—inconsistent with physicalism: the phenomenal quality 'quoted' may be a physical property, even though it is not revealed as such to the concept user.

Acquaintance physicalists do not give a constitutional account of all phenomenal concepts, but only of 'direct' phenomenal concepts: one deploys a direct phenomenal concept when one thinks about a given phenomenal quality by attending to it and thinking about it in terms of what it's like to have it.[4] Having formed a direct phenomenal concept of a certain kind of pain, I can then go on to judge that other people feel that way, or that I felt that way yesterday, and such judgements can clearly take place in the absence of pain (otherwise, one could not think that someone was in agony without feeling agony oneself). Indeed, arguably Mary in her black and white room has a concept of what it's like to see red in virtue of being in a linguistic community with people who have that concept.[5] But only a subject currently experiencing phenomenal quality Q can form a direct phenomenal concept of Q.

Of course, we cannot refute physicalism by just defining a notion inconsistent with it and calling it 'real'. However, I think we have good reason to think that we are

[3] Balog (2012); Papineau (2002).

[4] The notion of a direct phenomenal concept comes from Chalmers (2003).

[5] As argued by Tye (2009).

really acquainted with our phenomenal qualities, and that this in turn gives us good reason to think the conceptual dualism advocated by the phenomenal concepts strategists is inconsistent with a physicalist ontology. In the remainder of this paper I will (i) offer a detailed characterization of real acquaintance, (ii) argue for the real instantiation of real acquaintance so characterized, and (iii) present an argument against physicalism which starts from the premise that we are really acquainted with our phenomenal qualities.

4.2 An Account of Real Acquaintance

(In this section I will assume my view is true in order to vividly characterize it. In the next section I shall argue that it is true).

Real acquaintance is a natural relation which a subject bears to each of its phenomenal qualities. It is a special kind of intimacy in virtue of which the following two facts obtain:

Revelation: A psychologically normal subject can come to know the real nature of one of her phenomenal qualities by attending to that quality.

Phenomenal Certainty: A psychologically normal subject is able to put herself into a situation in which, with respect to one of her phenomenal qualities, she is justified in being certain that that quality is instantiated (where to be certain that P is roughly to believe with a credence of 1 that P).

A bird is really acquainted with its phenomenal qualities, but, being unable to attend to them, has no grip on their nature, and is unable to form beliefs about its phenomenal qualities. At all times I am really acquainted with each of my phenomenal qualities, but most of the time I, as it were, look through my phenomenal qualities to the features of the world they represent. When perceiving a red bus I attend not to what it's like to see red, but to the red quality of the bus itself. However, an advantage humans have over birds is that, with a slight mental effort, they are able to attend to and think about their experiences. Certain experiences, such as pain, anxiety, after images, are more apt for this kind of reflection. And when I attend to my phenomenal qualities, their real nature is directly revealed to me in such a way that I am justified in not entertaining the slightest doubt concerning their instantiation.

What is the 'real nature' of pain? It is clearly not the case that *all the properties* of pain are revealed to me when I attend to it. Pain might be instantiated a certain number of times in the world, but I am not aware of how many when I attend to my headache. A more plausible suggestion would be that all *necessary* properties of pain constitute its real nature. But even this is too much. Pain is necessarily such that $100 \times 127 = 12{,}700$, but it is not plausible that this is revealed to me when I attend to a throbbing in my shin.

Kit Fine distinguishes the modal conception of essence popular in contemporary metaphysics, according to which an essential property of X is a property X has in all possible worlds, from a definitional conception of essence, according to which an essential property of X is one that constitutes the *real definition* of X, that is, one that makes X the kind of thing it is.[6] Fine takes the notion of a real definition as primitive, but thinks it one we easily get a grip on by consideration of cases. In all possible worlds in which Socrates exists, he has the property of being either Socrates or the Eiffel Tower. But the property of being either Socrates or the Eiffel Tower does not plausibly contribute to making Socrates the kind of thing he is. The property of *being human* is a more plausible candidate. All properties that constitute the real definition of a thing are properties that a thing has necessarily, but the converse is not the case.

To make sense of the 'real nature' or 'essence' of pain, we need to be working with a Finean rather than a modal conception of essence. Pain is a property rather than an object, but it seems even more plausible in the case of properties that they have something like a real definition or nature. This is not to say that a property has some *other* property, which is its nature, as talk of properties 'having a real nature' might superficially suggest. Rather, regarding each property P, there is something to be understood regarding P, the understanding of which constitutes knowing what it is for P to be instantiated. Consider the property of sphericity. In knowing that for something to be spherical is for it to have all points on its surface equidistant from its centre, I know what it is for sphericity to be instantiated.

It is difficult to put the point unambiguously. With regards to any property one has a concept of, there is a sense in which one 'knows what it is for the property to be instantiated'. Suppose Jim has an indexical concept of the property of being gold. That indexical concept does not afford Jim an understanding of the real nature of that property. And yet there is a sense in which Jim can truly say, 'Of course I know what it is for something to be *that stuff*: it is for it to be *that stuff*', where he specifies by demonstration the condition an object must satisfy in order to count as gold.

However, perhaps even more so than in Fine's discussion of the real nature of objects, consideration of cases shows that there is a perfectly clear notion here. Suppose David and I are playing a fun game called 'Guess my favourite property'. I am trying to guess David's favourite property, which turns out to be sphericity. Contrast my understanding of David's favourite property before he tells me what it is—when I can only think of it as 'David's favourite property'—and my understanding of David's favourite property after he tells me it's sphericity. There is a clear sense in which I go from *not knowing what the property in question is*, to *knowing what the property in question is.*

Now, when I'm still guessing I could always be clever and say, 'Of course I know which property we're talking about: it's *David's favourite property*'. If I use the phrase

[6] Fine (1994).

'David's favourite property' as a rigid designator, then I am able to refer to the property in question (I pick it out in all possible worlds!). But it is only when I am able to think of it in geometrical terms that I grasp its nature, that I understand what it is for an object to have that property. The notion of a real nature is closely linked to the notion of a transparent concept that I have developed in other work; roughly, a transparent concept is one that renders a priori accessible the real nature of its referent.[7]

Talk of 'knowing what it is for a property to be instantiated' suggests that properties are universals. But I take it that this kind of talk is consistent with nominalism at a more fundamental level of analysis. If we identify properties with sets of tropes, then we can say that real acquaintance with a pain trope affords an understanding of what it is for a certain trope to be a pain trope. Even the austere nominalist, who at a fundamental level of analysis quantifies only over particular objects, can arguably analyse this notion. She can say that a pained subject, in virtue of being pain-acquainted, is afforded an understanding of what it is for her to be pained.[8]

As long as there's something to be understood about an object that constitutes knowing what it is about an object that fits it to satisfy some predicate 'N', then we can give some kind of analysis of talk of 'the real nature of property N-ness' whatever our ultimate metaphysics. There are perhaps some very austere forms of concept nominalism, according to which reality just consists of characterless blobs, which predicates apply to only as a result of our interests. Blobby nominalism of this kind could provide no analysis of talk of the real nature of properties.[9] But blobby nominalism of this kind is not very plausible. Surely it is a mind-independent fact that the planet Earth is such as to satisfy the predicate 'roughly spherical', and we can understand how the Earth can be such as to satisfy this predicate, even if its being so isn't a matter of the Earth's instantiating a certain universal.

Our fundamental metaphysics will make a difference, though, to what kind of things we may take the objects of real acquaintance to be. If we take properties to be Aristotelian universals, then we can say that it is the in res universal of pain with which I am acquainted, and which I thereby understand the real nature of. But on other views, it seems we cannot be acquainted with the property itself. For the Platonist, the universal of pain is outside of space and time. The austere nominalist and the trope theorist either do not believe in the universal of pain, or identify it with

[7] Goff (2011 and MS).

[8] One could give a meta-linguistic analysis of what it is in general to 'know what it is for a property to be instantiated'. I shall not attempt to do this here.

[9] Armstrong equates all forms of austere nominalism with blobby nominalism. However, if the austere nominalist takes it to be a fundamental fact about the world that objects are propertied, then, despite not believing in properties, she has a non-blobby picture of the world. Devitt (1980) and Lewis (1983) have argued contra Armstrong for the tenability of this kind of position. The austere nominalist who believes that objects are propertied has a more ideologically expansive view than the blobby austere nominalist, despite not having a more ontologically expansive view.

the set of pained things/pain tropes. In all these cases, it is difficult to see how we could make sense of the subject bearing a natural relation to pain. But in each case I think there is a natural candidate for the object of acquaintance.

The Platonist can say that the subject is acquainted with the state of affairs of her instantiating the universal of pain, and thereby understands the real nature of that universal. The trope theorist can say that the subject is acquainted with a pain trope, and thereby understands what it is for a trope to be a pain trope. The austere nominalist can say that the subject is acquainted with itself at a time when it is pained, and in virtue of this acquaintance knows what it is for a subject to be pained. Unless the trope or the particular object (at a given time) in question is blobby, there will be a way of understanding how the trope/object is such as to satisfy the relevant predicate, and we may suppose that such understanding can come from a real acquaintance with the trope/particular object at a time.[10, 11]

The final point I want to make about real acquaintance is crucial. Real acquaintance is not *defined* as the relation that guarantees the *Revelation* and *Phenomenal Certainty*. The concept of real acquaintance is a primitive notion, but one that turns out necessarily to have these implications. One might suspect I was cooking up this notion, were it not so intuitive, and so familiar from the history of philosophy. One easily latches onto the idea that one is 'so close' to one's experiences that their nature is laid bare and their instantiation certain. This is not to say that we really do stand in such a relation to our phenomenal qualities. My point is just that it is not plausible for my opponents to claim they haven't the slightest idea what I'm talking about.

4.3 An Argument for Real Acquaintance

Why should we believe that we are really acquainted with our phenomenal qualities? One reason is that we seem to be. The fact that there seems to be a table in front of me gives me some reason to believe that there is a table in front of me. The fact that I seem to stand in a peculiar type of intimate relationship with my pain such that its nature is directly revealed to me in such a way that I can be rationally certain of its instantiation, gives me some reason to believe that I really do stand in that relationship with my pain.

There is a further reason to believe in real acquaintance: the hypothesis that I am really acquainted with my phenomenal qualities explains a couple of very plausible

[10] To say that we are acquainted with 'a particular object at time t' is not to say that we are acquainted with t. We can say that by virtue of being acquainted with itself at a time when it is pained a subject can understand what it is for something to be pained, and by virtue of being acquainted with itself at a time when it is pleasured a subject can understand what it is for something to be pleasured. It doesn't matter that the subject is acquainted with something which is not essentially pained (or pleasured, or whatever), just so long as it is an objective fact about the world that it is pained at the time of acquaintance (which wouldn't be the case if the subject were blobby).

[11] I am grateful to Mike Martin for prompting me to think more carefully about the metaphysics of real acquaintance.

theses about our epistemic situation with regards to phenomenal qualities: *phenomenal certainty* and *phenomenal insight*:

Phenomenal certainty: A psychologically normal subject is able to put herself into a situation in which, with respect to one of her phenomenal qualities, she is justified in feeling certain that that quality is instantiated (where to be certain that P is roughly to believe with a credence of 1 that P).

Phenomenal Insight: We have rich a priori knowledge concerning our phenomenal qualities.

4.3.1 Phenomenal Certainty

We have already come across *Phenomenal Certainty* in characterizing real acquaintance. But it is an incredibly plausible thesis in its own right. Consider the following case. Suppose I am in agony, having just had my leg cut off. I attend to my agony, think about it in terms of how it feels thereby forming a phenomenal concept of the agony, and then deploy that phenomenal concept in judging that I am feeling *like that* ('*like that*' expresses the phenomenal concept). In normal circumstances, I can rule out any scenario in which that judgement is not true; I am justified in believing with total certainty that I feel *that way*.

This is not a kind of certainty we are capable of having regarding states of the external world. I have a justified belief that there is a laptop in front of me. That belief has a very high level of justification. It has enough justification to count as knowledge. Nonetheless, I am not justified in being certain that there is a laptop in front of me, as there is a very small chance I am in *The Matrix*, and what seems like a visual experience of a laptop is in fact an elaborate hallucination created in my mind by evil computers.

I am not saying that every time we form a phenomenal concept, we achieve rational certainty that the concept is satisfied. And I'm not saying we never make mistakes about our conscious experience. I'm just claiming that there are certain, quite familiar, circumstances in which such rational certainty is achieved regarding a judgement about phenomenal qualities, and that a normal human being is able to create such circumstances for herself.

It would be good to have a method for distinguishing the cases where certainty is reached from the cases where it isn't, and I am broadly sympathetic to that proposed by David Chalmers (2003). However, one doesn't need to do this work in order to accept *phenomenal certainty.* I take it as a datum that there are commonplace circumstances in which I have certainty regarding the instantiation of certain qualities in my conscious experience.

4.3.2 Phenomenal Insight

Phenomenal insight is the thesis that we have a priori knowledge of certain essential features of phenomenal states. Most uncontroversially, we can know a priori essential resemblances and differences between phenomenal qualities, for example, what it's like to see red is similar to what it's like to see orange. It is also plausible that we know a priori that pain is ceteris paribus a bad thing: I can move a priori from the fact that ϕing will cause someone to feel *like that* to the fact that I have strong reason not to ϕ. Another plausible example: we can know a priori the representational properties of phenomenal qualities, for example, the phenomenal concept formed when I attend to my visual experience of seeing a tomato characterizes it as an experience as of a red, round thing. In order to avoid getting into more controversy than is necessary, I'll stick to the case of essential similarities and differences between phenomenal qualities.

One might agree that we have knowledge of essential similarities between our conscious states, but be reluctant to class this knowledge as a priori. One's reasoning might be that we know such facts through the *faculty* of introspection, which makes it natural to class this knowledge as a posteriori. According to this line of reasoning, introspective knowledge is a kind of sensory knowledge accumulated through an inner sense.

However, the fact that this knowledge comes from introspection does not entail that it is a posteriori, because introspection and phenomenal concepts are essentially bound up with each other. We form phenomenal concepts through introspecting our phenomenal qualities. We can't go from the fact that we know a truth about phenomenal qualities through introspection to the fact that that truth is a posteriori, as we may well use introspection to form the relevant phenomenal concepts, and thereby discern the truth from the concepts.

The way to decide whether these truths are a priori is to ask whether or not their negations are conceivable. If the negation of a given proposition is inconceivable, it follows that its falsity can be ruled out by mere reflection on concepts. If both the truth and the falsity of a given proposition are conceivable, it follows that we are reliant on some faculty to work out which is the case, and hence the resulting knowledge is a posteriori. It is overwhelmingly plausible with regards to the propositions under consideration that their negations are inconceivable: we cannot conceive of a situation where phenomenal red is more similar to phenomenal green than it is to phenomenal orange. I conclude, therefore, that we have a priori knowledge in this case, and that *phenomenal insight* is true.

4.3.3 *Real Acquaintance,* Phenomenal Certainty, *and* Phenomenal Insight

Intuitively we stand in a peculiarly intimate relationship with our phenomenal qualities in virtue of which *phenomenal certainty* and *revelation* are true. Supposing that things are as they seem to be in this respect allows us to explain *phenomenal certainty* and *phenomenal insight*. It is of course part of the basic characterization of real acquaintance that it grounds *phenomenal certainty*. And we can explain *phenomenal insight* by saying that, in virtue of a real acquaintance with phenomenal red and phenomenal orange, the subject understands the real nature of each of those qualities, and it is thereby apparent that the two qualities have a similar nature. This might be understood analogously to our knowledge that triangularity and trilaterality are necessarily co-extensive. I know what it is for an object to have three sides, I know what it is for an object to have three angles, and it is thereby apparent to me that those two properties must go together. (I am not saying that we are really acquainted with these geometrical properties; the cases are analogous only in the sense that in both cases we have knowledge grounded in an understanding of real natures.)

The fact that the real acquaintance naturally and intuitively explains these facts about our epistemic situation gives us reason to believe in it. Our reason to believe in real acquaintance is somewhat similar to our reason to believe in the external world. We are justified in believing in the external world because (i) there seems to be an external world, (ii) supposing that, in this respect, things are as they seem to be explains the structure and coherence of our experience. We are justified in believing that we are really acquainted with our phenomenal qualities because (i) we seem to be really acquainted with our phenomenal qualities, (ii) supposing that, in this respect, things are as they seem to be explains two extremely plausible theses concerning our relationship to our conscious experience: *phenomenal certainty* and *phenomenal insight*.

How strong these reasons to believe in real acquaintance are will depend on the prospects for an alternative explanation of *phenomenal certainty* and *phenomenal insight* (just as the strength of our reasons for believing in the external world depends on the prospects for alternative explanations of the structure and coherence of our experience, for example, idealism). If we have two equally good explanations of *phenomenal certainty* and *phenomenal insight*, and only one of them is consistent with physicalism, then those who take themselves to have good reason to believe physicalism will take themselves to have good reason to favour the explanation consistent with physicalism. I will now argue that the prospects for the CPS physicalist providing such an explanation are bleak.

4.3.4 *Can the Physicalist Explain* Phenomenal Certainty *and* Phenomenal Insight?

I will try to show that there is a form of the phenomenal concepts strategy that can account for *phenomenal certainty* (or something like it), and that there is a form of the phenomenal concepts strategy that can account for *phenomenal insight*, but that there is no form of the phenomenal concepts strategy that can account for both *phenomenal certainty* and *phenomenal insight*. Indeed, I will give reasons for thinking that no form of PCS physicalism could account for both of these theses.

4.3.5 *A Physicalist Account of* Phenomenal Certainty

Proponents of acquaintance physicalism can account for the infallibility of certain phenomenal judgements. According to the acquaintance physicalist, a direct phenomenal concept of pain involves within its constitution the feeling of pain it refers to. Any subject judging that she is in pain by employing a direct phenomenal concept of pain must therefore be in pain: she must be feeling pain in order for that pain to constitute the direct phenomenal concept. Such a judgement, therefore, cannot fail to be true.[12]

I am not sure that this kind of infallibility can give us rational certainty. It is one thing to think that a judgement cannot fail to be true; it is another thing to think I can be *justified* in not entertaining any doubt about the judgement. To have rational certainty that p, a subject has to be in a position to rule out any scenario where p fails to be the case. Merely having a belief that cannot fail to be true does not entail that a subject is able to do this. However, I shall set this worry on one side, and suppose that the acquaintance physicalist has the resources to account for *phenomenal certainty*.

Whilst acquaintance physicalism may be in a good position with respect to *phenomenal certainty*, the same cannot be said of *phenomenal insight*. There are broadly speaking two ways in which it can be a priori that a certain description D (non-trivially) truly applies to a certain referent R thought about under concept C. Firstly, it could be the case that in deploying C we pick out R as 'the actual D', thus rendering it inconceivable that R thought of under C is not actually D. For example, we think about Julius as 'the actual inventor of the zip', and thereby render it inconceivable that Julius is not the actual inventor of the zip.[13] Secondly, it might be that, in deploying C we pick out R in virtue of being really acquainted with R, and our real acquaintance with R makes it apparent to us that D truly describes the real nature of R, or some fact that follows from the real nature of R. For example, it might be that I am really acquainted with phenomenal red, and really acquainted with phenomenal orange, and through grasping the real nature of these qualities it is apparent to me that phenomenal red satisfies the description 'has a similar nature to phenomenal orange'.

I can see no other way in which our substantive a priori knowledge concerning phenomenal qualities could be accounted for. Certainly we would not have such knowledge if the entity were thought of under a radically opaque concept, that is, a concept such that reference is wholly determined by facts which are not a priori accessible.[14] Some entity referred to under a radically opaque concept might be *associated* by thinkers with a certain description. For example, even if the reference of 'John' is determined by causal facts outside the head, it might be that speakers in our community associate the name 'John' with the description 'a cad not to be trusted'. However, because this description is not involved in reference-fixing, it will always be conceivable that it does not apply to John. This isn't a case of a priori knowledge; it's just a bad reputation.[15]

[12] This account of infallibility is defended by Papineau (2002) and Balog (2012).

[13] Kripke (1980).

[14] In Goff (2011) and Goff (MS) I distinguish a range of concepts from transparent to radically opaque (I give a slightly different definition of 'radically opaque').

[15] Probably most names are not radically opaque, and contain some descriptive constraints on reference. For example, if it turns out that the entity that 'John' is causally connected to is not a person, then arguably 'John' fails to refer. However, such descriptive constraints on reference may not be enough to

In order to account for our a priori knowledge of phenomenal qualities, phenomenal concepts would have to refer either by description or by real acquaintance. The acquaintance physicalist can take neither of these options. A phenomenal concept, on her view, picks out its referent not by description, but in virtue of being partly constituted by the referent. And this constitution relation between concept and quality cannot result in the subject's having real acquaintance with the quality, as real acquaintance is inconsistent with PCS physicalism (I will argue for this more thoroughly below). Therefore, the acquaintance physicalist is unable to account for *phenomenal insight*.

4.3.6 A Physicalist Account of Phenomenal Insight

Most forms of the phenomenal concepts strategy seem to construe phenomenal concepts as radically opaque. It is causal connections, or facts about the natural functions or material constitution of phenomenal concepts, which hook the subject up to its phenomenal qualities, not descriptions which are a priori available to the subject. Janet Levin and Robert Schroer, however, have proposed theories of phenomenal concepts according to which they are hybrids of descriptive and radically opaque sub-concepts.[16]

Levin's view mingles elements of analytic functionalism and the phenomenal concepts strategy. The reference of a phenomenal concept is determined in two distinct ways. On the one hand, a phenomenal concept picks out a conscious state by characterizing it in causal-functional terms and/or in terms of the similarities and differences between phenomenal qualities. On the other hand, a phenomenal concept picks out a state by being causally connected to that state in the right kind of way. This makes reference a little precarious, as both of these reference-fixing routes must be successful for the phenomenal concept to refer. If the phenomenal concept fails to be causally connected in the right way to anything, or if the thing the phenomenal concept is causally connected to doesn't have the relevant causal-functional/similarity properties, then reference fails.

Schroer thinks that phenomenal concepts are descriptive concepts that pick out conscious states in terms of their mode of composition from more basic phenomenal elements. The concept 'phenomenal orange 7', for example, characterizes its referent as being composed of phenomenal red hue and phenomenal yellow hue, as well as some specific degree of phenomenal saturation and phenomenal lightness. But the sub-concepts referring to the phenomenal elements are radically opaque: reference to phenomenal elements is determined by causal facts outside of what is a priori accessible. For Schroer, the phenomenal elements turn out to refer to physical

uniquely identify an object, and hence to wholly determine reference. Perhaps, then, names are a bit like the 'hybrid concepts' discussed below.

[16] Levin (2002), Schroer (2010).

properties, and hence the conscious state which the phenomenal elements compose turns out to be a composite physical state. Zombies are nonetheless conceivable, as there is no a priori information in the sub-concepts which would allow us to know that they refer to physical properties.

Both of these hybrid views can account for *phenomenal insight*, or at least our a priori knowledge of similarities and resemblances amongst phenomenal states. On Schroer's view it is stipulated by the description that determines the reference of 'phenomenal orange 7' that the state denoted involves phenomenal red hue, and it is stipulated by the description that determines reference of 'phenomenal red 8' that the state denoted involves phenomenal red hue. In virtue of this we can know a priori that these two qualities share a common element and thus resemble each other. On Levin's view the similarity is built directly into the descriptions.

However, neither view can account for *phenomenal certainty*. Suppose through introspection I am aware of a phenomenal quality which presents itself as falling under the concept 'phenomenal orange'. Assuming that quality is phenomenal orange, it is a priori that it resembles phenomenal red. But how do I know that that quality I am aware of is phenomenal orange? Neither Schroer nor Levin fill in the details, but presumably there must be some reliable sub-personal mechanism that gathers information about the quality, and ensures that I deploy the correct phenomenal concept, i.e. 'phenomenal orange' rather than 'phenomenal green', 'pain', or 'anxiety'.

This puts introspective beliefs about phenomenal qualities in the same epistemological boat as ordinary perceptual beliefs: reliant on the proper functioning of an information-gathering mechanism. My belief that there is a table in front of me is reliant for its truth on the proper functioning of my senses. Similarly, for Schroer and Levin, my judgement that I am experiencing phenomenal orange (as opposed to phenomenal green, pain, or anxiety) must be dependent on the proper functioning of some information-gathering mechanism involved in introspection. They are unable, therefore, to explain why the belief that I am currently experiencing phenomenal orange is not subject to doubt in the way that my belief that there is a table in front of me is.

4.3.7 *Physicalism Can't Account for Both* Phenomenal Certainty *and* Phenomenal Insight

In summary, we can offer the following argument against the possibility of a form of PCS physicalism which accounts for both *phenomenal certainty* and *phenomenal insight*:

(1) We pick out qualities in our experience in one of the following ways (a) by being really acquainted with those qualities, (b) by description, (c) with radically opaque concepts, (d) with some hybrid of descriptive and radically opaque sub-concepts.

(2) The PCS physicalist cannot go for option (a).

(3) If the PCS physicalist goes for options (b) or (d) then she cannot account for *phenomenal certainty*.
(4) If the PCS physicalist goes for option (c), then she cannot account for *phenomenal insight*.
(5) Therefore, the physicalist cannot account for both *phenomenal certainty* and *phenomenal insight*.

4.3.8 *Objection: Semi-Acquaintance*

Real acquaintance is defined as an all-or-nothing matter, in the sense that the complete nature of the object of acquaintance is revealed to the subject of acquaintance. But is there not logical space for a kind of relation between thinker and property that yields the thinker a *partial* grasp of the nature of the property thought about? Perhaps the physicalist could explain *phenomenal certainty* and *phenomenal insight* in terms of a commitment to *semi-acquaintance*, defined as a special kind of intimacy between a subject and its phenomenal qualities in virtue of which the following two theses are true:

Semi-Revelation: A psychologically normal subject can come to know *some aspect* of the real nature of one of her phenomenal qualities by attending to that quality.

Phenomenal Certainty: A psychologically normal subject is able to put herself into a situation in which, with respect to one of her phenomenal qualities, she is justified in being certain that that quality is instantiated (where to be certain that P is roughly to believe with a credence of 1 that P).

Obviously such a relation would account for *phenomenal certainty*. And the proponent of semi-acquaintance could perhaps account for *phenomenal insight* in terms of the partial grasp of the nature of phenomenal qualities afforded to us by the obtaining of *semi-revelation*.

It is important to note that semi-acquaintance can be of help to the physicalist only if it is of a very specific kind. In many cases, an aspect of a physical property is a physical property. Suppose pain were the combination of c-fibre and d-fibre stimulation. If a semi-acquaintance with pain revealed to us that pain involved c-fibre stimulation, this would be enough to make it a priori that pain is physical, contrary to what the PCS physicalist supposes.

In order to maintain the conceptual independence of the phenomenal and the physical, the PCS physicalist would have to suppose that semi-acquaintance affords us an understanding of merely structural or functional properties of phenomenal qualities. We can note that the facts about phenomenology that Levin and Schroer think are a priori available are all of this kind. Schroer thinks we can know a priori certain facts about the internal structure of phenomenal qualities. Levin thinks that we can know a priori certain causal and resemblance facts concerning phenomenal qualities. By restricting our a priori knowledge of phenomenal qualities to facts about structure or causal roles, it remains opaque whether or not phenomenal qualities are physical.

It seems that for semi-acquaintance to help the PCS physicalist it would have to be *structural semi-acquaintance*, defined as a special kind of intimacy between subjects and their phenomenal qualities in virtue of which the following two theses are true:

Structural Semi-Revelation: A psychologically normal subject can come to know certain facts about the internal structure and/or causal role of that quality.

Phenomenal Certainty: A psychologically normal subject is able to put herself into a situation in which, with respect to one of her phenomenal qualities, she is justified in being certain that that quality is instantiated (where to be certain that P is roughly to believe with a credence of 1 that P).

I submit that we have no intuitive grip on the notion of semi-acquaintance (of which structural-acquaintance is a kind). We can of course stipulatively define the notion. But there is a kind of disunity between the two aspects of its characterization, which can be appreciated by comparison with the notion of real acquaintance. The idea of real acquaintance is the idea of a certain kind of intimacy between a subject and each of its phenomenal qualities, in virtue of which (i) a normal subject can know the nature of those qualities, (ii) a normal subject can come to be rationally certain that those qualities are instantiated. The two aspects of the characterization of real acquaintance are unified around this particular notion of intimacy.

I would ask the proponent of semi-revelation whether or not on her view, for any given subject S and an arbitrary one its phenomenal qualities Q, S is intimate with *the whole* of Q, or with only *one aspect* of Q, call it A. There are two possible answers to this question:

Option 1: S is intimate only with A, and that's why she can only understand the nature of A, not the nature of the whole of Q. The problem with this option is that it's unclear how we can explain the fact that (in normal circumstances) S can be rationally certain that the whole of Q is instantiated, not merely that A is instantiated. A normal individual in agony can know for certain that she is in agony, not merely that some aspect of her agony is instantiated.

Option 2: S is intimate with the whole of Q, and can thereby be rationally certain that the whole of Q is instantiated. The trouble with this option is that it's unclear why S can come to know only an aspect of Q, rather than the whole of Q.

There seems no non-arbitrary way of deciding which of the above options the proponent of semi-acquaintance ought to go for. And the fact that it's not clear how to spell out the details in this respect suggests that the notion of semi-acquaintance is cooked up rather than part of the way things pre-theoretically seem to be.

There might be a concern that I am putting too much weight on what we intuitively have a grip on. But whilst the argument for real acquaintance must begin with how things intuitively are—intuitively I am epistemically intimate with my pain such that its nature is directly revealed to me in such a way that its instantiation is beyond rational doubt—it does not end there. There are very plausible theses about our epistemic situation, namely *phenomenal insight* and *phenomenal certainty* that are straightforwardly explained by this intuitive way things seem to be; and this gives us strong reason to believe that, in this case, the way things intuitively seem to be is the way things really are.

There is a more straightforward reason why the physicalist is going to find it difficult to make use of semi-acquaintance, which arises when we appreciate that doing so would require giving a physicalistic account of the semi-acquaintance relation. The physicalist cannot just take semi-acquaintance to be a primitive relation; rather she must give some physicalist account of it, explaining it in more fundamental terms.

Given that semi-acquaintance is characterized in terms of *semi-revelation* and *phenomenal certainty*, giving a physicalist account of semi-acquaintance will involve giving a physicalist account of *semi-revelation* and *phenomenal certainty*. And for similar reasons to those discussed in detail above, it is hard to see how the physicalist could account for both *semi-revelation* and *phenomenal certainty*. She might explain *semi-revelation* with reference to some descriptivist account along the lines of Levin and Schroer; but that will leave her unable to explain *phenomenal certainty*. She might explain *phenomenal certainty* by giving some acquaintance physicalist model, along the lines of Balog and Papineau; but that will leave her unable to explain *semi-revelation*. Once we realize that the physicalist can't take the semi-acquaintance relation as primitive, we can see that it offers no help at all.

4.4 The Acquaintance Argument against Physicalism

Now that we have support for the thesis that we are really acquainted with our phenomenal qualities, I can turn to the argument against physicalism itself:

Premise 1: We are really acquainted with our phenomenal qualities.

Premise 2: If (i) we are really acquainted with our phenomenal qualities, and (ii) our phenomenal qualities had a real physical/functional nature, then (iii) the real physical/functional nature of our phenomenal qualities would be accessible through introspection.

Premise 3: It is not the case that there is a real physical/functional nature of our phenomenal qualities accessible through introspection.

Conclusion: Our phenomenal qualities do not have a real physical/functional nature, and therefore physicalism is false.

Old school physicalists, such as analytic functionalists, may dispute premise 3, claiming it to be a priori that phenomenal qualities are certain causal role properties. I will not here argue against such views; my main target in this paper is PCS physicalism, which I take to be the view that (i) each phenomenal quality has a real physical/functional nature, and (ii) the nature of phenomenal concepts entails an epistemic gap between phenomenal qualities phenomenally conceived, and phenomenal qualities conceived of in terms of their real physical/functional nature. Such physicalists are committed to premise 3.

One view I certainly do not intend to argue against is Russellian monism. Galen Strawson calls himself a 'physicalist', but thinks that the real nature of fundamental physical entities is, at least in part, experiential. Physics characterizes properties in terms of their causal role: negative charge is whatever property plays the negative charge role, mass is whatever property plays the mass role. According to Strawson, the properties which turn out to play those roles, and hence turn out to be negative charge and mass, are at least in part, experiential. These fundamental forms of experience come together in the brain to constitute the conscious experience we associate with organisms.[17]

Strawson can, and I think would, agree that we are really acquainted with our phenomenal qualities. When I attend to my pain, its real 'physical' nature (according to Strawson's use of the word 'physical') is revealed to me, as how pain feels just is its real 'physical' nature, the real nature of that property we pick out by its causal role when we think of it as 'c-fibres firing'. Strawson's panpsychism is a form of Russellian monism, which I take to be the view that the real nature of (at least some of) the properties denoted by fundamental physics is phenomenal or protophenomenal, where protophenomenal properties are properties which are not phenomenal but (in certain combinations) a priori entail the existence of phenomenal properties, without doing so merely in virtue of realizing structural/functional properties.[18] Any Russellian monist who takes the real nature of c-fibres firing to be experiential, and chooses to call this nature 'physical', can also accept that we are really acquainted with the real 'physical' nature of c-fibres firing.

I take it that there is no privileged definition of 'physical' or 'physicalism' out there for us to discover. There are a number of ways in which we might define the word 'physicalism', and our choice should be shaped by pragmatic considerations. I prefer not to call Strawson's view 'physicalism', simply because the sides of the debate over the knowledge argument and the zombie conceivability argument don't line up nicely if we do. Those who draw metaphysical conclusions from the knowledge argument and the zombie conceivability argument thereby rule out more standard forms of physicalism, but do not thereby rule out Strawson-style 'physicalism' (although of

[17] Strawson (2003, 2006).

[18] See Russell (1927). For other examples of Russellian monists, see Eddington (1928), Feigl (1958/67), Maxwell (1978), Strawson (1994, 2003, 2006), Chalmers (1996), Griffin (1998), and Stoljar (2001).

course they may dislike Strawson-style physicalism for other reasons). It makes things easier to call those who draw such metaphysical conclusions 'anti-physicalists', and their opponents 'physicalists'.

I do not have space here to give a complete definition of physicalism, but I will stipulate that a 'physical' property, although it may be identical with a phenomenal property, has a real nature which can be grasped in non-phenomenal/protophenomenal terms (according to the above definition of 'protophenomenal'). Someone who believes in properties the real nature of which can only be grasped in phenomenal/protophenomenal terms does not count as a 'physicalist' by my lights. This is a terminological choice; the substantive point is that my argument is not aimed at the Russellian monist.[19]

4.4.1 *Objection: Dual Revelation*

The PCS physicalist is most likely to respond to my argument by denying that we are really acquainted with our phenomenal qualities, but I have given considerable support to this premise of my argument. Their only other option as far as I can see is to deny premise 2 by accepting what I call 'dual revelation':

> *Dual revelation*: For some property *F*, there are two conceptually distinct ways of knowing the real nature of *F* (i.e. knowing what it is for *F* to be instantiated).[20]

If the PCS physicalist accepts dual revelation with respect to phenomenal qualities, they can claim that the real nature of pain is available both from completed brain science and from introspection, even though there is no conceptual connection between these two ways of understanding its nature. They could then deny premise 2: the real physical/functional nature of pain is not introspectively accessible, even though the real phenomenal nature with which that physical/functional nature is identical is introspectively accessible.[21]

I find it difficult to make sense of dual revelation. Of course we can *refer* to a property in all sorts of ways: by description, by being causally connected to it, by possessing a concept the natural function of which is to track it. But it is quite another thing to suppose that we can *understand the nature* of a single property in two radically distinct ways. Certainly we don't seem to be in a position of dual revelation with regards to the most uncontroversial cases of properties we have an understanding of the nature of. For an object to be spherical is for all points on its surface to be equidistant from its centre. For something to be a prime number is for it to be a

[19] I give a full definition of 'physicalism' in Goff (MS).

[20] In Goff (2011) I rather uncharitably called dual revelation the 'Thesis of Dubious Intelligibility'.

[21] Nic Damnjanovic (2012) has explicitly defended the plausibility of this kind of PCS physicalism and, in conversation, Ned Block seems sympathetic. Shortly prior to the final submission of this paper Esa Diaz-Leon (forthcoming) and J. H. Taylor (forthcoming) had interesting attempts to make sense of dual revelation accepted for publication. I look forward to responding to these papers in future work.

number that can be divided only by itself and one. There seems no way of specifying the essence of a sphere or a prime number in a radically different way, such that there is no possibility of deducing the radically new definition from the old one (or vice versa).

To accept dual revelation is to accept that the world is, at least in some respects, radically unintelligible; there are some necessary connections which even a complete understanding of the world would not render intelligible. If there are such brute identities between, say, physical and mental properties, an omnipotent being with a complete understanding of the essence of pain and c-fibres firing would be surprised that she were not able to create one without the other.

I hasten to stress that I am not a supporter of the Chalmers/Jackson Canberra plan,[22] according to which all facts are a priori derivable from the fundamental facts. It may be that our ordinary descriptions of the world are littered with radically opaque concepts; blind pointers which afford no understanding of the nature of the features they denote. In this case, our ordinary sentences may be made true by the real nature of the world, without having any conceptual connection with that real nature. If phenomenal concepts were radically opaque, then I would have no objection to PCS physicalism. But the idea that there could be brute necessary connections even between descriptions which render transparent real natures is to suppose that the world as it is in and of itself is in certain respects unintelligible.

It will not be possible to build a completely satisfactory case for this thesis here,[23] but I suspect that any metaphysical or scientific investigation of the world is reliant on the assumption that reality is not radically unintelligible in the way that dual revelation would imply. Metaphysical and scientific hypotheses must not just fit the evidence, but must fit the evidence in a theoretically satisfying way. However, to the extent that reality can be radically unintelligible, anything goes, and our ability to constrain metaphysical and scientific theories with respect to theoretical virtues and vices is severely limited.

Consider the following example. Suppose I'm in a spooky forest, trying to decide whether or not I should believe in the spirit of the woodland, i.e. that beneficent spirit that lives in the trees and wishes them well. Imagine that I have some very weak reason to believe in the spirit of the woodland, perhaps some old wizened fellow wandered out of the forest and croaked in a mysterious voice, 'Oooo there's a spirit of the woodland in there me laddie'. The stranger's testimony, we can suppose, gives me a very weak reason to believe in the spirit of the woodland.

It is natural to think that this very weak reason is counterbalanced by the Ockhamist imperative not to add to our ontology without good reason. But if dual revelation is an option, I can believe in the woodland spirit without adding to my ontology, by identifying it with the bark of the trees. Of course there is no a priori

[22] Chalmers (2012), Chalmers and Jackson (2001).

[23] I expand on my defence of this thesis in Goff (MS).

connection between the scientific essence of bark, described as such, and the spirit of the woodland, described as a mental thing that cares about the forest and wishes it well. But I can claim that these are just two conceptually distinct ways of grasping the essence of a single thing. Without the constraint that identity statements couched in transparent (i.e. real nature revealing) concepts must be intelligible, it's hard to see what I'm doing wrong.

Wouldn't this be to believe that there is more to the nature of bark; that as well as its scientific essence it has certain mental properties? No; the suggestion is that the scientific essence *just is* the mentally defined essence: we have two different ways of understanding exactly the same nature. Of course I don't think this theory makes sense, because I don't think dual revelation makes sense. But if dual revelation is an option then there seems to be no way of using Ockham's razor to rule out the view.

It's not going to stop there. Dual revelation opens the door to all sorts of metaphysical indulgence that Ockham's razor can't touch:

- Suppose we think the normative force of genuine reasons cannot be captured in a naturalistic vocabulary. No worries, simply assert a brute identity between normative force and some natural property, e.g. identify *not to be doneness* with pain. We might even believe in real fire and brimstone moral properties, such as sin and evil, but just identify them with natural properties.[24]
- Suppose I believe in a world of quiddities, the nature of which can be completely captured in completely non-causal terms, but I'm worried that without real powers the continuing regularity of the world is just a massive cosmic coincidence.[25] No worries, just take the utterly non-causal quiddity descriptions, and your favourite full-blooded powers description, and claim that these are just two radically different ways of understanding the same properties.[26]
- Suppose you really want to believe in your guardian angel, ever near, loving you deeply. No worries; just identify her with your bedspread.[27]

In all these cases, there is a strong intuition that there's some cheating going on; ontology is being smuggled in without the proper price being paid for it. Perhaps the following analogy with tax avoidance is helpful. In tax avoidance, as opposed to evasion, one is sticking to the exact letter of the law whilst brazenly breaking its spirit. In the above cases the exact letter of Ockham's razor may be being respected, but its spirit is not.

[24] I am not ruling out the view that ethical properties are identical with natural properties. My point is just that the naturalist needs to do some work to make such identities intelligible, as is done for example in Frank Jackson's (1998) defence of ethical naturalism.

[25] This sort of worry is defended in Strawson (1987).

[26] Taylor (forthcoming) turns this specific comparison against me, arguing that the Heil/Martin (Heil and Martin 1998, Martin 2007) view that categorical and dispositional properties are identical is both plausible and consistent with dual revelation.

[27] As far as I know no one in the literature has defended this specific identity.

It is not that there will be no constraint from theoretical virtues once we commit to dual revelation. It will still be the case, for example, that the theory of evolution fits the empirical data better than a literal interpretation of Genesis. However, there will be unlimited possibility for 'adding' numerous whacky entities to the world, by identifying their essences with the essences of things we already believe in. Rational investigation of the world relies on the assumption that the world is minimally intelligible.

4.5 Conclusion

We are really acquainted with the qualities of our experience. When I attend to the reddish quality in my experience, the real nature of that quality is apparent to me. Nothing less than a commitment to real acquaintance can explain both my certainty that I am experiencing a reddish quality, and my phenomenal insight into certain essential features of that quality, for example, that it is similar to the orange-ish quality I am also experiencing. If that reddish quality had a real physical nature, then that real physical nature would be apparent to me in attending to the quality. But it isn't, so it doesn't.[28]

References

Armstrong, D. (1968), *A Materialist Theory of Mind* (London: Routledge and Kegan Paul).

Balog, K. (2012), 'Acquaintance and the Mind-Body Problem', in C. Hill and S. Gozzano (eds), *New Perspectives on Type Identity: The Mental and the Physical* (Cambridge: Cambridge University Press).

Block, N., and Stalnaker, R. (1999), 'Conceptual Analysis, Dualism and the Explanatory Gap', in *Philosophical Review* 108/1: 1–46.

Chalmers, D. J. (1996), *The Conscious Mind: Towards a Fundamental Theory* (Oxford: Oxford University Press).

Chalmers, D. J. (2003), 'The Content and Epistemology of Phenomenal Belief', in Q. Smith and A. Jokic (eds), *Consciousness: New Philosophical Perspectives* (New York: Oxford University Press), 220–72.

Chalmers, D. J. (2012), *Constructing the World* (Oxford: Oxford University Press).

Chalmers, D. J., and Jackson, F. (2001), 'Conceptual Analysis and Reductive Explanation', in *Philosophical Review* 110: 315–61.

Damnjanovic, N. (2012), 'Revelation and Physicalism', in *Dialectica* 66/1: 69–91.

[28] I am grateful to (in alphabetical order) Emma Bullock, David Chalmers, Paul Coates, Sam Coleman, Esa Diaz-Leon, Hedda Hassel Mørch, Geoff Lee, Mike Martin, David Papineau, Adam Pautz, Jonathan Simon, Henry Taylor, Julia Telles de Menezes, Michael Tye, and the participants at the 'Phenomenal Concepts' workshop at the Institute of Philosophy (London), the 'Nature of Phenomenal Qualities' workshop at the University of Hertfordshire, the 'Mind and Consciousness' conference at the University of Western Australia, and the 'Phenomenal Concepts' conference at the Federal University of Rio de Janeiro (where earlier versions of this chapter were given).

Devitt, M. (1980), '"Ostrich Nominalism" or "Mirage Realism"?', in *Pacific Philosophical Quarterly* 61: 433–9.

Diaz-Leon, E. (forthcoming), 'Do *a posteriori* Physicalists Get Our Phenomenal Concepts Wrong?', in *Ratio.*

Dretske, F. (1995), *Naturalising the Mind* (Cambridge, MA: MIT Press).

Eddington, A. (1928), *The Nature of the Physical World* (New York: Macmillan).

Feigl, H. (1958/1967), *The "Mental" and the "Physical": The Essay and a Postscript* (Minneapolis: University of Minnesota Press).

Fine, K. (1994), 'Essence and Modality', in *Philosophical Perspectives* 8: 1–16.

Goff, P. (2011), 'A Posteriori Physicalists Get Our Phenomenal Concepts Wrong', in *Australasian Journal of Philosophy* 89/2: 191–209.

Goff, P. (MS), *Consciousness and fundamental reality.*

Griffin, D. R. (1998), *Unsnarling the World-Knot: Consciousness, Freedom, and the Mind-Body Problem* (Minneapolis: University of Minnesota Press).

Harman, G. (1990), 'The Intrinsic Quality of Experience', in *Philosophical Perspectives* 4: 31–52.

Heil, J., and Martin, C. B. (1998), 'Rules and Powers', in *Noûs* 32 (S12): 283–312.

Hill, C. (1997), 'Imaginability, Conceivability, Possibility and the Mind-Body Problem', in *Philosophical Studies* 87/1: 61–85.

Hill, C., and McLaughlin B. (1999), 'There Are Fewer Things in Reality than Are Dreamt of in Chalmers's Philosophy', in *Philosophy and Phenomenological Research* 59/2: 445–54.

Jackson, F. (1998), *From Metaphysics to Ethics: A Defence of Conceptual Analysis* (Oxford: Clarendon Press).

Kripke, S. (1980), *Naming and Necessity* (Oxford: Blackwell).

Levin, J. (2002), 'Is Conceptual Analyses Needed for the Reduction of Qualitative States?', in *Philosophical and Phenomenological Research* 64/3: 571–91.

Levine, J. (1983), 'Materialism and Qualia: The Explanatory Gap', in *Pacific Philosophical Quarterly* 64/9: 354–61.

Lewis, D. (1966), 'An Argument for the Identity Theory', in *Journal of Philosophy* 63/1: 17–25.

Lewis, D. (1970), 'How to Define Theoretical Terms', in *Journal of Philosophy* 67/13: 427–46.

Lewis, D. (1983), 'New Work for a Theory of Universals', in *Australasian Journal of Philosophy* 61.

Lewis, D. (1994), 'Reduction of Mind', in S. Guttenplan (ed.), *Companion to the Philosophy of Mind* (Oxford: Blackwell), 412–31.

Loar, B. (1990), 'Phenomenal States', in *Philosophical Perspectives* 4: 81–108.

Loar, B. (2003), 'Qualia, Properties, Modality', in *Philosophical Issues* 13/1: 113–29.

Martin, C. B. (2007), *The Mind in Nature* (New York: Oxford University Press).

Maxwell, G. (1978), 'Rigid Designators and Mind-Brain Identity', in C. W. Savage (ed.), *Perception and Cognition* (Minneapolis: University of Minnesota Press), 365–404.

Papineau, D. (1993), 'Physicalism, Consciousness, and the Antipathetic Fallacy', in *Australasian Journal of Philosophy* 71/2: 169–83.

Papineau, D. (2002), *Thinking about Consciousness* (Oxford: Clarendon Press).

Papineau, D. (2006), 'Comments on Galen Strawson', in *Journal of Consciousness Studies* 13/6: 100–9.

Perry, J. (2001), *Knowledge, Possibility and Consciousness* (Cambridge, MA: MIT Press).

Rey, G. (1995), 'Towards a Projectivist Account of Conscious Experience', in T. Metzinger (ed.), *Conscious Experience* (Paderborn: Ferdinand Schöningh), 123–42.

Russell, B. (1927), *The Analysis of Matter* (London: Kegan Paul).

Schroer, R. (2010), 'Where's the Beef? Phenomenal Concepts as Both Demonstrative and Substantial', in *Australasian Journal of Philosophy* 88/3: 505–22.

Stoljar, D. (2001), 'Two Conceptions of the Physical', in *Philosophy and Phenomenological Research* 62/2: 253–81.

Strawson, G. (1987), 'Realism and Causation', in *Philosophical Quarterly* 37: 253–77.

Strawson, G. (1994), *Mental Reality* (Cambridge, MA/London: MIT Press).

Strawson, G. (2003), 'Real Materialism', in L. Anthony and N. Hornstein (eds), *Chomsky and His Critics* (Oxford: Blackwell), 48–88.

Strawson, G. (2006), 'Realistic Monism: Why Physicalism Entails Panpsychism', in Anthony Freeman (ed.), *Consciousness and Its Place in Nature* (Exeter: Imprint Academic), 3–31.

Taylor, J. H. (forthcoming), 'Physicalism and Phenomenal Concepts: Bringing Ontology and Philosophy of Mind Together', in *Philosophia*.

Tye, M. (2009), *Consciousness Revisited* (Cambridge, MA/London: MIT Press).

SECTION II

Perception and Phenomenal Qualities

5

Moore's Dilemma

M. G. F. Martin

I want to consider here a curious turn in the development of the original sense-datum tradition, presented in G. E. Moore's Presidential Address of 1918, 'Some Judgments of Perception' (hereafter, 'Some Judgments') (Moore 1918). This announced a fundamental alteration in his views about what philosophy could establish concerning the nature of sense perception, and it is a position that he officially held from 1918 all the way to 1953, only repudiating the new option he introduced in 'Some Judgments' in his final piece of writing on perception, 'Visual Sense-Data' (Moore 1957). Although Moore's shift in this paper has been cited as a source of the theory of appearing, and in its own right has had some commentary on it, what is really puzzling about the official position advanced in the paper, and the significance of Moore's stance, has been rather overlooked. The point is of interest in making sense of early analytic philosophy, but it also offers morals for us to learn concerning moves made in discussion of sense experience in recent debate too.

Moore introduced the term 'sense-datum' in 1910–11 in a set of lectures at Morley College, only published in 1953 as *Some Main Problems of Philosophy* (Moore 1953). The term itself was popularized by Russell in *The Problems of Philosophy* (Russell 1912) and it is from that publication that most contemporary critics came to focus on the new-fangled sense-datum theories of perception. As Moore introduced the term, and continued to guide his readers about it, it is to stand for 'whatever is given as the object of sensory awareness'. This makes explicit that Moore does not define 'sense-datum' to mean something non-physical, or even mental, which is to act as an intermediary between us and the ordinary objects we suppose ourselves to perceive. Rather, Moore takes it as the task of philosophers once they have identified their targets, the ultimate objects of sensory awareness, to go on to ascertain the nature of sense-data. Of course, that is not to say that framing matters in this way does not bring with it other questionable assumptions: notably that all cases of sensory awareness or sense experience involve an actually existing object of awareness; and also, and less obviously, that objects that one picks out purely relationally, as that which one stands in the relation awareness to, might nonetheless have something interesting in common such that we should talk about the nature of these things together. (Compare: suppose we collect all the things that a toddler has managed to put into his or her mouth and then ask about their common nature, the nature of the stomachum datum.) So it is no part of the definition of 'sense-datum' that the object of awareness should be mental or should be non-physical.

But the common idea that sense-datum theorists suppose that we are only ever aware of non-physical entities is a deserved reputation. Already in the Morley College lectures, Moore makes clear that he thinks 'the accepted view', that sense-data exist only as long as we are aware of them (and hence are not identical with any environmental objects), is probably correct. In 1914, in 'The Status of Sense-Data' he appeals to considerations about varying appearances in support of the non-identity of sense-data with anything environmental (Moore 1914: 371–3). His elaboration of these concerns is more ponderous and careful than Russell's breezy introduction in *The Problems of Philosophy*, but it works in much the same way. Let us call this approach 'the Traditional Sense-Datum Theory', TSD for short. It combines two key assumptions: (i) Moore's commitment in the very definition of the term 'sense-datum' to the idea that there always is an object of sensory awareness whenever one has sense experience; and (ii) the denial that any such objects of awareness are identical with the ordinary medium-sized objects, or even parts of those objects, that we encounter in the environment around us.

'Some Judgments of Perception' turns away from this doctrine. Moore introduces a new theory of sense perception in this paper, what Broad came to christen, 'the Multiple Relation Theory of Appearing', hereafter MRTA.[1] But Moore does not endorse this theory (or at least does not wholeheartedly endorse it), either at this point, or explicitly at any time after this. The advertised point of introducing MRTA in 'Some Judgments' is not to recommend it over TSD. It is not the theory to be preferred, to be thought correct, or more likely correct, nor as one better supported by argument or the evidence at hand. Moore's point is more modest and restricting than that: he thinks that MRTA is both the alternative to TSD, and one which philosophers lack the evidence to rule out as false. Rather than offering us a definitive view of sense perception, 'Some Judgments of Perception' offers us a dilemma: we are allegedly entitled to conclude that either TSD or MRTA is correct, but we cannot rationally choose between them.[2] And this position of indecision is repeated by Moore six years later in 'A Defence of Common Sense', and the same moral is drawn there (Moore 1925). Moore repudiates the idea that MRTA is coherent only in

[1] See Broad (1923: 237ff). See also Broad (1925: 178–208) for further discussion.

[2] Moore had already canvassed the contrast between 'seems' and 'is' as early as the Morley College lectures (Moore 1953: 39), where he considers the idea that regions of space might only seem to be filled with a given colour without actually being so, as a possible way of defending the idea that we perceive sense-data as located in public space. The idea is also raised in passing in 'The Status of Sense-Data' and offered as a reason to be less than fully confident of the traditional view. Nonetheless 1918 is the first time Moore both sets out in some detail the alternative and also underlines the dilemma.

his last writings on sense perception, 'Visual Sense-Data', written in 1953, although only published in 1957.

Some discussions of Moore's second thoughts in 1918 suggest that Moore is re-thinking the appeal of the argument from illusion, and is in some way endorsing, at least partially, MRTA. From this perspective, his later repudiation of this option is seen as a falling back from the insights he had partially gained some thirty-five years before. On the other hand, other readers have suggested that this alternative theory is introduced only in a half-hearted way, and that Moore's real commitment is to the traditional theory, which he returns to as swiftly as he can.[3] Both readings reflect aspects of things that Moore says in this paper, and in other places. But while they are tempting as strategies to clean up Moore's discussion, both go beyond the strict letter of his texts. He is careful to offer MRTA simply as a possibility, one which the evidence cannot rule out. In none of his writings does he ever seek to argue from the truth of MRTA to any other claim. In common between 'Some Judgments of Perception' and 'A Defence of Common Sense' is the idea that we can be certain that we make perceptually grounded judgements about the humdrum environmental objects around us, even though we cannot be certain of the correct philosophical analysis of these judgements. Without strong reason to the contrary, then, it is best to stick with Moore's explicitly expressed intent and to take him to have established a dilemma: we know that either TSD is correct or MRTA is correct, but we cannot know which.[4]

It is this dilemma which forms the central concern of our discussion here. What form does it take? As we shall see, Moore offers positive characterizations of both horns of the dilemma, so it should be a substantive question why our options are limited only to these two. In addition, as we will see in more detail shortly, the salient contrast between TSD and MRTA is that of a sense-datum *being* blue versus a sense-datum *seeming* blue, where it is granted that something may seem some way without being so. Commentators have applauded Moore's recognition of the 'seems'/'is' contrast, but the outline they then go on to offer of MRTA is typically somewhat murky. For some, Moore should be read as an advocate of the theory of appearing, associated with Dawes Hicks's criticisms of sense-data.[5] On the other hand, in a

[3] See Baldwin (1990: 238, 240, 243–4). Contrast Robinson (1994: 37–40) who presents a Moore who is all along committed to the traditional sense-datum view but cannot see how to refute the 'seems' analysis. Snowdon (2007), on the other hand, avoids attributing to Moore a preferred side in his discussion of 'Some Judgments'.

[4] In addition to 'Some Judgments' and 'A Defence', consider Moore's contribution to a symposium discussing Broad's views of perception in 1926, 'The Nature of Sensible Appearances' (Moore 1926). Moore reiterates here again that we cannot be certain what is the correct view, but indicates that he finds probability in favour of the traditional view that Broad is inclined to, for which Broad's label is 'the sensum theory'.

[5] The assimilation of Moore to Dawes Hicks here is originally proposed by Broad, see above cited page from *Scientific Thought* (1923). Chisholm (1950) also identifies what Broad discusses under the heading 'Multiple Relation Theory of Appearing', as what he labels 'the theory of appearing' and otherwise associates with Dawes Hicks and other critics of sense-datum theories. Baldwin suggests that Moore has

context where some claim that merely to recognize a significant contrast between appearance and reality is to commit to the presence of intentional contents in experience, one might try to interpret Moore as offering an early sketch of a representational or intentional theory of perception.[6]

If we leave our current preconceptions to one side, and look instead at the bundle of commitments Moore carries round with him during this period, we can see his concern with the contrast between appearance and reality in a different light. The concern is not quite the same as that which obsesses many proponents of intentionalism: the need to give a general explanation of how things can appear a certain way while failing to be so. Rather, we'll see, one makes better sense of Moore's stance when one considers it in terms of what one can know about things considered independently of one's experience. For Moore, I'll suggest, the key contrast is between two modes of uniting terms in a proposition: treating *seeming* as a mode of copulation and one which contrasts with *being* allows Moore to acknowledge the possibility that an object of awareness might be united with blue only relative to my current experience. It is Moore's scrupulous concern with what we can know simply on the basis of our experience, together with his commitment to thinking of sensing as a form of knowing which generates the dilemma. Or so I will argue below.

This offers us a solution to our dual puzzles about the vagaries of early analytic philosophy: what did Moore's change of heart consist in in 1918, and how should we make sense of his recantation in 1953? But the ultimate terms of this debate ought to have a wider echo. Moore's principal focus in all of these debates is what he can know about seeing just from reflection on his own case, when he stares at the inkstand, or his hand, or a tree in mid-distance. Moore wants to spell out the nature of sensory experience through relying to a greater or lesser extent on introspective reflection. The resurgence of interest in debates about sense perception and phenomenal consciousness has brought with it a concern with introspective knowledge of our experience no less intense than Moore's. Lessons from Moore are lessons for this enterprise more generally. Moreover, Moore's theories raise questions both about how to understand experience as being intentional and what it might be for experience to be subjective or objective in character.

taken over Dawes Hicks's analysis of perception, in his discussion of 'Some Judgments'. Langsam (1997) refers us back to Moore, as well as Chisholm in his defence of the theory of appearing.

[6] Note that the theory of appearing is commonly identified as an alternative to representational or intentional theories, however. Jackson (1977) discusses the multiple relation theory of appearing (distinguishing between Broad's account and Chisholm's) as a competitor to a sense-datum theory, but does not identify it as a form of representationalism.

Langsam introduces the theory of appearing as a way of trying to block the argument against direct realism. Alston (1999) takes the theory of appearing to be an alternative to the representational theory of mind. Byrne (2009) treats both as offering a theory which is intended as a rival to intentionalism. Byrne concludes (appealing to concerns Broad expressed many decades before) that the theory will either be inadequate or a simply an alternative formulation of intentionalism.

In the first section of the chapter, I lay out a little more the context and argument of 'Some Judgments of Perception', how it first leads up to Moore's dilemma. The second section raises three interpretative puzzles about the way Moore introduces the dilemma. The most common readings of that dilemma to be found in the small literature on Moore and sense-data, that Moore is inclined towards endorsing some form of the theory of appearing, is tackled in the third section. In the fourth, I explore the extent to which Moore can be understood as offering a form of intentionalism about perception. Although there is some merit in this reading and it avoids some of the problems associated with the theory of appearing, I argue in the fifth section that we do better to place this discussion in a wider context of Moore's commitments concerning on the one hand the nature of sensory awareness, and on the other the nature of universals and predication. This offers an understanding of the paper which avoids the problems of the standard reading and also makes sense in part of his later rejection of the position. I explain in the sixth section why this ultimately tells against treating Moore as offering a form of the intentional theory, and in the concluding section I draw connections between Moore's discussion and some more recent debates about the objectivity of sense experience.

1. Moore's focal concerns in 'Some Judgments of Perception' are on what are now often called perceptual demonstrative judgements, or thoughts. He begins with some examples of sentences which can be used to express such judgements, 'That is an inkstand', 'That is a tablecloth', 'This is a finger', 'This is a coin'. But the lexical form does not on its own indicate the kind of judgement had in mind. As Moore makes clear, we should narrow our concern to those judgements that are judgements about what one currently sees or feels, and 'based upon' something which one perceives about the object in question. But he notes that these conditions alone will not single out narrowly the class of judgements on which he intends to focus.

Clearly demonstrative expressions such as 'this' and 'that' used either on their own or as part of a complex phrase, 'this overbearing supreme court justice', 'that ski slope', have both a deictic and an anaphoric use, as do most pronouns and indexical expressions. Why is Moore unsatisfied with the restriction to uses prompted and based upon what one currently sees? He doesn't offer any further elaboration, but one possible thought is that one's judgement may be prompted by what one sees, but nonetheless not be solely grounded in one's perceptual experience. For example, Moore himself takes judgements such as 'that clock has stopped' to be more complex than a judgement of perception. That is, he accepts that one makes the judgement because it has been prompted by perception, but thinks we should understand it as a complex judgement which contains a judgement of perception as a proper part, namely that which we might express with the sentence, 'that is a clock'.

In fact all of Moore's examples of judgements of perception are identification judgements: containing a bare demonstrative, the copula, and then an indefinite noun phrase; 'that is a clock', 'that is an inkstand', 'this is a finger', and so on.[7] In taking such examples as instances of judgements of perception, Moore is already putting himself at odds with Russell's discussion of these matters: in *The Problems of Philosophy*, Russell uses the label of 'judgement of perception' for judgements which are strictly about sense-data: 'there is such and such a patch of red' for a simple such judgement or 'that patch of red is round' and 'this is to the right of that' all made about the current sense-datum or sense-data seen, and the sensible qualities or relations among them apprehended (1912: 114).

One element of this implicit disagreement between them is Moore's attraction to a kind of common sense realism. This stance is further elaborated in 'A Defence of Common Sense' and 'Proof of an External World' (Moore 1925 and 1939), and somewhat later in the paper 'Certainty' (Moore 1959). He is at pains to point out that it is natural to suppose such judgements as he is concerned with involve a commitment to realism, the existence of ordinary objects in a world independent of us. This realism is to be contrasted with the idea that the world might be no more than the permanent possibility of sensations. And it leads Moore to draw a contrast between what our ordinary commitments are, and what the correct philosophical analysis of them should be. While common-sense commitment to ordinary objects should remain a fixed point across philosophical theories, theories may nonetheless disagree about what the correct logical analysis of these judgements may amount to.

Moore carefully distinguishes between seeing an object and being in a position to make one of these identificatory judgements about it: one may see too little of an object to be in a position to single it out, he suggests. At the same time, Moore is certain that when it comes to opaque, medium-sized, visible objects such as inkstands, coins, or hands, one can be said strictly speaking to see at best only the facing surface of the object and not the object itself. Given this, Moore takes there to be a certain indirection in judgements of perception, such that, although their topic is some suitable environmental object, one makes a judgement about the environmental object through singling out something distinct from it: there is a *this* or a *that* to which the object in question is related such that we should understand the form of these identificatory judgements along these lines:

(1) This is an inkstand

(1A) $\exists x \forall y\, [[R\,(\textit{this}, \mathrm{y}) \leftrightarrow \mathrm{y} = \mathrm{x}] \wedge \mathrm{x} \text{ is an inkstand}]$.

The *this* in question will be what Moore defined as a 'sense-datum', whatever it is that is given in one's current sensory awareness, and which one has singled out in making the identificatory judgement. Variously this will be what one strictly speaking sees, or

[7] We might be tempted to extend the class to include such examples as, 'That is John', 'This must be the book John was talking about', involving proper names or definite descriptions.

the ultimate object of sight, or the ultimate object of judgement. For Moore, the fundamental question about such judgements of perception, the question of their philosophical analysis, turns on specifying what the relevant relation *R* is, and concurrent with that determining the nature of the *this* or *that* which is to be *R*-related to the ordinary object of perception: in the case of vision, is it a part of the surface of the object, or is it something wholly distinct from the object, but somehow perceptually standing in for it? (Note that Moore's discussion makes clear that the identified topic of the judgement is uniquely related to the ultimate object of perception, as this logical form indicates. If one adopts with Frank Jackson a recursive definition of what it is to be the immediate or direct object of perception, then there will be no guarantee of uniqueness here (suppose TSA correct, both the surface of the hand and the hand itself might count as *R*-related to the sense-datum). That suggests Moore would need to consider a sequence of relations R_1, $R_2 \ldots R_n$ in which indirect objects of perception are related to the ultimate object, rather than their ancestral *R*.) This provides the context in which Moore first goes on to discuss the argument from illusion and then introduce his new alternative to it.

Moore offers no explicit argument or rationale for the claim that we see hands only by seeing their surfaces. And Moore's contention here has led to some debate. Perhaps the deepest and most intriguing commentary on this is Thompson Clarke's 'Seeing Surfaces and Physical Objects'.[8] But because our concern is with the argument from illusion, and so mainly with aspects of predication, I'll refrain from any comment on this first move in Moore's paper; although it involves many interesting features, they can for the most part be set aside for the interpretative concerns we have here. It is interesting to note, though, that the kinds of identificatory judgements that Moore singles out do seem to combine the introduction of some environmental object with a certain indirection. This is highlighted (without reference to Moore) in a recent paper by Friederike Moltmann who notes the singular status of the bare demonstrative in such judgements. It is perfectly proper to say, 'That's John', on hearing the front door open, or 'This is a beautiful woman', pointing to the cover of this week's *Elle*. In contrast one cannot say, 'Mary is going to the opera with that', pointing to John (rather than 'Mary is going to the opera with that man') or 'Esther used to live with this' (rather than 'Esther used to live with this woman').[9] Moltmann suggests that we should understand the bare demonstrative as singling out a trope, where the identified person or perceptual object is intimately related to that demonstratum. Even if one does not accept Moore's general approach to perception, then, there may be something about the judgements he happened upon which invites us to think of them as involving indirection.

If we leave these questions aside, Moore offers us the following framework for his debate: in all cases of visual or tactual awareness, there is some object which is strictly

[8] In addition to Thompson Clarke (1965) see Chisholm (1957: 156), where he discusses Moore's first introduction of this idea in *Some Main Problems of Philosophy*.

[9] Moltmann (2013).

seen or felt and is the *ultimate object* of judgement. In the case of vision this object is never to be identified with an opaque, three-dimensional solid, but only ever at best a proper part of such an object: its facing surface. So it is to be taken as certain that judgements of perception concern ordinary environmental objects, but that this topic of concern is introduced somewhat indirectly or through deference via the ultimate object of judgement. A full discussion of the nature of such judgements therefore needs to settle what the ultimate objects are, and together with that what the relation *R* might be that ultimate objects stand in to those things that we are certain the judgements concern, such as inkstands, fingers, or trees.

Moore starts out with the presumption that the ultimate object of judgements of perception is a part of the surface of the inkstand or tree, and hence that the relevant relation *R* should be thought of as a part–whole relation (though Moore does not think that any part–whole relation will lead to the transmission of judgement—recall that Moore takes some seeings of parts to be too small to count as seeing the whole; the availability of the judgement of perception and our counting as seeing the object go hand in hand for him). But at this point Moore introduces a form of the argument from illusion as the most serious consideration against this presumption.

Moore is clearly at some pains to state this argument as explicitly and carefully as he can. Again we have here a contrast with the cavalier way in which Russell first formulates matters in *The Problems of Philosophy*. That said, as careful as Moore intends to be, the argument is less perspicuous than one might hope. Moore is focused on the questions when can we identify things in perception which have been perceived on different occasions, and when can we tell them apart. As he puts it, he is concerned with perceptible difference. So he notes that commonly we do keep track of objects and judge that one thing is identical with that which has been perceived before. Moreover, such an identification is consistent with acknowledging change in the object—his examples concern a child's balloon altering in size as it is blown up, and a rubber doll changing in shape as it is stretched between one's fingers. But this is to build up to a case in which he wishes to suggest that we can judge of perceptible difference even though we have perceived no change in an object.

Moore offers familiar examples of conflicting appearances: one sees a tree in the near distance and then views the tree again much further off; one sees a coin face on, and then looks again at an oblique angle to it; one views the surface of a wall without and then with blue-tinted spectacles; I now feel a coin through touch and without looking, whereas earlier I looked and did not touch. And Moore takes the following to be true, or seemingly to be true:

> It seems, therefore, to be absolutely impossible that the surface seen at the later time should be identical with the object presented then, and the surface seen at the earlier identical with the object presented then, for the simple reason that, whereas with regard to the later seen surface I am not prepared to judge that it is in any way perceptibly different from that seen earlier, it seems that with regard to the later sense-datum I cannot fail to judge that it is perceptibly different from the earlier one: the fact that they are perceptibly different simply stares me in the face. (Moore 1918: 22)

The form of argument here is somewhat complicated to unpack because Moore's discussion moves back and forth between questions of numerical identity and questions of qualitative difference. In the circumstance, the subject is supposed to know, though not, or not solely, on the basis of perception, that the facing surface of the tree at time t_1 is identical with the facing surface of the tree at time t_0. Two things which are identical are not different from each other. But, of course, in a circumstance of change, the surface as it is at t_1 might differ from the surface at t_0 without failing to be identical, just through having changed: being qualitatively different over time without being numerically different. In the circumstances with which we are concerned, though, we have both identity of the surfaces, and knowledge that there has been no change in them. Nonetheless, Moore emphasizes that with respect to the sense-data seen at t_0 and t_1 the fact of variation stares one in the face. Here the relevant perceived difference is not, initially at least, one of non-identity, but difference in quality.

Moreover, the terms that Moore uses might mislead one into thinking that the subject's concern is solely with the question whether there are differences, without necessarily focusing on the specific differences. Compare this to the kind of competition once popular in certain newspapers, 'Spot the Difference'. Starting out on this nugatory exercise confronting two very similar photographs, one might notice that there is something different about the left image with respect to the right, but as yet have no sense of what that difference is. This would be a case of perceiving difference, but nothing more than difference. Given the context of his discussion, it should be clear that Moore does not have this merely general knowledge in mind. Taking the lead from his use of the adverb 'perceptibly', we might rather focus on the question what one can know on the basis of vision in this situation. We might then represent Moore's claim as that there is some way the later presentation is of which one knows that it differs from the earlier presentation in that respect. Using '*e*' as a term for the object present at t_0 and '*l*' the term for the object present at t_1, Moore's claim is that in respect of some quality or other, one knows that *e* has it, and *l* lacks it; or *vice versa*; and we might symbolize it so:

(2) $\exists F \exists G\, [K\, [F(e) \wedge \neg F(l)] \vee K[\neg G(e) \wedge G(l)]]$.

That gets us to the starting point of Moore's argument, but it still doesn't help us get to his intended conclusion. At this stage of the argument, Moore is attempting to offer a compelling argument for TSD's commitment that we are always aware of non-physical sense-data, and hence that *neither* sense-datum is identical with the surface of the tree. But it is really unclear how he can get there just on the basis of (2). One route might go as follows. *Ex hypothesi* the surface has not changed between t_0 and t_1, so consider the supposition that the surface is identical with *e*. Either the surface is *F* at t_0 in which case, since it has not changed, it is also *F* at t_1, and so we conclude that the surface is not identical with *l*; or the surface is not *G* at t_0, but then, since it has not changed, it is also not *G* at t_1 and hence, again, given our supposition, is not identical with *l*. Now run the reverse supposition that the surface is identical with *l*, by parallel reasoning we get the conditional conclusion that it is not identical with *e*. Discharging our assumptions gets us to the conclusion that the surface is either not identical with *e* or it is not identical with *l*. So, for at least one of the presentations, the 'ultimate object of perception' is not identical with the surface. This gets us the ontologically inflationary conclusion that there must be non-physical objects of awareness in addition to the surfaces of objects, but it doesn't get us the negative conclusion that in our example the surface of an object is *never* the object of awareness. To get to the stronger conclusion, Moore requires the non-identity for both occasions.[10] And he doesn't make explicit any reasons to make that further move.[11]

Nevertheless, even if one cannot reconstruct the argument validly to get to the conclusion that one never directly or strictly sees the surface of any opaque object—that surfaces are never the ultimate objects of sight—that is the conclusion that Moore takes the argument to set out to show. And in the remainder of his discussion in this paper, and in his later discussions, the assumption is made that TSD would be the correct position to endorse but for the assumption that he now questions. This does not flow from the *aporia* that we have just indicated, but rather engages with questions about the move from 'seems' to 'is', and it is this which first offers the dilemma.

So we have now surveyed the context in 'Some Judgments' in which Moore first introduces MRTA and the dilemma. Having set up TSD, and offered an argument in its favour, he suggests the argument rests on an assumption which can be rejected and an alternative theory offered in its place. Although many commentators have taken it to be obvious what assumption is in play and what alternative is on offer, as we'll see below, this turns out to be more elusive than one might have supposed.

2. Moore's discussion of perceptual identification judgements, and his survey of the argument from illusion, have set the context in which he presents the dilemma which forms the centrepiece of his presidential address. Having presented the argument for TSD in as strong a form as he can (and leaving our worries to one side), Moore confesses that while he finds this an argument with 'considerable force', it is

[10] Sticking closer to the terms in the text, one might rather try to reconstruct the argument in terms of reasoning about pairs: on the one hand we have the pair of the sense-data, [*e*, *l*], and on the other the pair of the surface of the tree at t_0 and the surface of the tree at t_1, [s_0, s_1]. The former pair exhibits difference, the latter pair does not—'difference' can be interpreted either in terms of the pair instantiating the relation of non-identity or in terms of variation in quality between the pair. So there is a property which the former pair exhibits lacked by the second. Hence the pairs are non-identical. But again, this won't get us further than the non-identity of the surface with one of *e* and *l*, for it is surely sufficient for pairs to be non-identical that one member of a pair be non-identical with some member of the other.

[11] A familiar move made by those tempted by TSD is to appeal to an indistinguishability thesis at this point, particularly in the context of a spectrum argument. (See, for example, Ayer 1940, Foster 1985, and Robinson 1994); a similar such argument, though not for sense-data, is surprisingly to be found in Johnston (2006). Typically, proponents of such arguments do not take them to be demonstrative—they are intended, at best, to offer a plausibility ground for the general conclusion. This clearly would not suit Moore's purpose at this stage, since he is concerned to show that modulo the assumption disputed by MRTA, TSD would be the philosophical theory of which we could be certain.

nonetheless not conclusive. According to Moore, the argument rests on an assumption which, however plausible, can be challenged, and once challenged, an alternative option opens up:

> it rests on an assumption, which, though it seems to me to have great force, does not seem to me to be quite certain. The assumption I mean is the assumption that, in such cases as those I have spoken of, the later presented object really is perceptibly different from the earlier. This assumption has, if I am not mistaken, seemed to many philosophers to be unquestionable; and I own that it used to be so with me... What now seems to me to be possible is that the sense-datum which corresponds to a tree, which I am seeing, when I am a mile off, may not really be perceived to *be* smaller than the one, which corresponds to the same tree, when I see it from a distance of only a hundred yards, but that it is only perceived to *seem* smaller; that the sense-datum which corresponded to the penny, when I was straight in front of it, but is only perceived to *seem* different—that all that is perceived is that the one *seems* elliptical and the other circular... the kind of experience which I have expressed by saying one *seems* different from the other... involves an ultimate, not further analysable, kind of psychological relation, not to be identified either with that involved in being "perceived" to be so and so, or with that involved in being "judged" to be so and so; since a presented object might in this sense *seem* to be elliptical, *seem* to be blue etc., when it is neither perceived to be so, nor judged to be so.
>
> (Moore 1918: 23–4)

I think one's first impression on reading this passage is that it is fairly clear what Moore is concerned with: the gap between things *seeming* a certain way, and their *being* that way. The problem with the traditional sense-datum theory is just that it thinks that it can close that gap. If we question that assumption, then we end up with a view on which we recognize visual experience as a matter of pure seeming. And commentators have typically understood Moore in just this way, ascribing to him a provisional rejection of the sense-datum theory together with an endorsement of some alternative which emphasizes appearances over private objects.

But Moore is no clearer here, despite his best intentions, than in his initial discussion of the argument from illusion. There are a number of problems. First, the assumption Moore ascribes to TSD does indeed seem to be the principal premiss of the argument he has been discussing over the few pages before. To that extent, at least, he does not change the subject. But precisely because it is the key premiss of the argument, it should leave us puzzled what position we are in once the assumption is questioned. For TSD used just this description of the situation to fix for us the particular case we are to be considering. If the assumption is false, then having rejected the TSD description of the case, we have as yet offered nothing in its place which provides common ground among the parties.

This issue ought to be particularly pressing for Moore, given that his conclusion is supposed to be that we have to remain strictly undecided between TSD and MRTA, both of which remain possibly correct as accounts of sense experience. What characterization can we offer of our evidential position in being undecided between the two? The disjunction of the assumption and its negation will simply give us a tautology, and so fail to indicate anything specific about the situation one is in when regarding the tree, and then, along with Moore, taking five steps back.

The most obvious way to address this concern is to appeal to something we can do in any situation in which our perceptually prompted judgements are challenged. If, looking across the lawn I surmise, 'That is a redwood', and you question the propriety of my opinion, for example by questioning whether there are any redwoods in this part of California, I can retreat to the judgement, 'Well, it looks like a redwood'. And, more generally, we can offer a judgement about how things seem, or appear, or that things are just as if, and then go on to give the description we were originally inclined to offer. Whatever the correct analysis of judgements of seeming or appearing turns out to be, pragmatically they weaken one's conversational commitments to truth of a perceptually based description and even one's commitment to the existence of what otherwise one would be talking about. Moreover, such judgements seem expressive of aspects of our sensory or perceptual reaction to the world. And, at the limit, may be taken as no more than a report of such a sensory state. And typically philosophical discussions of sense perception liberally use such sentences as 'It seems/appears/looks to Moore as if...' as reports of a perceptual state.

Typically, such revision and withdrawal occurs in relation to discussion of some environmental feature and one's perception of that. But we might extend the manoeuvre so as to employ it in debate with the sense-datum theorist, and the description they wish to give of the situation. After all, the proponent of TSD supposes that his audience finds intelligible the description of the course of experience in which one first stands close to the tree trunk, and then carefully stepping backwards from it, considers how the tree is now. The least committal description here presumably would be in terms of how things seem or look at the earlier time, and how they seem or look at the later time. So the description in terms of looking or seeming we might then take as a neutral description of the situation which both the proponent of TSD and his sceptical audience can agree on as fixing the subject matter of their disagreement. If we agree with Moore at the end that we are rationally unable to decide between theories, then we can stick with this subjective description of the situation.[12]

Describing matters in this way does not directly conflict with Moore's own explicit description of the situation. That we can retreat to a judgement about how things seem when our description of the world is challenged does not by itself show that we

[12] To be fair, one might well wish to reject even the description in terms of how things seem or look. After all, Moore seems insensitive to the facts of size and shape constancy in vision. As Reid (1997/1785) had already complained in relation to Hume (1975/1748), it is just not true that as you step back from the tree it seems to get smaller. One has the visual sense (and not just the background knowledge) that there is no alteration in size. While there is something about the visual experience which answers to the description seeming small, or seeming elliptical, there is equally an aspect which reflects the constancy. This indicates, yet again, how for all Moore's care, he barely advances the cause of offering a rigorous statement of the argument from illusion.

were relying on a judgement about how things seem all along. Just as a sceptical challenge about your current perceptual judgements is not enough to show that all such judgements rest on judgements about one's own perceptual experience, so too conceding the possibility that one can challenge the sense-datum theorist's description of the situation, does not commit one to supposing that the sense-datum theorist always argues first from a claim about the nature of sense experience.

But if we make explicit the dialectical position in this way, namely by retreating to a position in which we describe the situation just in terms of how things seem, then we face another interpretative puzzle. For now the description of the situation which is, strictly speaking, neutral between the sense-datum theorist and his opponent actually sounds a lot like the view that Moore ascribes to the opponent. For, in characterizing the common ground with the opposition, the sense-datum theorist points out that we agree that it seems as if the tree is smaller, or that the coin is elliptical. But this just sounds like the terms in which Moore goes on to characterize the opposing view, as opposed to what both sides can agree on.

So, what then is Moore's dilemma? Understood one way, it simply takes us back to the question whether the traditional sense-datum view is correct. Suppose we grant for some case that the sense-datum theorist's description of how things seem in that situation is correct. What, then, follows from this? The choice we face is that of either endorsing TSD, or refusing to. But that is not the only way of understanding Moore here, nor yet the most natural way of taking what he says after this and beyond. The alternative to the sense-datum theory does seem, in Moore's hands, itself to be some kind of theory, and not merely the philosophical Bartleby, refusing to join in the affirmations of the under-cautious sense-datum enthusiast. In that case we face the interpretative task of explaining what is added in Moore's discussion of seeming beyond the merely neutral starting point, and then raising the question what would warrant Moore in smuggling in the extra material in the first place.

3. In effect, Thomas Baldwin's account of the evolution of Moore's approach to perception treats Moore's dilemma as involving the first of these options: as sticking with the subjective judgement. He suggests that in allowing sense-data just to seem smaller or elliptical without being so, Moore is articulating a view of perception to be found in Dawes Hicks and others, 'the theory of appearing'. And Chisholm in his influential paper 'The Theory of Appearing' glosses the key move involved here as follows:

> One fundamental question, then, concerns the inference from statements such as *A* [There exists something which appears diamond-shaped], in the language of appearing, to statements such as S [There exists something which *is* diamond-shaped], in the sense-datum language. We may call this the *sense-datum inference*. And we may say that the *sense-datum theory* is the view which countenances this inference, whereas the *theory of appearing* is the view which does not.
>
> (Chisholm 1950 in Swartz 1965: 173)

There are two notable difficulties with this interpretation of Moore's discussion. The first concerns Moore's attitude to the objects of sensory awareness. Once we introduce the language of seeming or appearing, then we can talk about our sense experience without committing to anything being small or being elliptical. But likewise, it appears, we can avoid commitment even to the existence of something which appears small or elliptical. There is no reason why the bracketing device of indicating this was how things struck me perceptually should not go ahead of any of the statements one uses to characterize the situation, and just as one has avoided the need for the statements to be strictly true, so too one can avoid the commitment to the existence of those entities needed to make them true. As Chisholm summarizes the theory of appearing, it seeks to avoid the ontological inflation of objects of awareness. Yet Moore steadfastly insists that for all acts of sensory awareness, there must actually be some object of which one is aware. So if Moore in 1918 is recognizing the force of Dawes Hicks's position, then he is only dimly aware of its potential consequences. Note that this problematic aspect of his position is recognized by most commentators who see Moore as taking this path; clearly they do not see this as decisive ground against the interpretation.

The second concern connects with Moore's eventual repudiation of this option in 'Visual Sense-Data'. Moore's point at that stage revolves round after-images and other sensible objects which, he assumes, must be the way that they appear. This, he suggests, shows that MRTA as he introduced it in 'Some Judgments' is unworkable. Baldwin and Snowdon both think that Moore simply begs the question against his imagined opponent at this point. But that is to miss what is really puzzling in Moore's position. The fact that things seem a certain way is typically not inconsistent with them being so. The mistake in the sense-datum inference is to suppose that things must always be the way that they appear. Why should it be a problem for the rejection of this inference if sometimes the way things are is just the way that they appear?

Taking Moore to endorse the theory of appearing, at least as that is later understood by Chisholm and some recent writers, doesn't make enough sense of Moore's position. It doesn't explain how he can recognize the epistemic limits of our knowledge of seeming and yet insist that there always is an object of awareness; and it doesn't explain why he comes to think that supposing some objects must just be as they appear is inconsistent with the theory in the first place. Of course, Moore's thoughts some thirty-five years later may have been confused, so seeking consistency across the two papers may not be a requirement of an adequate interpretation. Nonetheless, this puzzle does offer some evidence that Moore finds more content in the alternative approach than Chisholm's gloss on the theory of appearing provides. How then might we interpret it, and how might that help with the puzzle?

4. Before offering an account which meets these desiderata, I want first to turn to the second interpretative strategy: making sense of MRTA as offering a positive account

of the perceptual situation in terms of seeming. What could such an account amount to? One potentially attractive option here is to see Moore as offering an intentional theory of sense experience, one that treats our sensory states as possessing a representational content. Take our neutral description of the visual experience, say of the back of Moore's hand. Moore might report this as 'it seems to me as if there is a pinkish expanse with five segments extended from it'. According to TSD, this report is made true by the existence of an object which actually is pinkish, and it is this object's being pinkish which determines the correctness of Moore's subjective report. By contrast, an intentional theory of sense experience, one which supposes that the experience possesses a representational content, will insist that the subjective report is made true by the representational properties of the sense experience: it is the hand's being represented by the experience to be pinkish, or one's experientially taking the hand to be pinkish which make it correct for Moore to report his experience in the way he does. And in that case, the experience possessing such a content does not entail that the hand, or anything else, actually is pinkish.

Now one line of thought which recommends this interpretative strategy rests entirely on general considerations. Given the kind of first-personal enquiry Moore is engaged in in 'Some Judgments' and at the end of 'A Defence of Common Sense', it is reasonable to interpret his concerns as being about the nature of sense experience and TSD and MRTA as presenting contrasting accounts of this. Recent discussions of the grounds for endorsing intentional or representational theories of perception have suggested that once we recognize the possibility that things can appear in ways that they are not, we thereby have to recognize the role of intentional content in sense experience. Moore's challenge to TSD is naturally read, on this line of thought, as just his recognition of the intentionality of visual awareness.[13]

Consider Moore's inspecting his hand in the context of a suitable visual illusion. Perhaps the lighting has been altered or Moore has been drugged, and now that he stares intently at the back of his hand, it seems to him as if there is a somewhat greenish expanse before him, even though his hand has not altered in colour at all. On the sense-datum interpretation of this situation, there is actually something green which Moore is aware of, and since the surface of his hand is not green, we can conclude that the ultimate object of awareness is something other than the surface, albeit something in virtue of which he counts as seeing the hand. If we reject TSD, and suppose that the object merely seems green without being green (as in Moore's initial characterization of MRTA), how else might we describe the situation? Well Moore is presented with the sensible quality greenness, so the colour green is 'before his mind'. But since nothing is green in the situation, neither his hand nor any putative non-physical sense-datum, this must also be a case of the absence of green. How can we make sense of the seemingly contradictory state of affairs: of green as

[13] See, for example, Siegel (2010) and Byrne (2009).

both 'present' and 'absent'? A long line of thought takes this combination not to be a contradiction but simply the mark of the intentional. To think of the experience, with respect to greenness, as an instance of presence in absence, is to think of experience as an intentional phenomenon. The experience simply exemplifies the formal conditions of intentionality: the mind is directed on some suitable intentional object, some specific shade of green, without there being any actual material object which coincides with this. Our recognition that experience can present qualities without these being instantiated by any object of awareness is a recognition that sense experience is thereby intentional in nature.

If we leave these general considerations about appearance and reality, presence and absence, to one side, there is still further evidence in favour of this line of interpretation. For Moore's own texts offer support for an intentionalist interpretation. The further things Moore says about MRTA in 'Some Judgments' are strongly reminiscent of his earlier discussion of belief and judgement in *Some Main Problems of Philosophy*. There Moore rejects the idea that belief and judgement are directed on a distinctive kind of entity, namely propositions. And Russell, in joining Moore in this negative verdict, sought to provide a contextual elimination of propositions as entities, and instead to treat the relation of judging as a 'multi-grade' relation which relates the subject who makes the judgement with a variable number of other entities which together comprise the terms of the judgement together with an ordering. On this view, to judge that this hand is green is to stand in the judging relation to: (i) this hand; and (ii) the property of being green. The distinctive unity that propositions manifest which contrasts with mere lists is here explained in terms of distinctive relation of judging which binds terms together in a manner that can correspond to facts.

Now the passage makes clear that Moore rejects any reduction of seeing, or any other sensory state, to judging. He offers the familiar observation that one may distrust one's senses, and so see things a certain way but not judge them to be that way. But that does not rule out interpreting Moore here as exploiting an analogy with what the judging relation does. Just as the act of judging should be thought of as bringing together terms so that subjects may judge the world to be now this way and now that, so too seeming may be thought to bring together terms, so that sensory episodes can present to the subject ways the world may be judged to be. We might, then, think of each visual experience as determined by a suitable sensory proposition which exhibits the object of sensory awareness and predicates of it the sensible qualities it seems to have. Moore eliminates the proposition as an entity in favour of the multi-grade relation of seeming between perceiver and terms, but this complex will occupy perfectly the functional role of propositions and propositional attitudes. Hence, the account of seeming would appear to do no other than treat sensory experience as a kind of propositional attitude. To the extent that we think of propositional attitudes such as belief, or mental acts such as judgement, as paradigms of intentionality, then, that will reinforce the impression that Moore is offering here an equivalent intentional or representational gloss on acts of sensory awareness.

Note that it in no way undermines this interpretation to point out that Moore remains committed to the actual existence of objects of awareness. It is true that the majority of writers who seek to establish the intentionality of sensory experience do so in order to finesse away the need for the actual or material existence of objects of awareness: Anscombe, for example, talks of the intentionality of sensation in order to contrast 'intentional objects' of sensation, which are not a kind of entity according to her, with material objects of sensation.[14] It is one thing to exploit aspects of intentionality in seeking to explain away apparent commitment to entities, and another to make a criterion of intentionality the avoidance of any such commitment. Russell's and Moore's conception of propositions and then judgements make such entities and such acts dependent on the terms of the proposition in question: if some entity really is the subject of one's judgement (and not merely the witness to the truth of some quantified proposition), then one can judge in that manner only given the existence of that entity. By parity, even if Moore insists that the content of perceptual states is available only given the existence of the object of awareness, that still leaves open the thought that these states should be thought of as representing the objects to be some way, given that the tree's seeming small is consistent with it either being small or not.

So there is quite a compelling case to be made for attributing to Moore a nascent form of the intentional theory of perception, when he offers MRTA as one half of his dilemma. And this better fits what he has to say than assimilating him too closely to Dawes Hicks, or what Chisholm and others go on to make of the theory of appearing, since it is entirely consistent with his commitment (however puzzling we may find it) to the actual existence of objects of awareness. Be that as it may, the intentional gloss on Moore fares no better than the theory of appearing interpretation in making sense of Moore's final rejection of MRTA. Why should the assumption that after-images exist and really are coloured or shaped pose a fatal problem for MRTA?

On an intentional construal of sense experience, we take our visual states to represent the objects of awareness to be some way. In Moore's version of this, this is for us to stand in the relation of seeming both to the object of awareness, in this case an after-image, and some sensible quality, bluish-white or circularity. The intentionalist insists that one's experience can present an entity as being blue or circular without it having to be the case that the object is either blue or circular. Now clearly the existence of round, blue after-images would be quite consistent with this constraint. That experience admits of the possibility that objects be presented as ways they are not is not equivalent to saying that no experience can present things as they are. Why shouldn't our after-image experiences be guaranteed always to be veridical?[15]

[14] Anscombe (1965).

[15] Note that in stressing just this point, in one of his discussions of intentionalism, Byrne argues that we should think of sense-datum theories as consistent with intentional accounts, see Byrne (2001).

So neither the interpretation of Moore which emphasizes appearances without ontological extravagance nor that interpretation which sees him recognizing the appeal of the intentionality of sensation can really make sense of why Moore's obsession with after-images leads him back to the traditional sense-datum account. This might be taken just to show that despite their striving for clarity, early twentieth-century theories of perception and knowledge are much less coherent than we might wish. Such a conclusion is too pessimistic, though. Once we leave aside our current preoccupations with the nature of perception, we can make better sense of the movement in Moore's thought. While Moore isn't very explicit in 'Visual Sense-Data', I think we can reconstruct the line of reasoning which rules out MRTA. Once we do so, however, we'll see that the way Moore construes seeming is inconsistent with the way of thinking of experience common among many proponents of intentionalism.

5. The key issue for Moore, I suggest, concerns our sensory knowledge of after-images. That is, the key shift in his opinions in last writings is that in 'Visual Sense-Data' he accepts not only that after-images have certain sensible qualities, but that we are aware of the sensible qualities of after-images through the sense experiences we have of them.

To see the significance of this concession, we need to look at the original motivation for MRTA in a different light. We have to start back well before 'Some Judgments', with one of the fundamental threads that runs through Moore's discussions of sensory awareness, at least from 'Refutation of Idealism' (Moore 1903). Moore insists that sensory awareness is a mode of knowledge, and that knowledge must always be a relation to something entirely independent of that knowledge, and hence that idealism is false. In effect, for Moore, the refutation consists in drawing his opponent's attention to the example of sensory awareness, and then drawing from that example the general morals he wishes us to learn: that sensing adds nothing to its objects, and that its objects exist and have the qualities they do independently of that sensing.

Note that Moore is well aware that it is more common to think of acts of sensation as being subjective, and as having a content which is internal to the act of awareness, and so internal to the mind. But he rejects that view of experience as mistaken, and continues to insist that we need to think of sensory awareness as a form of knowledge. (Critics, in turn, complain that since sensation so obviously is subjective, it is a mistake to assimilate sensory awareness to knowledge—this is what H. A. Prichard (1938) called 'the sense-datum fallacy'.) So even if the argument from illusion succeeds in showing that we are never aware of environmental objects such as the surfaces of trees or hands, it does not lead us to the point of positing mental objects, or entities which exist within our minds or experiences. For Moore and Russell (prior to his flirtation with neutral monism), sense-data are non-environmental, and non-physical, but not mental.

This is not to say that Moore or Russell deny that sense-data are private to each perceiver: they are happy to accept that whichever sense-data I come to be aware of when I step back from the tree, these are entirely disjoint from the sense-data that you enjoy. Nor is there any commitment to the persistence of these entities across occasions of sense experience. Moore does not believe that pains, for example, exist waiting for us to discover them, even though he would insist that in pain experience we are aware of a sense-datum which exists independently of that awareness. Both Moore and Russell concede that sense-data may be dependent for their existence and for their character on the operation of each subject's nervous system. This concession is nonetheless entirely consistent with the hypothesis that the entities exist independently of the act of sensing, even if their existence is maintained by a causal process which coincides with that awareness.[16]

In the context of this conception of experience, the traditional sense-datum theory brings with it a certain commitment concerning the information that sense experience provides us with. In having the visual experience of the sense-datum *R*-related to the surface of the tree, the subject is acquainted with the sense-datum and thereby knows it to be brown or small, or whichever sensible qualities characterize the visual experience in relation to this sense-datum. What one knows, in knowing 'This is brown' or 'This is small', is that the object in question is that way independent of one's current act of sensing. Of course, if we acknowledge the privacy of these objects, and concede that their existence is dependent on suitable activity of the nervous system, then the item of knowledge is limited in scope to the interval during which one has the awareness. We cannot assume that the datum in question is going to carry on existing with that same character beyond our momentary awareness. But that does not undermine the claim that the object of knowledge is utterly objective: what we know, given their utter independence of our awareness, is that either they remain so or there is some genuine change in the world.

Against this background consider the question how sense experience can really provide us with evidence of a world independent of it, and hence be properly objective. This concern is often associated with Hume and Kant, though the most

[16] Baldwin suggests that Moore is not unwavering in this commitment, since in the discussion of sense-data in *Some Main Problems of Philosophy* he concedes that the accepted view that sense-data are dependent and private is probably correct (see Baldwin 1990: 40–3). But this, I think, is not decisive. In that discussion, Moore is eager to emphasize that such dependence is not equivalent to being 'in the mind' or having the kind of status that our own thoughts or acts of awareness do. We might then think that the key change between 1910–11 and 1914 is the way in which Moore comes to characterize the dependence he does not wish to question: in 1914, he emphasizes that this need be no more than dependence on our nervous system, a way of putting things Russell adopts in 1912, but that this is not sufficient to show that there is any psychological dependence, i.e. that awareness itself has any object which is dependent on it. Likewise, while in recent discussion it is natural to associate the privacy of sense-data with their mind-dependence (for on the assumption that an object's existence is constituted by one's awareness of it is a straightforward explanation of why only one person could be aware of it), in much of the early twentieth-century discussion, privacy is separated from and treated as a further matter on top of the question whether objects are mind-dependent.

developed discussion of these issues is to be found in P. F. Strawson and his students.[17] Ironically, Strawson targets 'the earlier sense-datum theorists' (1966: 99), as people who think of sense experience as purely subjective in its import: presenting simple sensible qualities whose instantiation could be exhausted in the occurrence of experience itself.[18] Were such sense experience really possible, Strawson hypothesizes, then the judgements that such experience would warrant could concern no state of affairs beyond the occasion of the experience itself. Strawson's concern at this point is with the idea that unless experience can provide grounds for self-ascription of such experiences by the subject, then such experience cannot be conscious. Now experience, according to Strawson, can ground such judgements only if it provides the materials for drawing the distinction between how things seem to the subject and how they are. In turn, for it to do that, experience needs an objective import which takes us beyond what is solely given in an experience by itself. The problem with the sense-datum theory as conceived by Strawson, then, is that its conception of experience fails to have any such objective import: the information that a subject can derive from the experience does not suffice to distinguish between the experience itself and the object of that experience. At various points, Strawson suggests that the problem can be addressed if we recognize that our experience presents objects as located in a space independent of us: we draw the contrast between objects of experience and experience by recognizing the possibility that an object may be present but unperceived because we are not in a suitable relation to it to have an experience. Evans supplements Strawson's various discussions with the idea that our conception of body and shape play a distinctive role in this understanding of how the objects of experience can exist independently of our awareness of them.

The view that Strawson associated with the earlier sense-datum theorists looks very much like the kind of subjectivism which Moore repeatedly criticizes. Moore would agree with Strawson that subjective experience, were it to occur, could not issue in knowledge. But Moore does not explicitly address the kind of general concern that Strawson raises: how could sense experience, just in presenting us with objects and sensible qualities, provide us with information about a world which exists independently of that presentation? Indeed, where Strawson and Evans seem to assume that sense experience would be subjective in character were it to lack the kind of spatial and causal content they insist on, Moore instead seems to suppose that our recognition that sensory awareness is knowledge is sufficient ground to establish the objectivity of sensory awareness.

Nonetheless, I suggest, Moore's introduction of MRTA involves some recognition of these issues, albeit put in rather different terms from those that Strawson and Evans use many years later. For, the best way to understand Moore at this point is to

[17] See, particularly, Strawson (1966: 89–112); but also Strawson (1959: Ch. 2). For further discussion of these concerns, see also Evans (1980) and Cassam (1997).

[18] Strawson most likely has in mind Ayer as his target; compare his explicit discussion of Ayer and sense-datum language in Strawson (1979).

see him as acknowledging the force of the question whether we should simply assume that experience can provide us with information that goes beyond the experiential situation itself. And in his reconstruction of the argument from illusion, the assumption that we know the objects of awareness in themselves plays a key role. So this offers us a slightly different understanding of the dilemma posed in 'Some Judgments'.

The argument to show that the object of awareness cannot be the surface of the tree assumes that the sensible quality, e.g. the size of the sense-datum, conflicts with the objective size of the surface of the tree. This would be the correct assumption if our sense experience reveals to us the way things are in themselves, independently of how we experience them. But there is an alternative understanding: that our sense experiences simply present objects united with sensible qualities relative to our sense experiences. So to propose that perception reveals only how an object *seems* and not how it *is* is to propose that sense experience only provides us with knowledge of objects relative to the occasion of our sense experience, and not independently of that.

In effect, Moore's version of MRTA provides for the same restriction on our knowledge of the world that would be a consequence of a pure subjectivist understanding of the contents of sensory consciousness, without thereby endorsing a subjectivist construal. In recent discussions of sense perception and the argument from illusion, the key lack of modesty is an ontological one: the sense-datum theorist seems to posit a whole new realm of objects for us to be related to in having experience. There is no evidence that Moore is ever worried by such profligacy. But there is another immodesty here: an epistemological one. TSD supposes that sensory acts themselves give us knowledge of how these sense-data are. MRTA claims instead that we only ever perceive how sense-data seem, and one cannot infer from this how they are. The key virtue of MRTA can then be seen as its being epistemologically more modest.[19]

Clearly there is more to be said about this way of understanding MRTA, and the bearing it has on the proper interpretation of Moore's original dilemma. But our urgent purpose is to make sense of Moore's ultimate repudiation of MRTA in 'Visual Sense-Data' and, more specifically, to make sense of why after-images should be thought such a problem for the view. Note from Strawson's perspective, after-images are not likely candidates for creating a problem about a view which limits the objective import of our sense experience, as MRTA does. After-image experience is

[19] One should add one further rider on the points made here. The discussion here requires that we think of how acts of awareness relate to their objects as involving predication, or variations on predication: and hence as involving both particulars and universals. Moore himself emphasizes this element in his disagreements with Stout over universals and tropes. Moore's position would not be available if one supposed that sense experience was of particularized qualities, or tropes, as Stout supposes, and Moore left open as a possibility in his earliest writings; or it contained just colours as universals, without these being predicated of anything, as Moore concedes the possibility of in some passages in *The Commonplace Book*.

often taken as a paradigm of subjective sense experience: if after-images really are entities, then they are entities which depend on our awareness of them. So much more of a reason, many critics of sense-datum theories suppose, to insist solely on the existence of after-image experiences, and not in addition to the after-images as objects of sensory awareness in such experience. But, in fact, TSD can acknowledge the privacy and lack of independence of after-images as long as this is understood in terms of their dependence on our nervous systems, and not that sensory awareness brings them into existence. On Moore's conception of such experience, then, we are aware of how the after-image is in itself, that is bluish-white and vaguely circular, even if what we know about will cease to obtain when we no longer have the experience.

In denying that after-images are strictly speaking in the mind, TSD can affirm that our ordinary sensory awareness of such items provides us with knowledge of the ways that sense-data are. And, one might think, there is indeed some plausibility to this thought in just common-sense terms, if one has already granted the thought that after-images exist, and not just that experiences of after-images happen. And this provides the ultimate stumbling block for MRTA: according to Moore it cannot acknowledge that we have an awareness of after-images which provides us with the knowledge that such images possess the sensible qualities that we ordinarily attribute to them.

That, at least, I suggest, is the best gloss we can offer on Moore's brief summary of the nonsensical position:

> Until very recently I had thought that, though some of the arguments that purported to show that it cannot were strong, yet they were not conclusive, because I thought that, e.g. in the case where you directly see an 'after-image' with closed eyes, it was just possible that the after-image only looked to have certain colours and shape and size, and did not really have them...
>
> (Moore 1957: 210)

MRTA is not committed on any construal to deny that after-images have particular colours, or shape, or size. Moore's concern here is rather that the only grounds that we have for attributing some specific shade of bluish-white to a given after-image, or a squashed circular shape to it is that that is how the after-image appears to us. Yet, according to MRTA, appearing in itself only indicates how the object is relative to our sense experience, not how it is in itself.

This concern is not specifically one about reliability or certainty. When Moore embraces his dilemma, he is still prepared to insist that he is certain that he has a hand, or that he is standing up, even though he admits that he cannot give a philosophical account of how he comes to be certain of these matters. Neither TSD nor MRTA would explain Moore's knowledge of his handedness or his posture through direct experiential encounter. So Moore is never inclined to suppose that the only route to knowing about things in the world is through some form of direct awareness. It is no accident, then, that Moore chooses the example of after-images to press his concern in 'Visual Sense-Data'. For after-images are private entities, each of us directly encounters only his or her own after-images. Hands, bodies, mountains and stars may all have a larger role within the world which we may come to track and so come to be certain of, even if we cannot directly encounter them in experience. Among the phenomenal ephemera of life, the only reasons we have to credit after-images with specific colours or shapes are the visual experiences we have of them.

According to MRTA, the character of our sense experience is accounted for through objects seeming to have certain sensible qualities. And seeming to be bluish-white is consistent with not being bluish-white. According to Moore, MRTA does not take the colour that the after-image actually is to play any role in explaining the visual experience one has of the after-image. So our visual experiences of after-images give us no direct knowledge of the qualities that after-images possess. Moore takes that to be absurd. Once we grant that after-images exist, it is implausible to ascribe to them any qualities other than the ones we experience them as having. And so some visual experience at least must provide us with knowledge of the way some things *are* and not just the way they *seem*.[20]

Note that, as Moore reports matters in 'Visual Sense-Data', what he changes his mind about is the question whether we can live with the opinion that after-images merely seem bluish-white or round without us thereby having sensory awareness of them as actually being this colour or shape.[21] There is no reason to suppose Moore is concerned in 1918 with how we justify going beyond subjective reports, as Chisholm's gloss on the theory of appearing would suggest, nor yet that he has convinced himself in 1953 that he now can make that move. Despite the various narratives on offer from commentators, Moore does not shift fundamentally in his views about the nature of sense experience between 1918 and 1953. He simply revises his attitude towards the evidence on offer.[22]

6. Seeing MRTA in this light not only explains the rationale for Moore's final change of heart. It also puts us in a better position to evaluate the traditional interpretation that Moore here endorses a form of the theory of appearing, and the alternative suggestion we made above, that Moore here offers a kind of intentional theory of perception. Moreover, as I'll argue below, the contrast that we need to draw between Moore's dilemma, given this understanding of it, and how it has commonly been

[20] Note a certain ambiguity here. One might hold that sense experience acquaints us with sensible qualities. That sense experience might have such a distinctive role has been canvassed by Johnston (2004) and Pautz (2010). Moore's MRTA could endorse this proposal, if the kind of acquaintance required did not involve the seeming predicative unity of the quality with some object. But the empiricist thought that sense experience is special in providing us with acquaintance has typically been expressed in terms of the idea that we are acquainted with a quality in its being exemplified by sensible objects of awareness, and it is this combination which MRTA as Moore conceives of it is ruling out.

[21] One might, of course, question whether this plausibility really meets the standard of certainty that Moore is clearly so keen on in 1918 and 1924. It does not seem inconsistent to suppose that we know after-images only as they appear to us, and not as they are in themselves.

[22] In fact the various discussions of sensory awareness, sense-data, and after-images throughout *The Commonplace Book* (Moore 1962) suggest at various points that Moore concedes for some objects that we can draw no distinction between how they seem and how they are. The earliest such example is in relation to sounds.

presented before underlines some morals for us more generally about the aims of philosophical theories of sense experience, and reliance on introspective reflection offered in support or against some account of perception.

Above I raised the puzzle of how we should characterize the epistemic position of the subject caught in Moore's dilemma. If we stick simply with the observation that the subject is to question the assumption made by the traditional sense-datum theorist, we do not have any material to specify what is distinctive of being in the situation in which one confronts the bark of a tree from middle distance, or the back of one's hand close up, or some suspicious patch of colour on the wall opposite. In discussing the theory of appearing, we suggested that Moore could retreat simply to the subjective report about his experience, 'That this seems small', or 'It looks to me as if there is a bluish-white expanse'. And the idea that the debate about sense experience concerns moving beyond the report just of the mental state itself is part of how Chisholm initially characterizes the theory of appearing.

But in fact, in the end, this is not how Moore himself presents the dilemma. As we stressed above, the claims made by the sense-datum theorist are substantive claims, but so too are the claims made by MRTA. So the disjunction of these two claims is not a tautology. Moore takes the neutral position to be one in which one is presented with an object of awareness, and one is thereby aware of some sensible quality which relates in some manner or other to that object. In the course of his discussion, what he assumes is that there are exactly two ways in which the qualities can relate to this object. On the one hand, the object may simply instantiate the quality and in having the experience one thereby can come to know that the object is that way. On the other hand, sense experience may provide one with no knowledge of what is the case independently of this experience occurring, and in that situation one thereby can come to know that the object seems that way. Hence Moore's slightly awkward phrasing when he talks of us perceiving the object to seem small.[23] So, against his background assumptions, Moore has managed to characterize the uncertainty one has in terms of a disjunctive claim concerning the objects of awareness. The dilemma concerns quite how much knowledge one has of these objects. And in turn, Moore has no need to step back further and just consider the knowledge one has of one's psychological state. From Moore's perspective knowledge of how things seem is not the same as simply knowledge of what psychological state one is in.

We have already noted that from the perspective of the theory of appearing, Moore's failure to recognize the commitment to an actually existing object of awareness is problematic. Now we can also see that the conception of what the subject ought to be in a position to know is different between the two approaches. How then, does the intentionalist theory fare, as a gloss on Moore's MRTA?

In one way, there may be no determinate answer to this. Although it has been common in recent discussion to talk of *the* intentional theory of perception, or

[23] An awkwardness noted in Alan White's discussion of Moore's views of perception, see White (1958: 173).

representationalism, or *the* content view, there is little consensus on what the essential commitments of an intentional approach to perception should amount to. Understood in at least one minimal way, the analogy we have already pointed to between the multiple relation theory of judgement and the multiple relation theory of sensing is sufficient to treat MRTA as an intentional theory of perception. Moore's multi-grade relations of judging and seeming occupy the functional role needed for treating psychological acts as relations to propositions, or proposition-like entities. On such a view there is no more interesting condition which needs to be met for sense experience to count or fail to count as an example of an intentional state or even a propositional attitude.

Typically, however, writers have advertised the intentional theory of perception as providing a key advantage over sense-datum theories as being consistent with the thought that sense experience provides us with a direct or immediate contact with the perceived environment. And so one can ask whether Moore's MRTA meets this additional desideratum of an intentional account. Our reconstruction of Moore's objection to his own view involves the assumption that, given MRTA, being aware of the way an object seems is never tantamount to being aware of the way an object is. Even in situations where how an object is coincides with how the object seems, being aware of how it seems does not amount to being aware of how it is. Only given this assumption can Moore be justified in claiming that MRTA is inconsistent with our awareness of the after-image being bluish-white. And, in the interpretation we have offered this assumption is closely connected with the idea that even if sense experience relates one to an object independent of one's awareness, it cannot really provide one with knowledge of anything that goes beyond the experience itself.

This way of interpreting Moore's thought fits well with the account he offers of judgement. Moore insists that in matters of contingent fact, what one judges could have been false even if true, but one's act of judgement would have in that situation been the same. So Moore takes the plurality of terms one is related to in judgement to be distinct from the facts which make the judgement true, when the judgement is true. This commitment of Moore's has come under scrutiny and some criticism among 'identity' theorists of truth.[24] Its consequence in the case of perceptual experience takes Moore's account in a direction away from what many writers find attractive about the prospect of intentionalism.

The attractive case for intentionalism focuses on what we say about the illusory case: the sense-datum theorist supposes that there must be a suitable bearer of the sensible quality at hand. This demand leads to the ontological inflation, positing suitable non-environmental objects of sensory awareness. If instead we claim that the quality is before the mind without having to be instantiated, then we can avoid that inflation. Consistent with this, one may well insist that in the case of veridical perception, one is not only aware of the object of perception but also of the way

[24] See Cartwright (1987), Hornsby (1997), and also McDowell (1994).

that it is. That is to say, it is an attractive doctrine to suppose that one can both hold that an object can be represented to be some way that it is not, and that when it is represented to be some way it is, such representation can count as being aware of the object's being that way. One sees the patch and it looks green when it is not: green enters in the experience as represented, but nothing in fact need be green. One sees the patch when it is green: green enters the experience as represented, but also, in this case one thereby counts as being aware of the patch as being green. If Moore's MRTA is a version of intentionalism, then it doesn't allow for this combination of commitments. For Moore, one is forced to choose between a view on which sense experience reveals the way something is with a view on which experience merely reveals a way in which it appears.

This highlights a certain irony in Baldwin's criticisms of Moore. In interpreting Moore as partly endorsing the theory of appearing, Baldwin takes Moore to be returning to a kind of direct realism about sense perception. And, to some extent that must be right, since Moore does take it as a virtue of MRTA that it allows the ultimate objects of perception to be parts of environmental objects; and this is reiterated even at the very end of 'Visual Sense-Data' when he has finally rejected it as incoherent. But Baldwin hypothesizes that Moore is kept back from a full-blown direct realism about perception through the mistaken assumption that there must always be an existing object of awareness. Given the gloss that we have put on MRTA here, however, we can see that Moore's acknowledging that something may merely seem to be *F* in experience without *being F* leads him to consider the possibility that we are never aware of the way things actually are. This puts him even further away from the charms of direct realism.

7. I want to close with two morals that we can draw from looking this intensely at Moore in 1918 and trying to make sense of the dilemma he then posed his audience. Both derive from an observation I made at the outset: Moore's dilemma presents us with the choice between two substantive theories of sensory experience. And once we recognize that fact, it becomes unclear on what ground we should be restricted to choosing just between these two options.

The first, and in many ways most obvious, point is that we really don't face Moore's dilemma: we are not restricted just to the choice of accepting TSD or MRTA when we stare at the backs of hands and wonder what is involved in us being so aware. And that is underlined for us in the contrast that we drew in the last section between standard intentionalism and Moore's MRTA. If we stick to Moore's assumptions, then what we are at least certain of is this: there is an object of awareness and there is some sensible quality to which the experience unites it. What is uncertain, according to him, is how that object and sensible quality are united.

Now when we think of an example of perceptual illusion, precisely the focus of the argument leading up to the dilemma, it is tempting to think that our problem boils down to the question: does the object of awareness have the quality or not? TSD is the theory which claims that it does (and then draws as a consequence the non-identity of the object with the surface), MRTA is the theory which claims it does not. Assuming that we are concerned with a case which is not borderline, that we are concerned, for example, with a determinate shade of very pale blue, a bluish-white, it may well seem that there really are only two possible options. Either the object is bluish-white or it is not. If the choice could turn on just this question, then there really would only be two options.

But in fact we've seen that there are at least two ways in which the illusory experience might fail to involve the object's being bluish-white. On the one hand, the experience might involve representing the object as being bluish-white, relating us to a possible but non-actual state of affairs in which the object is bluish-white. This is the way many intentionalists are inclined to describe the situation. And this is what would lead us to talk of this as a case of presence in absence. Moore's theory, on the other hand, invites a different gloss. The object of awareness is united with bluish-white only relative to the experience, it is bluish-white in experience, but not in itself. On this view of the illusory experience, there is nothing in it which directs us towards the non-actual state of affairs of the object's being bluish-white.

That suggests that Moore's dilemma is not the same as the intentionalist's dilemma. So even if we do find ourselves in the situation Moore is concerned with, aware that we are suffering an illusion, but otherwise uncertain of the correct view of the matter, his is not the only option on the table. One could side with what is now the standard form of intentionalism, and suppose that object and quality are united merely representationally.

But this isn't only a point against Moore. Earlier, I highlighted a question about whether and how sense experience can inform us about the world independent of that sense experience. In the most prominent discussions of this question, in Strawson and Evans, for example, the issue becomes one of what properties can be thought to be presented to the subject in experience: typically emphasis is laid on the status of primary qualities such as figure and size, and the role that these play in our understanding of the causal conditions that give rise to sense experience in the first place. Moore's alternative to sense-datum theories offers another way in which sense experience might fail to be fully objective. Even if the sense experience presents a mind-independent object (which, as we have stressed, Moore supposes it always must) and even if it presents a property, such as shape, which an object could have only independently of the mind, still the experience might fail to present the objective state of affairs of that object having the property. For Moore we are to think of the experience as revealing the object as being round only relative to this current experience of it.

It is tempting for the intentionalist to look for evidence in favour of the doctrine just from reflection on our sense experience. In a case of illusion, the object is not bluish-white but still bluish-white is present to the mind. If we are reluctant to join with the sense-datum theorist and affirm that something else is indeed bluish-white, how else are we to explain the experience than in terms of its representing the object to be bluish-white? But the apparent coherence of Moore's conception of MRTA blocks this piece of reasoning, just as this intelligibility of this conception of experience undermines Moore's conception of the dilemma. We might dismiss Moore's conception of what it is for objects to seem bluish-white as ultimately making no sense. Or we might independently and antecedently have reason to think of our perceptual experiences as representational states, and so to make best sense of what we can introspect of them as indicative of that representational nature. But if we start out as Moore does just by reflecting on what we can tell from our experience, then we can no more endorse the intentionalist understanding than we can Moore's MRTA. The possibility of illusion on its own doesn't seem to offer us a determinate enough picture to settle anything.

The second moral takes us back to the contrast between the theory of appearing and Moore's MRTA. The conflation of Moore's position with that of Dawes Hicks goes back to C. D. Broad. In Broad's hands, this means treating Dawes Hicks's position as no different from Moore (in *The Mind and Its Place in Nature*, Broad (1925) considers together the multiple relation theory and the 'multiple inherence theory' as close alternatives to his sensum account—the multiple inherence theory rejects the assumption that the apparent properties conflict, and so objects are taken to possess multiple colours or shapes at the same time; in seeing a close affinity between this view and MRTA, Broad is taking MRTA along the lines we sketched above. No such construal is appropriate for Dawes Hicks, however). In later authors, as we noted, the assimilation goes in the other direction.

One thing this indicates is that it can be hard to distinguish whether in talking of how things seem we are talking about the subject's psychological state, or we are rather talking about something that the subject can know about the world on the basis of his or her experience. It is difficult to hear any real import in the move between: 'It seems to Moore as if the tree is small' and 'The tree seems small to Moore'. Or rather, it looks as if the key contrast would concern the existential commitment, whether there really must be an object which seems some way whenever Moore has an experience. And given that Moore assumes this, apparently on entirely independent grounds, then the movement and back and forth appears innocuous.

Once we spell out Moore's version of MRTA, we see that this can't be so. Moore assumes that the sense experience in question, whether TSD or MRTA is eventually shown to be correct, involves a relation to a specific sensible quality. When it seems as if there is a bluish-white patch before one, Moore supposes we know that either you stand in a relation of acquaintance to the colour bluish-white, as instantiated by the sense-datum, or you stand in a relation of seeming to the shade in question. And this is to assume that the character of the experience is just a matter of which sensible quality the subject is related to through that experience. This assumption is surely not in play simply through us granting the subjective fact that it seems to Moore as if he is confronted with a bluish-white patch.

Now Moore seems to have made this kind of assumption about sensible experience from the beginning of his realist period. The famous discussion of the diaphaneity of sensible experience in 'A Refutation of Idealism' introduces the idea that the relation of sensible awareness adds nothing to the discernible character of one's experience:

> the moment we try to fix our attention upon consciousness and to see *what*, distinctly, it is, it seems to vanish: it seems as if we had before us a mere emptiness. When we try to introspect the sensation of blue, all we can see is the blue: the other element is as if it were diaphanous. Yet it *can* be distinguished if we look attentively enough, and if we know that there is something to look for.
> (Moore 1903: 450)

I mentioned earlier Moore's intended refutation as a demonstration of how we have knowledge of that which is entirely independent of us. Were consciousness something that added character to the objects of awareness, then one could question whether we could ever know those objects in themselves, independent of the taint that consciousness adds to them. So, although Moore thinks it important that we recognize that consciousness takes the form of a relation to something (and hence can be distinguished in the experiential circumstances), it is also important to emphasize that nothing is added by it. With that commitment in place, the character of acts of sensory awareness is taken always to derive from the objects of awareness. If two acts of consciousness differ in their character, then Moore will assume, they must differ in some respect in their objects, in what he later comes to call the sense-data, or the sensible qualities which those data exhibit.

With this assumption of *diaphaneity* in play, Moore will simply assume that there could be nothing more to an experience than what objects or qualities are given in it. For him, the move from its seeming as if there is a bluish-white patch before one, to bluish-white seeming some way, will indeed be a trivial move. For he has already assumed that if there is a determinate way one's experience is when things seem some way to one, then that in turn must amount to a sensible quality or some sensible qualities together being presented to the subject.

But what possible grounds are there for this assumption? One way of seeing it, I suggest, comes out of the understanding of sense perception as a means we have to acquire knowledge of the world around us, and what the connotations are of the idea of sensible or observational qualities. One might think that, at least in ideal circumstances, our senses can reveal to us ways that objects are. And, moreover, that in such circumstances one can come to know about the sensible qualities of such objects in the best possible way that one can. For example, one might suggest that really the best way to come to know about some determinate shade of colour, say a bluish-white, just is to view a sample under optimal viewing conditions: against a neutral background under strong Northern midday sunlight.

Now, even if we think that sense perception can distinctively provide us with knowledge in this way, at least for the sensible aspects of objects, still on its own that will not get as far as Moore's strong assumption about sense experience in general. After all, we not only suppose that we can know about objects through sense perception, but we know that the conditions for coming to know about objects vary, and hence our experiences can vary too. One can see the bluish-white sample under rather less good conditions—under artificial shop lights, or in the fading light of a late afternoon; against one strong background colour, or another. All of these experiences will be different from each other. And, I would suggest, it is unclear whether they should all have some distinctive qualitative aspect in common which is the presentation of bluish-white.

When we think of the variety of circumstances under which we can confront the colour or the shape of objects, then we are much less likely to assume that there is one distinctive way of experiencing the colour or the shape. Suppose that I see and can recognize roughly the shade of bluish-white both in the ideal viewing conditions and in the shadowy afternoon. Are both experiences to be understood as being presented with the quality in question, either as TSD supposes or as MRTA? Or is only one of these experiences genuinely a visual experience of the bluish-white?

Likewise, even if it seems to me that there is a patch of bluish-white before me, does that show that I am thereby related to bluish-white, rather than to some other colour, which in the circumstances strikes me in relevantly the same way as bluish-white would under ideal circumstances? What would rule out conceiving of the situation in this way? That might suggest that we understand the subjective reports, such as that it seems to Moore as if there is a bluish-white patch there, as indicating a salient similarity between this experience and one in which he confronts an instance of bluish-white.

That this isn't just a trivial matter is reflected in the rather different attitudes that Dawes Hicks evinces on these matters, and Russell's tart response back. In his review essay on *The Problems of Philosophy*, Dawes Hicks complains about Russell's use of the argument from conflicting appearances in the following way:

> Suppose, for the sake of argument, that colour is inherent in the table, suppose the table has in reality a specific colour. Then, surely, there would be nothing to conflict with this supposition in the fact that such real colour will present a different aspect if another colour be reflected on upon it, or if a blue pair of spectacles intervene between it and the observer, or if it be enveloped in darkness rather than in daylight. The reasoning would only be valid on the assumption that if the table is really coloured, the real colour must appear the same in darkness and in daylight. (Hicks 1912: 401)

Russell's response to this is a form of incomprehension (in correspondence he complains of Dawes Hicks being 'muddle-headed'):

> This brings me to what Dr Dawes Hicks says on the subject of colour and shape. He suggests that 'the real colour will present a different aspect if another colour be reflected upon it' (p. 401). But surely we cannot speak of a colour 'presenting an aspect'. A colour which presents a different aspect is a different colour, and there is an end of the matter. (Russell 1913: 79)

I suggest that here we find Russell making just the same assumption that is present in Moore's discussion, in respect of colour experience at least: Russell supposes that diaphaneity holds. If one's visual experience is different in character from one occasion to another, then that difference must be a difference in its object. Rather than allowing that colours may appear differently, Russell assumes a difference in the character of colour experience can only be a difference in what colour is experienced.

Whatever the merits of Russell's or Dawes Hicks's views on colour, the disagreement between them can hardly be settled just by fiat. But Moore's presentation of his dilemma seems to presuppose that the matter has been settled, and settled in Russell's favour. This again gives us reason to question the grounds under which he sets the dilemma up initially.

At the outset of *Sense and Sensibilia* J. L. Austin (1962), in somewhat schoolmasterly tones, lays out an assessment of the two failing pupils in the school of English philosophy, the sense-datum theory of perception and the argument from illusion. Sense-data, he characterizes as a mere phantasm of philosophers' speculation; they are no part of the grit of reality. The argument from illusion on the other hand is argument only in name: a piece of pseudo-reasoning, recognized as spurious even by those most adept at shuffling its cards. Whether the lessons Austin wanted to impart have really been taken by his readership is a nice question, but there can be no doubt that the negative affect in his scorn did leave a lasting impression. One aspect of his attack that lasts is the sense that somehow the sense-datum theory and the argument from illusion are intertwined in their bad reputation: there is a thought that one of the bad things about the sense-datum theory is the manner in which it rests on the argument from illusion; and that what is problematic with the argument from illusion is that it leads to a commitment to the existence of (non-physical) sense-data.

What our inspection of Moore teaches us, though, is that there is something more problematic in the argument from illusion than just that. In some circumstances at least we are inclined to accept a close association between sense perception, things being apparent to us, and our knowledge of them. But Moore's assumption goes well beyond this: it requires that all sense experiences amount to knowledge of sensible qualities. What could justify this generalizing move? Moore never tells us. And it is difficult to see what could show one that it should be accepted.

Above, I argued that we should not conflate Moore's dilemma with the question that intentionalists about sense experience are inclined to press on us: is this a case of something's genuinely being bluish-white, or is this simply a case of bluish-white being before the mind, without being instantiated? Even if the two sets of question are not the same, they both seem to adopt a questionable framing assumption. That when it comes to sense experience and sensible qualities, we can talk about types of experience in terms of the qualities we experience. And hence that it makes sense for us to ask about a range of experiences, visual experiences of bluish-white, say, and what it takes for such an experience to occur. Unless we have made Moore's simplifying assumption, as Russell has, that there is only one way to experience a given shade, then we cannot start out with just that assumption.

What does Moore and his dilemma teach us in the end? On the one hand, from our perspective there are odd and idiosyncratic commitments threaded through Moore's whole discussion. Not least, there is the peculiarity in Moore assuming that all sensory awareness must involve an actually existing object of awareness. In addition, Moore assumes that sensory awareness is necessarily a form of knowledge, and as a consequence is always awareness of something independent of that awareness. As we have seen repeatedly, this added assumption of Moore's imposes substantive constraints on the form a theory can take. At the same time, one might feel that the terms in which Moore is debating these matters is just too far removed from the concerns of contemporary neuroscience. Moore might be aware that our sensory experience is dependent on the operation of the nervous system, but his whole discourse seems much more distanced and cloudily connected to anything that we now know about how the activation of the visual system leads us to see that tree, or this hand, or that patch of colour. We have added together strange assumptions about what sense perception must involve with unattractive ignorance of crucial physiological and neurological facts. Is it a wonder if the theory which results should look so strange to us now?

On the other hand, Moore's ambitions are to start with matters that are the most basic and obvious to him, and should be so in turn to his readers. And his strategy then, from these manifest starting points, is to work matters through as carefully as he can, and to avoid any speculation. The key assumption in all of this is that there are questions for us to raise about the nature of sense perception which require us to adopt the first-person perspective, the point of view of the person who is staring at the tree, their hand, or the patch on the wall. And that having raised these questions, we should continue to pursue them through such careful, reflective attention. While Moore's specific assumptions about consciousness seem idiosyncratic, the idea that debate about sense experience and phenomenal consciousness should begin from what we all know in reflecting on what it is like to see a hand or taste a pineapple is still very much alive. At the very least, then, seeing what we can make of Moore's enquiry tells us something about the limits of this kind of first-personal enquiry into the nature of sense experience.[25]

References

Alston, W. (1999), 'Back to the Theory of Appearing', in *Philosophical Perspectives* 13 Epistemology: 181–203.

[25] This chapter derives from a discussion initially focused on recent attempts to revive the argument from illusion. That was presented at the original workshop in Hertfordshire in 2011, and at colloquia at Warwick, Irvine, Chicago, and Oxford. I'm grateful to audiences at all these occasions for questions and comments. The idea that Moore might be presenting a form of intentionalism was originally suggested to me by Fraser Macbride, and I'm grateful to him for extended discussion of Moore's metaphysics and epistemology. Thanks also for written comments to Paul Coates and Véronique Munoz-Dardé.

Anscombe, G. E. M. (1965), 'The Intentionality of Sensation: A Grammatical Feature', in R. Butler (ed.), *Analytic Philosophy*, 2nd Series (Oxford: Blackwell), 158–80.

Austin, J. L. (1962), *Sense and Sensibilia* (Oxford: Clarendon Press).

Ayer, A. J. (1940), *The Foundations of Empirical Knowledge* (London: Macmillan).

Baldwin, T. (1990), *G. E. Moore* (London: Routledge).

Broad, C. D. (1923), *Scientific Thought* (London: Routledge and Kegan Paul).

Broad, C. D. (1925), *The Mind and Its Place in Nature* (London: Kegan Paul).

Byrne, A. (2009), 'Experience and Content', in *Philosophical Quarterly* 59 236: 429–51.

Cartwright, R. (1987), 'On a Neglected Theory of Truth', in *Philosophical Essays* (Cambridge, MA: MIT Press), 71–95.

Cassam, Q. (1997), *Self and World* (Oxford: Clarendon Press).

Chisholm, R. M. (1950), 'The Theory of Appearing', originally in Max Black (ed.), *Philosophical Analysis* (Englewood Cliffs, NJ: Prentice Hall); reprinted in R. J. Swartz (ed.), (1965), *Perceiving, Sensing and Knowing* (New York: Anchor Books), 168–86.

Chisholm, R. M. (1957), *Perceiving* (Ithaca: Cornell University Press).

Clarke, T. (1965), 'Seeing Surfaces and Physical Objects', in Max Black (ed.) *Philosophy in America* (London: George Allen), 98–114.

Evans, G. (1980), 'Things without the Mind', in Z. van Straaten (ed.), *Philosophical Subjects: Essays Presented to P. F. Strawson* (Oxford: Clarendon Press), 76–116.

Foster, J. (1985), *A. J. Ayer* (London: Routledge).

Hicks, G. D. (1912), 'The Nature of Sense-Data', in *Mind* 21 83: 399–409.

Hornsby, J. (1997), 'The Presidential Address: Truth: The Identity Theory', *Proceedings of the Aristotelian Society* 97 1: 1–24.

Hume, D. (1975/1748), *Enquiry Concerning Human Understanding*, 3rd ed., edited by L. A. Selby-Bigge and revised by P. H. Nidditch (Oxford: Clarendon Press).

Jackson, F. (1977), *Perception: A Representative Theory* (Cambridge: Cambridge University Press).

Johnston, M. (2004), 'The Obscure Object of Hallucination', in *Philosophical Studies* 120: 113–83.

Johnston, M. (2006), 'Better than Mere Knowledge? The Function of Sensory Awareness', in T. Gendler and J. Hawthorne (eds), Perceptual Experience (Oxford: Oxford University Press), 260–90.

Langsam, H. (1997), 'The Theory of Appearing Defended', in *Philosophical Studies* 87: 33–59.

McDowell, J. (1994), *Mind and World* (Cambridge, MA: Harvard University Press).

Moltmann, F. (2013), 'Tropes, Bare Demonstratives, and Apparent Statements of Identity', in *Noûs* 47 2: 346–70.

Moore, G. E. (1903), 'The Refutation of Idealism', in *Mind* 12 48: 433–53.

Moore, G. E. (1914), 'The Status of Sense-Data', in *Proceedings of the Aristotelian Society* 14: 355–81.

Moore, G. E. (1918), 'Some Judgments of Perception', in *Proceedings of the Aristotelian Society* 19: 1–29.

Moore, G. E. (1925), 'A Defence of Common Sense', in J. H. Muirhead (ed.), *Contemporary British Philosophy*, 2nd Series (London: George Allen and Unwin), 193–223.

Moore, G. E. (1926), 'The Nature of Sensible Appearances', in *Aristotelian Society Supplementary Volume* 6: 179–205.

Moore, G. E. (1939), 'Proof of an External World', in *Proceedings of the British Academy* 25: 273–300.

Moore, G. E. (1953), *Some Main Problems of Philosophy*, Muirhead Library of Philosophy, (London: George Allen and Unwin).

Moore, G. E. (1957), 'Visual Sense-Data', in C. A. Mace (ed.), *British Philosophy in Mid-Century* (London: George Allen and Unwin), 205–11.

Moore, G. E. (1959), 'Certainty', in *Philosophical Papers* (London: George Allen and Unwin), 227–51.

Moore, G. E. (1962), *Commonplace Book 1919–1953* (London: George Allen and Unwin).

Pautz, A. (2010), 'Why Explain Visual Experience in Terms of Content?', in Bence Nanay (ed.), *Perceiving the World* (Oxford: Oxford University Press), 254–309.

Prichard, H. A. (1938), 'The Sense-Datum Fallacy', in *Aristotelian Society Supplementary Volume* 17: 1–18.

Reid, T. (1997/1764), *An Inquiry into the Human Mind on the Principles of Common Sense*, edited by Derek Brookes (Edinburgh: Edinburgh University Press).

Robinson, H. (1994), *Perception* (London: Routledge).

Russell, B. (1912), *The Problems of Philosophy*, 9th ed. (Oxford: Oxford University Press).

Russell, B. (1913), 'The Nature of Sense-Data: A Reply to Dr. Dawes Hicks', in *Mind* 22 85: 76–81.

Siegel, S. (2010), 'Do Visual Experiences Have Contents?', in Bence Nanay (ed.), *Perceiving the World* (New York: Oxford University Press), 333–68.

Snowdon, P. F. (2007), 'G. E. Moore on Sense-Data and Perception', in S. Nuccetelli and G. Seay (eds), *Themes from G. E. Moore: New Essays in Epistemology and Ethics* (Oxford: Clarendon Press), 119–39.

Strawson, P. F. (1966), *The Bounds of Sense* (London: Methuen).

Strawson, P. F. (1979), 'Perception and Its Objects', in G. F. Macdonald (ed.), *Perception and Identity* (London: Macmillan), 41–60.

Swartz, R. J. (1965), *Perceiving, Sensing and Knowing* (New York: Anchor Books).

White, A. R. (1958), *G. E. Moore: A Critical Exposition* (Oxford: Basil Blackwell).

6

Projection, Revelation, and the Function of Perception

Paul Coates

6.1 Introduction

According to the standard view, phenomenal qualities—qualities such as the red colour that appears to a normal human observer who looks at a ripe strawberry in broad daylight, the taste of mint, the smell of coffee, and so on—are picked out by reference to consciousness. Perceptual and other kinds of conscious experiences, such as the awareness of a pain, essentially involve the immediate presence of phenomenal qualities to the subject. The term 'immediate' here connotes the fact that such qualities are present in the subject's conscious awareness in a *sensory* manner, as opposed to merely intentionally, as in thought: when I veridically see something red, the immediate consciousness of the red phenomenal quality is very different from the type of consciousness I have when I only think about that quality. The presence of phenomenal qualities accounts for the what-it-is-like-ness aspect of perceptual and other experiences—that is, for their phenomenal character. This way of identifying phenomenal qualities is independent of claims about the precise structure of experience, and is not intended to rule out the possibility that certain phenomenal qualities are identical with observable features of physical objects external to the experiencing subject—that is, with their sensible properties; such is the view of Direct Realism, as I elaborate below.[1] However, I shall be arguing for a different position: the phenomenal qualities present in perceptual experience belong to *inner states* of the experiencing subject. They are not located in the non-sentient world, but are properties that belong to the mind or brain.

[1] Perceptual terminology varies. By 'Direct Realism', I include disjunctivist views, naive realism, and the relational account, these being versions of the general position which holds that the sensible properties of external physical objects can be immediately present to the subject in veridical perception, and which rejects the idea that perceptual experiences are inner states. Different versions of this view are defended in Snowdon (1981 and 2005), Smith (2002), Campbell (2002), Martin (2002 and 2006), Johnston (2004), Fish (2009), and Logue (2011), to cite but a few advocates.

To conceive of phenomenal qualities as belonging to inner states points towards a causal analysis of perception. According to the Causal Theory (as I shall refer to the view), veridical and hallucinatory experiences are not just phenomenologically indiscriminable, they also share a common ontology. Veridical experiences are inner states, and are only distinguishable from hallucinatory cases extrinsically, by reference to the distinctive ways in which they are caused. When I perceive a red apple on the table before me, in some manner to be explained by reference to facts about the appropriate pattern of causation involved, I make perceptual contact with that particular apple, and not to others that may resemble it. My experience is *of* that apple, but it is not present as a *phenomenal* constituent of my experience.

The Causal Theory aims to do justice to the phenomenological directness of perception by distinguishing between two dimensions of perceptual consciousness. As we noted above, experiences are distinguished from other mental episodes by the fact that they involve the *sensory awareness* of the phenomenal qualities present in consciousness, qualities which are manifested in a non-conceptual manner. But there is a further aspect to experience. Its intentional nature needs to be accounted for. To perceive an object is to be aware of it as a thing of a certain kind. I may see an object as an apple, or more minimally, simply as some reddish thing over there. In experiencing a mind-independent object *as* an object of a certain sort, the subject also represents the perceived object directly through the exercise of concepts of at least a low-level classificatory kind, in addition to being presented with phenomenal qualities. Arguably, these two dimensions of experience, though closely linked, are logically independent of each other.[2]

According to the critical realist version of the Causal Theory, experiences thus have a complex, two-fold nature. In the normal perceptual situation, the non-conceptual awareness of phenomenal qualities is combined with a second component, referred to as 'the perceptual taking'. This taking is an intentional state causally prompted by the inner states that bear the phenomenal qualities. However, we do not normally represent our own experiential states *as such*. The perceptual takings are directed at objective features of the local environment, and not at the phenomenal states that guide and accompany them.[3] It is by virtue of the taking component that perceptual experiences are targeted directly, without inference, upon external, mind-independent objects and events. The subject entertains concepts, and directly takes the external objects to belong to familiar, easily recognizable, kinds.[4] External objects

[2] Views on this question differ. See, for example, Millar (1991) and the discussion in the Introduction to this collection.

[3] Throughout, I defend a critical realist version of the Causal Theory: see Drake (1920), W. Sellars (1975: Lecture I), and also my own Coates (2007) for a more detailed exposition. The two-component model of consciousness adopted here for visual experience is close to the theoretical position advocated, on the basis of experimental work in psychology, in Lambie and Marcel (2002).

[4] Such concepts may be low-level, and their exercise does not entail that the subject is self-aware. Thus the account would be applicable to perceptual processes in non-human animals.

occupy the subject's attention and form the focus of potential action. The perceived public object is, we might say, *phenomenologically* present, even though the *phenomenal* qualities of which we are immediately aware turn out, upon philosophical reflection, to belong to our own private inner experiences. In distinguishing an inner aspect of experience from the object at which the subject's intentional states are directed, the critical realist theory retains many of the advantages of the sense-data view while at the same time avoiding its more problematic features.

It is therefore misleading to describe the Causal Theory as claiming that perceptual experience is indirect. Imagine that I look at a red apple on a tree in front of me, seeing it *as* an apple. In being *immediately* aware, non-conceptually, of a red phenomenal quality—a quality that belongs to my own inner state—my perceptual thoughts focus spontaneously on the apple I see before me. I do not reflect upon my subjective experience of the red phenomenal quality. Without drawing inferences from any prior occurrent state, I *directly take* the apple to be objectively red, to share some physical surface property with other red physical items. Nevertheless, the sensory non-conceptual state of phenomenal consciousness forms the background of my perceptual consciousness of the apple.[5]

The upshot is that when we perceive, phenomenal qualities belonging to inner states are projected onto the physical objects we take to be present in the environment. The notion of projection deserves careful phenomenological investigation. Here I shall confine myself to some brief preliminary remarks, before taking up the main issue with which this chapter is concerned, the relation between the function and the analysis of perception. Properly understood, projectivism does not lead to paradoxical consequences that conflict with our central intuitions about perception. In seeing a reddish apple on a tree, I am aware, in a non-conceptual manner, of subjective colour qualities belonging to my inner experience, but I do not attend to them or conceptualize them *as such*. It follows that normally, in seeing the red apple, I do not explicitly compare the red quality that I am immediately aware of with the objective colour properties of the red apple I take to be present. Non-conceptual phenomenal awareness causally guides cognitive episodes in which I perceptually categorize aspects of the external physical environment, distinguishing and classifying their objective higher-level features. This phenomenological point is evidenced by phenomena such as colour constancy, listening to speech, and indeed very many of our ordinary perceptual transactions with the world. I directly see the red apple on the tree as ripe, and potentially separable from the branch on which it hangs; I see the sadness in a friend's face; I see the skater spinning round in three-dimensional space.

[5] It is of crucial importance in the analysis of perceptual experience to note the distinction between the epistemic notion of *directness*, which has to do with what the subject is non-inferentially yet conceptually aware of, and the metaphysical notion of *immediacy*, which has to do with what is contained in (or present to) the subject's perceptual consciousness. Despite differences in terminology, the position I advocate here is in agreement with that defended in Strawson's contribution to this collection, and in particular with the points that he makes in his section 17.

I do not draw any inferences based upon a cognitive awareness of what is immediately present in my conscious experience. My perceptual thoughts are causally guided by the non-conceptual awareness of phenomenal aspects of my own inner visual states.[6] In the usual case, I do not go on to form any further, more explicit, beliefs about the nature of an object's observable properties and how these relate to such immediate awareness.[7]

It follows that projectivism does not require that I entertain any positive beliefs about the relationship between my inner sensory states and the properties of the external objects I perceive. The model does not imply that I entertain erroneous beliefs about the location of the phenomenal qualities I am aware of when I perceive an external object. Projection arises by virtue of the *absence* of any explicit belief contrasting the subjective appearance of an object with its objective nature. I simply take there to be physical things located in my immediate surroundings, things that belong to familiar kinds, and that have objective qualities such as colour and shape.[8] Understood in this light, a projectivist account of perceptual experience can be seen to be compatible with our common-sense beliefs about the nature of the objects we perceive.

Many philosophers reject the Causal Theory, and the projectivist account that belongs with it. One main alternative view, upheld by Direct Realists, comprises two related claims:

(1) In normal veridical perception, subjects are immediately aware of entities distinct from their own mental states—they are aware of the external mind-independent physical objects themselves; such objects are present as phenomenal constituents in the perceiver's conscious experience.
(2) Introspection of one's veridical experiences reveals nothing in addition to the external objects perceived.

[6] An illustration of how we are able to project the awareness of structures at one level onto the objects we perceptually engage with at another level is provided by Minimal Invasive Surgery; I discuss this, and other aspects of a sophisticated projectivist account of perception, in Coates (2007: Ch. 9).

[7] A good question is how it is that the subject's inner phenomenal state leads to higher-level cognitive takings aimed directly at objective features of the external environment. A full answer to this would appeal to considerations about how the cognitive systems of higher-level creatures have evolved, and the kinds of training they receive. It is of relevance to this answer that the human visual system has developed to involve a number of processing stages which convert the sparse two-dimensional information received at the retina into rich representations—of different kinds—relating to a three-dimensional environment.

[8] For this reason the worries expressed in Tye (2000: 165–6), that projection inevitably leads to nonsensical beliefs about the properties of sensations, are misplaced. My visual beliefs normally relate directly to the external objects, *simpliciter*. Taste is perhaps a somewhat different matter. Wide variations in our gustatory preferences may incline us to reflect on possible differences between the objective flavour qualities of the things that we sample, and the subjective qualities they present when tasted. This raises a problem for any account of perception. For more on why projectivism need not entail an error theory see Egan (2010).

According to the metaphysics underlying Direct Realism, an immediate experiential relation holds between the perceiver's consciousness and the external object perceived. This relation of experiential inclusion is *sui generis*, and irreducible.[9] It is not possible to analyse perception further, into more basic elements. In the veridical case the subject is immediately aware of phenomenal qualities. However, these belong to the external object itself, and not to the subject's inner state. There is no common ontological kind shared by veridical and hallucinatory experiences. Veridical experiences are *non-inner* states. Since nothing mediates the subject's perceptual awareness of an object, what is immediately present to perceptual consciousness is one and the same as the external, mind-independent object directly perceived.

From the standpoint of Direct Realism, the Causal Theory fails to account for a central feature of experience, the fact that normal perception reveals something of the *intrinsic nature* of external physical objects, so that we can come to understand aspects of the world around us. Supposedly, Direct Realism captures what is right in the claim that in normal circumstances we perceive objects as they really are. The Causal Theory is alleged to be opposed to common sense: genuine knowledge of the nature of the external world, it is claimed, would be rendered impossible on that account. The objection to the Causal Theory is that it postulates an inner veil of sensory states, which cuts us off from the outer physical world.

In this chapter I explore this general line of thought in more detail. By examining the way that perception fits into our lives, I shall show that this objection to the Causal Theory is unjustified. Upholding the Causal Theory does not have the consequence that knowledge of the world is rendered problematic. It is the Direct Realist's conception of the link between knowledge and our perceptual engagement with the world that needs to be re-assessed. Direct Realism rests upon a misleading picture of perception. It fails to appreciate the central function of perception in our lives. In consequence, it puts forward a mistaken account of the kind of knowledge that perception yields. More fundamentally, it is unable to account for the central fact of perception: that in having an experience the subject is perceptually connected with some particular objects in the environment, but not with others.

I shall argue for this as follows. I first describe the general *pictures*—to be understood in the sense used by the later Wittgenstein—that underlie the two opposed views about the nature of perception. I then spell out in more detail the various different *roles*, or *functions* of perception, and show how the Causal Theory provides a satisfactory account of these. I suggest that, to a significant extent, Direct Realism is motivated by a false picture of what perception is for, and faces a serious difficulty in accounting for what I shall refer to as the individual content of veridical and illusory experiences. I aim to show, in particular, how the immediate awareness of phenomenal qualities in perception contributes only indirectly, and in a limited

[9] See Hobson (2013).

way, to our acquisition of knowledge concerning objective reality. We can defend the view that phenomenal qualities belong to inner states without embracing any paradoxical conclusions about our understanding of reality.

6.2 Motivating Pictures and the Analysis of Perception: Direct Realism

For the purposes of the main argument in this chapter, we need to distinguish between three different notions connected with the concept of perception: *theories*, *functions*, and *underlying pictures*. I start by saying something about the Direct Realist theory and the picture that underlies it.

Acceptance of the Direct Realist theory is often encouraged by a certain conception of the nature of perception and the basis of our knowledge of the world. According to this conception, normal perception involves the subject's *openness* to the world.[10] The guiding picture is one in which a perceiver is immediately *confronted* by an external object, without the mediation of any intervening entities. The object is present as a constituent of the subject's consciousness, and hence nothing prevents the subject acquiring direct knowledge of at least some sensible properties of the mind-independent objects perceived. Perceiving involves an immediate awareness of properties that belong *intrinsically* to the external physical objects perceived.

I call this picture 'the Confrontation Picture'. It involves the idea that when subjects are perceptually confronted by external, mind-independent, physical objects, at least some of the intrinsic properties of those objects are *revealed*, so that something of the very nature of the object as it is in itself is made immediately present to the subject's consciousness.[11] This picture is thus connected with the view that experience is *transparent*: perceivers are confronted in experience by the objects themselves, and not merely by their effects. The idea is not simply that perception is direct, in the sense that through perception the subject acquires non-inferential knowledge of a basic set of the properties belonging to the objects in the vicinity. Direct Realism makes a stronger claim, that certain of an object's properties are immediately present in experience; the perceptual object becomes a constituent of the subject's consciousness. According to Snowdon's formulation of disjunctivism, 'the experience in a perceptual case in its nature reaches out to and involves the perceived object'.[12]

[10] For more on the idea of openness, see Valberg (1992: Ch. 2).

[11] I would have used the expression 'the Revelation Picture' (rather than the Confrontation Picture), had it not been for the fact that the term 'revelation' is already in use to describe a distinct (though closely related) thesis, concerning the folk concept of colour. Compare Strawson (1989), Johnston (1992), Jackson (1998), Menzies (2004), and Allen (2011). 'Revelation' as used in the present chapter implies a thesis about our perceptual knowledge of physical objects, rather than one about our concept of colours as such.

[12] Snowdon (2005: Section III). A somewhat similar elucidation is provided in Johnston (2004: 139), where it is claimed that 'seeing goes all the way out to the things seen'.

Because subjects have an unmediated awareness of the—observable—features of external mind-independent objects, they are able to understand what some of those objects' intrinsic properties are like. The understanding thus gained forms the basis for further knowledge of reality. The immediate acquaintance of mind-independent objects in perception is held to be necessary in order for the subject to be able to make demonstrative reference to them. How the knowledge gained from perception is utilized by the subject is taken to be of rather less consequence.

According to the Confrontation Picture, if we did not construe perception as yielding an immediate awareness of the intrinsic nature of things, then it would be unclear how our beliefs about the world could have content. It is because external objects are 'immediately present to the mind' that, according to McDowell, we are able to make judgements about the objects we engage with, and about their features. It is supposed that the Causal Theory is unable to explain how experience 'purports to be *revelatory* of the world we live in'.[13] In this chapter I shall be questioning these claims, and offering an alternative account of the nature of our perceptually based knowledge of external reality. I shall focus upon issues concerning the status of the objective colour properties of physical objects.

I first say a little more about what is involved in the Confrontation Picture, illustrating it through quotations that capture its essential features. Mark Johnston (2004) has summarized some of its main elements. In language reminiscent of Wilde's Lady Bracknell, he criticizes projectivism, and the Causal Theory, as leading to

> a dreadful kind of Kantian Relationalism about experience.

According to Johnston, the problem for this alternative view is that

> All the senses reveal about external objects is how they affect us; they show nothing of how such objects are in themselves.

Johnston's own preferred account treats phenomenal qualities

> as intrinsic, non-relational features of sensible particulars. The senses can make manifest how things are in themselves.[14]

In outlining his theory of Colour Impressionism, Colin McGinn also defends a position that incorporates the key elements of the Confrontation Picture. According to McGinn (1996: 545, 547):

[13] The quotation is from McDowell (1986: 152, italics added).

[14] These three quotations are from Johnston (2004: 175–6). In an earlier paper, Johnston (1992: 257) is more equivocal about the idea of revelation, yet states that the senses provide 'access to the natures of those features of external things that are colours'. In a subsequent paper the senses are likened to 'open windows' (Johnston 2006: 285n).

> Colour properties themselves are categorical, simple, monadic, intrinsic features of objects

and

> the nature of colour is revealed *in* how coloured objects look.

According to McGinn's impressionism, colours are properties that supervene upon those properties discovered by physics. Colours are irreducible, and belong to 'a further set of properties that objects may instantiate', further, that is, to the range of properties that appear in the scientific story about spectral reflectances.[15]

The key thesis of the Confrontation Picture, as it relates to observable properties such as colour, is the claim that the subject's perceptual awareness reveals intrinsic properties of the mind-independent objects perceived. The picture locates perceptual phenomenal qualities in the external world of mind-independent objects. In one form or another, this view is upheld by a number of writers on perception. A view similar to McGinn's is expressed by John Campbell (2002: 116):

> when you see the thing, you are confronted by the individual substance itself

and

> The phenomenal character of your experience...is constituted by...which particular objects are there, their intrinsic properties such as colour and shape.[16]

In trying to explain what it is to be in a visual relation to the things around one, Campbell invokes the analogy of seeing through windows that are *transparent*: in seeing, the mind is immediately confronted by the external world. In a similar vein, Heather Logue claims that 'our experiences are windows on the world'. No inner state or other kind of intervening entity mediates the subject's awareness of the external physical world.[17] Neither commentator expresses any concern over the circularity in these attempts at elucidation.

As these quotations illustrate, central to the Confrontation Picture is the idea that, in visual perception, the subject is immediately aware of the *intrinsic* properties of objects, *not merely of their effects*. The metaphors of confrontation and openness connect, somewhat obscurely, with spatial notions: nothing intervenes between the

[15] McGinn (1996: 545). McGinn's colour impressionism is very close to what has been called 'Colour primitivism': see Menzies (2004) and also Byrne and Hilbert (2007).

[16] Essentially the same view is defended in Travis (2004).

[17] Logue (2011: Section 3). The version of Naive Realism that Logue defends is atypical in allowing some contribution from the subject to the phenomenal character of experience.

subject and what is physically present in the surrounding scene; nothing prevents the external object itself entering the subject's consciousness.[18]

This picture pervades much contemporary writing about perception: the idea is that when I look at a ripe tomato in normal conditions, the redness I am aware of does not belong to my inner experience. It is as much an objective property of the tomato as its physical shape, mass, and chemical constitution. The idea is not that *every* aspect of the objective physical colour property is revealed in experience, but rather that, to the extent that the subject is immediately aware (in normal conditions) of a sensible property such as colour, then what they are aware of is an intrinsic feature of the external object. The phenomenal quality of redness is properly located in the external world. It is not a private quality belonging to the subject's inner state.

What can it mean to say that our experiences of qualities such as colours reveal the essential nature of a subset of the intrinsic properties of physical objects? We have an intuitive notion of an *intrinsic* property as a property belonging to a given object X, such that X has that property independently of the way things are outside of X. This intuitive notion proves hard to pin down precisely, but for the purposes of this chapter I shall assume that we have a good enough handle on what it entails.[19]

We need here to distinguish between three types of intrinsic property relevant to the debate about what we can perceive or know of the nature of physical objects. The *first* type of property to which the intuitive notion of intrinsicality applies is that which I shall call—loosely—a *scientific* property. This type includes properties such as mass, and also the complex properties that (on a Kripkean view) determine natural kinds such as gold, sugar, or being a cat. The scientific intrinsic properties that belong at one theoretical level of explanation—for example, being made of water—can be analysed in compositional terms down to lower levels, in which an internal complexity of structure is revealed. On some accounts, ultimately only structure and bare objects (propertyless things at the basic level) exist; there is no need for irreducible intrinsic properties to be posited.[20]

According to the view defended by Rae Langton, and also by David Lewis, there is a *second* type of intrinsic property; this relates to the type of properties that exist at the lowest level of analysis. Such are the *fundamental* intrinsic properties, upon which all other intrinsic properties supervene.[21] Langton and Lewis argue that we are forever precluded from knowing the nature of such fundamental intrinsic properties. Against such a view, it can be argued that we do know about them just

[18] It is worth noting that many intentionalists advance similar claims. Tye, for example, states that 'The phenomenal character of an experience, then, is out there in the world... In being aware of the external qualities, we are aware of phenomenal character. We are *confronted* by it' (Tye 2009: 119). Tim Crane (2011) puts forward a related view, arguing that 'central to the ordinary conception of experience seems to be the *presentation* of an object distinct from the state of mind itself'.

[19] Compare the discussion in Lewis (2009) and Weatherson and Marshall (2013).

[20] The notion that higher-level properties can arise from pure relations between bare particulars is contentious; however, see Esfeld (2003) and Esfeld and Lam (2011).

[21] Langton (1998) and Lewis (2001).

by virtue of knowing the causal relations that hold between the objects that instantiate them.

Independently of debates about the intrinsic properties that may or may not characterize the fundamental level of physical reality, we can grasp a good deal about higher-level scientific intrinsic properties through our understanding of the relations between physical things, how they causally interact with each other and with our senses, and through our theorizing about such matters. Nevertheless, the important point—for my purposes here—is that the essential inner natures of the type one *scientific* intrinsic properties are not directly observable. When I look at and bite into the apple, its DNA structure is not present in my experience in the way that its colour and flavour are.[22]

According to the Confrontation Picture illustrated by the quotations given above, there is a *third* type of intrinsic property belonging to physical objects, in addition to the two characterized above. These are the *sensible* intrinsic properties, which are, it is claimed, immediately revealed in experience. In normal perception, the phenomenal qualities I am aware of—such as the apple's redness and sweetness—are sensible intrinsic properties instantiated by the external physical objects I perceive. They are primitive and irreducible, and distinct from (though plausibly supervenient upon) the scientific properties discovered through empirical investigation.[23]

According to the Direct Realist view, there is no common factor shared by veridical and hallucinatory cases of experience. Veridical experiences form a special class. When I see a ripe tomato, it is a constituent of my non-inner experience. I am connected to it by a unique experiential relation. The phenomenal redness that I am aware of belongs intrinsically to that tomato, and not to an inner state of mine. Confrontation thus leads to revelation. Veridical perception informs us about the sensible intrinsic nature of the objects we encounter.

6.3 Problems for Direct Realism and the Confrontation Picture

There is a real problem about whether it is possible to make clear sense of the Confrontation Picture, and of the Direct Realist view it motivates. Not everyone agrees that experiences are non-inner, and that our perceptual experiences of

[22] With the appropriate background learning and set, a subject may directly (and defeasibly) perceive such properties to be present, in spontaneously exercising the corresponding concepts. However—according to one well-established tradition—such scientific properties are not immediately present in experience in the manner that the sensible properties are. My awareness of redness is at a sensory level, and requires no prior learning, whereas I can only come to be aware of spectral reflectances cognitively, through empirical discovery.

[23] Though for completeness, it is worth noting the claim that sensible intrinsic properties might be identified with the fundamental intrinsic properties (see Armstrong 1961: Ch. 15).

phenomenal qualities, such as colour, immediately reveal something of the sensible intrinsic properties of mind-independent physical things.

Many writers have argued on phenomenological grounds for the correctness of the Direct Realist view. But the projectivist version of the Causal theory has an answer to this objection. It is true that there is a directness to our perception of the world about us. However, as we noted at the outset, this is compatible with the fact that our cognitive grasp of perceptual objects is mediated by an awareness of phenomenal qualities belonging to inner experiences. The existence of deceptive hallucinations shows that the phenomenology of perception cannot be taken on its own to establish ontological claims about its structure.[24]

Moreover, facts about the nature of hallucinations have suggested compelling arguments in favour of the opposing view, the Causal Theory. Jonathan Lowe has defended the common factor conception of experience on the basis of what he terms 'the cut-off argument'. This argument appeals to two connected premises: first, the existence of hallucinatory experiences shows that the subject's brain states are sufficient for experiences *as of* external mind-independent objects; second, in the case of a veridical perception, the causal sequence of events leading from the object perceived to the subject's experience seems to involve the same type of subvening physical brain state that occurs when the subject hallucinates. In association, they strongly suggest that the character of a veridical experience does not depend *constitutively* on states of the environment external to the subject. Veridical, illusory, and hallucinatory experiences are inner states that form a common kind. They differ only in their causal ancestry.[25] To arrive at a positive account of perception, we should look to what is distinctive about the causes of the experiences that arise when we are perceiving the world around us. Arguably, the distinguishing feature of genuinely perceptual inner experiences is that they are caused by external objects in the appropriate way, so that they match (in an isomorphic sense) those objects to a certain degree, *and* also that such matching enables the subject to initiate activity making use of the objects. I say more about this dynamic positive account of perceptual experience in section 6.4.

The argument from hallucination for the Causal Theory has been the subject of much discussion in recent literature, and I shall say no more about it directly in this chapter. But there is a more fundamental problem for Direct Realism, a problem that is often overlooked: it is by no means easy to formulate a positive account of the Direct Realist position.

[24] The existence of complex (Charles Bonnet syndrome) hallucinations is a now well-established fact. See Manford and Andermann (1998) and also the papers in Macpherson and Platchias (2013: Part I).

[25] See in particular the defence of the Causal Theory elaborated in Lowe (2008). A version of the cut-off objection was originally developed and examined in great detail in Valberg (1992). Robinson (1994) puts forward a closely related argument. For some critical discussion see Martin (2004 and (2006), Smith (2002), Fish (2009), and Siegel (2008).

What is it for an experience to be non-inner? What can it mean to say that a conscious experience 'reaches out to and involves the perceived object'? The *metaphysical objection* to Direct Realism is that the view is unable to provide any coherent account of the experiential relation that, supposedly, is instantiated when a subject's consciousness makes contact with an external object through perception.

Introspective access provides us with some understanding of two different ways in which we can be conscious of things. The first is in sensation. Each of us has a moderately clear grasp of what it is for a feeling, for example of pain, to be a phenomenal constituent of our own experience. Pains are immediately present to consciousness. However, they are also private and subjective. Unlike the physical objects we perceive, pains are essentially mind-dependent. The phenomenal qualities attaching to one's awareness of sensations are very different in kind from the properties that belong to the physical objects we perceive.

In a different manner, through the exercise of intentional states such as thoughts, we can be cognitively conscious of mind-independent objects, items which are public and objective. But when I think about some particular external item, that item is not, *ipso facto*, present in my consciousness as a *phenomenal* constituent. The intentional object of my thought does not have any *actual* existence in my consciousness, in the way that a toothache has when I experience it. There is no real relation by virtue of which I am conscious in thought of a mind-independent item. The external, material object is only a constituent of my conscious thought in a *formal* sense, in so far as it contributes to the determination of its content. It need no longer even be in existence at the time that I entertain thoughts about it.

The upshot is that neither paradigm of conscious awareness can help us to understand the Direct Realist claim about perceptual consciousness, where some real entity is, allegedly, both phenomenally present in consciousness, yet also mind-independent. It is not at all clear how these two disparate features can be unified.

The only response open to the Direct Realist is to argue that the experiential relation distinctive of perception is irreducible, and *sui generis*. But this is a weak defence. It is simply unclear what kind of relation could fit the bill. How can an external physical thing, something mind-independent and objective, be included as a constituent in an individual subject's consciousness, in the phenomenal sense intended? The claim is tantamount to an appeal to magic. Something more needs to be said on the positive side, if Direct Realism is to lay any claim to being a plausible account of perception.

There is a further, more specific, difficulty for Direct Realism that arises in connection with the metaphysical argument. The Direct Realist faces an intractable problem in explaining how the perceptual object of an experience is to be determined. It is an essential feature of perception that the subject is related through experience to some particular object (or set of objects), and not to others. For this reason we distinguish veridical and illusory cases of experience, where there is some object perceived, from cases of hallucination, where there is no object with which the subject is in perceptual contact. As Grice pointed out (1961), the mere presence of an item X of kind F, together with the fact that the subject has experience as of an F, do not suffice to constitute a perception of X by that subject. It is incumbent upon any theory of perception to explain what further necessary condition is required. When I actually see a red apple on a tree nearby, I make visual contact with *that* particular apple, and not to others like it, however closely they may match my visual experience.

It will be helpful here to have a way of referring to this central feature of perceptual experience. Since the expression 'singular content', when applied to an experience, usually carries the implication that the experience has representational content, in an intentional sense, I need to use a less committal label.[26] Accordingly, I will speak here of the *individual content* of a non-hallucinatory experience. To speak of the individual content of an perceptual experience E is to specify *which* particular object in the subject's environment that experience E is *of* or *about*, if it is *of* anything, but in a manner that carries no presuppositions about the precise nature of perceptual content in general.

The issue I am concerned with here is what grounds or determines the individual content of a given experience. What principled reasons are available that justify us in claiming, in any given situation, that it is one particular object X that the subject S sees, or otherwise perceives, and not some similar-looking nearby object Y? For the Causal Theorist, there is a substantive answer to the question. In cases of vision, the subject sees the particular object X that is causally connected with the subject's experience in a dynamic way that could support successful navigational behaviour leading to beneficial use of that object X, in a manner that I sketch out further in the next section.

According to Direct Realism, questions about the determination of the individual content of an experience are to be answered by reference to the unique experiential relation. If it looks to me as if I see a red apple, then I am making perceptual contact with whichever apple I am connected to by the unique experiential relation involved in seeing. However, since we are unable to elucidate what the experiential relation amounts to, we are left none the wiser as to which object this is. I shall now show that no matter from which perspective we reflect upon the issue, the Direct Realist is unable to answer the metaphysical question about what it is that grounds individual content.

Consider, to begin with, the first-person perspective on experience. There is nothing manifest in experience that shows what is distinctive about the fact that I am seeing some *particular* ball X. Nothing that I am cognitively aware of enables me to discriminate a first case where it is the red ball X that I see, from a second in which I see a distinct, though similar red ball Y, or a third where I am hallucinating, and see nothing genuine at all. Therefore, what is available for me to grasp when I experience

[26] The question of whether or not perceptual experiences have singular contents is explored at some length in Tye (2009: Ch. 4).

a case of veridical perception is no different from what is revealed to my consciousness in a matching hallucinatory case. It follows that there is no relation to any item in the external world that I am able to grasp from the subjective point of view, which can inform my understanding of the alleged perceptual relation. In other words, although I am aware of what-it-is-like to have an experience *as of some* red ball, subjective experience yields no understanding of the nature of the which-it-is-of relation that connects me to *the particular* red ball X I actually am perceiving. First-person experience is, of course, essential to a grasp of the general phenomenology of the different modes and types of perceptual experience, but provides no insight into its ontology.

There is a temptation here, encouraged by the Confrontation Picture. This is to assume that we can arrive at an understanding of the experiential relation simply by reflecting upon our own situation in veridically perceiving an object. The reasoning starts from the premise that I know what it is like to be seeing some particular red ball when, for example, there is a red ball X directly in front of me, in broad daylight, and so on; when all the conditions for normal perception hold good. Since I am not aware of anything intervening between me and the ball X, I must know what it is like for X to be immediately present in my consciousness. Therefore I can arrive at an understanding of what it is for my experience to contain an external object.

But this line of thought rests on a confusion. The notion of experience appealed to here is one that presupposes a first-person perspective on my perception of an object. I certainly have an understanding of what it is like to have an experience type *as of* a red ball when I perceive one veridically; but this is indiscriminable from the understanding I have of what it is like to have an experience of merely hallucinating a red ball. I may be confronted by a red ball in a *purely spatial* sense, as an object present in my surroundings. But that fact on its own carries no implications about the nature of my subjective experience. As considerations concerning Gricean cases show, facts about the qualitative nature of my experience do not determine whether or not it is veridical, nor do they determine which object I am experientially related to—there may be several red balls in my vicinity. To adopt a sense of 'confrontation' that implies that the particular object physically confronted is a *phenomenal* constituent of the perceiver's experience is to presuppose a conception of experience for which there is, as yet, no entitlement. All that visual experience informs us about are the general appearance types of the objects we see. The first-person perspective cannot help us to understand what grounds individual content. Hence the first-person perspective does not provide any route to an understanding of Direct Realism.

To determine the material object of perception—an experience's individual content—we have to switch to an alternative standpoint, in which experiences are considered from a third-person perspective. In determining the object of perception in the case of a third party, we look to the *causal* factors relevant to the generation of his or her experience. The considerations that determine which external object an experience is *of*, which particular object is perceived in having that experience, are essentially causal. Most importantly, the conception of experience appealed to is that of an experience type, and *not* of an experience constitutively tied to any particular external object. The third-person perspective throws no light on what the unique experiential relation connecting a subject's consciousness to an external object could possibly be. It fails to suggest a genuine alternative to the causal theory of perception. Even when assessing my own case, I need to begin by considering my experience as a potentially independent occurrence, identified by its subject—myself—and its qualitative kind, and therefore as something possibly distinct from its perceptual object.

Let me illustrate these points by an example. Suppose that I have the experience of hearing a (single) humming noise when working in my study, and I try to work out what it is that is disturbing me. It turns out that there are several pieces of electronic equipment in neighbouring rooms, each creating some sort of humming sound. It may at first prove difficult for me to ascertain in any simple manner precisely *which* of the different objective sounds I am really hearing. Nothing that is subjectively available in my consciousness can resolve this issue on its own.[27] I am able to refer demonstratively to the sound as 'that humming noise', but from a purely first-person perspective I am unable to integrate my experience of the noise with any objective feature of the situation.[28]

In the end, following a painstaking process of turning switches on and off, I am able to determine which device is the source of the actual noise I am hearing. What I discover are objective facts about the causal origins of my experience, facts that are ascertained independently of knowledge of the ontological status of my experience. The causal relations between external events and the resulting neurophysiological processes in my brain—processes intimately connected with my experiences—are what determine that I am genuinely hearing an object, and not merely hallucinating. Crucially, they also determine *which* object I am hearing, allowing a specification of the individual content of my auditory experience. No appeal is made to any supposed direct experiential relation of the kind that the Direct Realist upholds. Knowledge of the causal factors that determine the perceptual object is independent of knowledge of any such relation. Such knowledge proceeds from a grasp of the experience *type*, one that is logically independent of the particular object perceived. (It has to be taken as independent: until we identify the relevant causal connections, we cannot determine which is the perceived object.) The basis upon which, in practice, we identify the perceived object supports the Causal Theorist's common-factor conception of experiences as inner states.

The Confrontation Picture and the associated ideas of transparency, and of open windows, throw no light on the Direct Realist account of individual content. They do not explain how the object of perception is to be identified, independently of causal

[27] And nothing subjectively available shows whether or not I am hallucinating.

[28] Evans presents an argument for this point (1982: Ch. 6), but it is often overlooked. In Coates (2009a), it is argued that considerations relating to demonstrative reference cannot support Direct Realism.

considerations.[29] Nor does the accompanying idea of revelation help to resolve the problem, in the absence of a principled basis for determining *which* features, of *which particular* objects, are revealed in the subject's experience. There is no clear, positive, non-causal account of what it is to be in direct perceptual contact with an object.

The upshot is that there is a serious problem for the Direct Realist in answering the metaphysical argument in favour of the causal theory. The Direct Realist account does not even begin to provide a coherent account of perception. Neither the first-person, nor the third-person, perspective on experience enables us to grasp the nature of the unique experiential relation that lies at the heart of the account. Unless it can be shown that there is some other way of grasping the experiential relation to the particular object perceived, the Direct Realist account must be dismissed as seriously flawed. There is no clear content to the view: it is unable to resolve the problem of determining the perceptual object. Direct Realism therefore threatens to become superfluous to any real understanding of perception. The theory ends up as *parasitic* upon a causal analysis of perception. In the remainder of this chapter I shall show, in addition, why it is *unnecessary* to appeal to the notion of an irreducible experiential relation and the accompanying idea of revelation.

6.4 An Alternative: The Navigational Picture

There is a lacuna in the Confrontation Picture that underlies Direct Realism. It fails to give any serious consideration to the question of what the knowledge gained through perception is *for*. The central function of perception is assumed to involve the acquisition of knowledge concerning sensible qualities, understood as a subset of the intrinsic properties of mind-independent objects. Such knowledge may support demonstrative reference to objects and some of their features, but the point of acquiring it is left open. The problem for the Confrontation Picture is that the analysis of perception is divorced from any consideration of the kinds of actions it typically generates. Spatial properties apart, knowledge of the intrinsic sensible properties of an object *as such* does not necessarily confer any advantage on the perceiver. Why should it matter to me whether an object is red or green, in itself? A red strawberry is sweet and nutritious; but a red berry from a different plant such as a yew tree, or a red-skinned frog, may be highly poisonous. It is only because of learned, *contingent*, associations between the way things appear and their causal properties that perceptually based knowledge about objects can be put to any constructive use.

There is an alternative picture, which points to a different conception of the role that perception plays in our lives. According to this second picture, perception is essentially connected with action. Perception helps us get around the world, and to

[29] For an excellent discussion of why the so-called transparency of perception is compatible with the conception of experiences as inner states, see Kind (2003).

act appropriately so as to increase our chances of surviving in it. It is true that for human beings, the awareness of phenomenal qualities of some kind is an essential feature of perception. This seems to be a deep contingent fact about our nature. However, this does not mean that phenomenal qualities should be equated with the sensible properties of external objects; rather, they belong to our inner states. All that is required for normal perception is that there exists a suitable degree of isomorphism between inner experiences and external objects, subject to the constraints I shall shortly spell out.[30] The role of perception in our lives is not to provide an immediate revelation of mind-independent properties, as the Confrontation Picture assumes, but to enable us to move safely through our surroundings and locate the objects we need, so as to make beneficial use of them, and hence to stay alive.

According to what I call the Navigational Picture, perception has the primary function of enabling the subject to *navigate* through the world, and to interact with the objects in it.[31] There are further, related, functions, which I shall come on to shortly; but it is the navigational function that is central. Distal modes of perception such as vision allow creatures to locate sources of nourishment and evade predators, to move around and to negotiate obstacles, and to single out objects in the environment for their own use (and also to avoid harm). In so far as perception leads to knowledge, that knowledge has its roots in practical activity.

For human beings, and other creatures capable of engaging in planned action-sequences, perceptually based knowledge need not be complete in all respects, so long as it enables us to steer through the world, arrive at moderately accurate beliefs about the location and usefulness of objects we encounter, and is conducive to successful action. As Sellars noted, the function of perception is to enable a creature to find its way around in a hostile environment.[32] Perception is essentially connected with the satisfaction of needs. It does not require the immediate revelation of the intrinsic qualities of objects of the kind envisaged on the Confrontation Picture.

I need to emphasize that I am not advocating a complete reduction of perception in terms of functional notions. Nor, it is important to note, am I endorsing the models put forward by defenders of the sensori-motor, or enactivist, theories of perception. Such theories find it difficult to account adequately for the subjective aspects of experience. Perceptually based navigational behaviour is, in the paradigm case, triggered by an object that causes the perception of it, which in turn leads to extended patterns of action focused upon that object. I see an apple in a tree, climb

[30] Sellars (1967), and more recently, Jonathan Lowe (1995: Ch. 3), have both emphasized the point that veridical perception (strictly, what we call 'veridical perception') only requires a certain degree of isomorphism between inner experiences and external objects.

[31] 'Function' is to be understood here as relating to what the subject is *currently* capable of, independently of evolutionary history. I have elaborated the navigational account more fully elsewhere, in Coates (2007: Ch. 7) and (2009b). The Navigational Picture has some affinities to the Causal Picture of experience outlined in Valberg (1992: 10–11).

[32] Sellars (1982).

up, reach for it so that I can then eat it. But this process is essentially mediated by distinct *inner* states, involving the (possibly irreducible) awareness of phenomenal qualities. Such states of awareness also occur where there is no disposition to act, and are not to be explained away by reference to our grasp of patterns of sensorimotor dependencies.

One obvious advantage of concentrating upon the navigational role of perception is that it helps us to appreciate the continuity between the perceptual processes of higher mammals and those of creatures further down the phylogenetic scale. From a biological point of view, it is clear that the effective use of perceptual processes, especially in distal perception, enhances the chances of survival to maturity. The development of sense organs has in consequence had an enormous effect on evolution. One current account emphasizes the central role, in more simple organisms, of the formation of perceptual systems enabling the detection of light. The development of rudimentary forms of vision around 540 million years ago, it has been argued, was the crucial driving force behind the Cambrian explosion of new life forms.[33]

So long as a creature can navigate through its surroundings so as to reach food sources, and avoid harm, it increases its chances of staying alive and reproducing. Complete and accurate knowledge of the surface properties of objects is not required for successful *action*. We may not fully understand the nature of the sensible properties that we take objects to manifest, nor grasp all of their intrinsic properties. But this does not prevent us from directly recognizing the categories to which the familiar objects that we interact with belong. It does not limit the success of our everyday perceptually based actions in moving around the world. What is essential to the experiences that issue in perceptual knowledge is that they contain information about the *locations* of objects in egocentric space, their *spatial structure*, and their *kinds* (natural or artificial), in so far as those kinds produce effects relating to our well-being. Subjects can still acquire useful knowledge of the surrounding world, even if they do not have an immediate phenomenal awareness of the intrinsic qualities of external objects. All that is necessary for knowledge leading to successful action is a suitable degree of isomorphism between our inner states and the external objects in our surroundings. What mattered when our ancestors saw a ripe fruit was that they recognized that it was edible, not that they grasped the real nature of the colour it displayed.

The isomorphism between the properties of inner visual states and external physical objects is of two kinds. There is an isomorphism relating to the spatial structure and layout of physical objects in our surroundings, and an isomorphism relating to the qualities of the surface structures of objects. For reasons of space I am not going to say much in this chapter about our awareness of spatial properties. I shall assume that we have an (implicit) a priori understanding of the nature of some

[33] For a development of this thesis, see Parker (2003).

simple formal geometrical concepts. I shall also be assuming that our inner visual experiences have a spatial structure, at least to the extent of allowing us to make sense of descriptions of their spatial characteristics. Formal spatial concepts have application to both the inner and the outer realm: (inner) visual experiences share a degree of spatial isomorphism with the external structures we perceive.[34] On introspecting, and also in theorizing about inner experiences, we can therefore apply our grasp of spatial concepts to experiences themselves. This grasp is what enables subjects, for example, to understand descriptions of certain typical kinds of migraine visual aura as 'crescent-shaped'.

Normally, however, we do not think of our inner visual states as such. In getting about the world, we do not attend to them, nor do we reflect upon their nature. More usually, the non-conceptual, phenomenal awareness of the spatial features of inner states causally guides the direct application of spatial concepts to external structures, when we arrive at perceptual beliefs about the objective layout, structures, and kinds of objects in our environment with a fair degree of accuracy. I see the uniform red colour of a folded gown without attending to the subtle differences in appearance of light and dark shades which the painter takes advantage of in portraying a likeness of the material in a convincing manner on the canvas. Looking at a table top from an angle, I directly see that it is rectangular, without reflecting upon the perspectival shape presented in the appearance. But it is the spatial character of my inner visual experience that guides my perceptual beliefs about shapes and positions of the things I see. There are issues here that require fuller discussion, but an elaboration of these ideas about the spatial structure of experiences is a task for another occasion. Here the main focus is upon colour qualities.

If these ideas about the navigational function of perception are correct, two things follow about our awareness of monadic phenomenal qualities such as colours. Firstly, different perceivers could, in theory, be aware of different shades of colour in perceiving the same objects; yet each of them would still be able to interact with the world as successfully as any of the others. Secondly, it leaves open the possibility that the sensible qualities of non-sentient objects can be given a full explanatory account in terms of the primary qualities that are discovered through detailed scientific investigation. It becomes plausible to claim that there is nothing more to objective physical colour than wavelength reflectance patterns, nor anything more to objective sound than rapid vibration, and so on.[35] In the next section I develop these ideas more fully.

[34] It is arguable that the Bela Julez random dot stereograms support the view that this shared spatial surface structure has a two-and-a-half dimensional form: visual hallucinations can have depth, even though they lack hidden surfaces.

[35] In an important series of papers, Grover Maxwell began developing an account of perception and structural realism consonant with this general view: see, e.g., Maxwell (1970) and (1972).

6.5 The Independence Claim

According to the Navigational Picture, the immediate revelation of the intrinsic nature of the surface properties belonging to physical objects is not necessary for our practical dealings with the world. The qualities immediately present in experience are in fact distinct from the physical qualities of the physical objects we perceive. Even if we were radically mistaken about the real nature of objective qualities such as physical colour, it would make no difference to the success of our everyday actions. This means that the Navigational Picture is committed to the following Independence Claim (IND), that:

(1) The phenomenal quality instantiations that we are immediately aware of in perception are not identical with the instantiation of any intrinsic qualities belonging to the external physical objects that we take to be present.[36]
(2) So long as there is a sufficient degree of correlation between inner experiences and physical things in the local environment such phenomenal qualities may differ in significant respects from the intrinsic properties of external physical objects, without affecting our ability to interact successfully with the world.

I shall now present three arguments in order to vindicate IND so far as concerns the colour qualities present in experience.

6.5.1 *The Inverted Spectrum and Connected Examples*

Prima facie, we seem to be able to make sense of standard inverted spectrum examples. Different conclusions have been drawn from this. The relevant point for my purposes in this chapter is that such inversions make no difference to the successful navigational actions of subjects. This follows immediately from the fact that in the standard examples, spectrum inversion is supposed to be undetectable: there are no behavioural differences between my inverted spectrum twin and myself.

Consider a simple model example. I see a tree from which there hang some apples of a certain kind, beyond my reach. By the red appearance of the apples, I judge that they are ripe and would be good to eat. So I find a stick, use it to knock the branch from which the apples hang, and cause some apples to fall so that I can select one and eat it. In order for me to carry out this extended action, there only needs to be an isomorphism between the properties and locations of the surrounding objects, and the properties of my experience—that is, the sensed colour qualities of inner experiences need only be the *counterparts*, in Sellars's sense, of the colour properties of external physical things. My inverted spectrum twin will be as successful as I am in obtaining the apple. For the purposes of achieving our practical ends, nothing is lost

[36] The focus here is on phenomenal qualities such as colour, corresponding approximately to Kant's intensive magnitudes.

if our inner experiences do not match. Knowledge of the real nature of physical colour properties is not required for action, so long as the experience of colour enables us to successfully track the objective properties of the objects we interact with.[37] Perception has developed in order to subserve a subject's needs, not to reveal the intrinsic properties of things.

One response to this argument is to deny the intelligibility of undetectable inverted spectrum possibilities, as Peacocke has done.[38] I don't think that such replies succeed, but I shall not press the point here, for we can also appeal to a case similar to the one that Ned Block discusses.[39] In a variant of the scenario imagined by Block, mad scientists operate on a subject—call him Casper—and place inverting lenses in his eyes. We can imagine this takes place at a very early stage in Casper's life. He grows up not realizing that his colour experiences are inverted relative to everyone else's. We could indirectly detect that his visual experiences differ in some way from ours, but only through the use of invasive procedures or sophisticated scanning techniques. Yet Casper can do all the things that we can do. He can perceive that there is an apple on the tree, and that it is ripe. Using his vision, he is able to select a stick to knock the branch from which it hangs, and so on.

This example provides the basis of a reply to a criticism voiced by Mark Johnston. He objects to the view that phenomenal colours belong to inner states on the grounds that this would lead to the 'incredible consequence' that I and my inverted twin could both 'immediately know just by looking that a German flag is red, yellow and black', despite having quite different experiences of it. He goes on to claim that:

> If external things are coloured, then their colours must be tightly connected to the qualities which visual awareness alone reveals ... perceptual judgements seem to predicate those very sensed qualities of environmental items. (Johnston 2006: 263)

There are really two criticisms conflated here. The first concerns the content of our attributions of physical colour properties. Johnston is perhaps assuming that the meaning of an objective colour term is necessarily connected with the way that samples of it are identified. But since Kripke's work, we have been aware that this model does not always hold good. Casper and his normal-sighted associates make identifying references to the same objective colour properties, but via the immediate consciousness of different phenomenal qualities belonging to inner states. There is no incredible consequence here.

The second point raised by Johnston's remarks concerns questions in the psychology and phenomenology of vision. It is indeed true that our perceptual judgements

[37] Wright argues for a similar point (Wright 2003: Section 5). I do not, however, accept Wright's intentionalist account of experience.

[38] In Peacocke (1988).

[39] Compare Block (1990).

about colour seem, in some sense, to attribute the phenomenal colours that we are immediately aware of to external surfaces. But this by itself cuts no ice. The same phenomenon of external attribution occurs in deceptive hallucinations. Macbeth *projects* the inner image of a dagger onto the world before him, into a space which lacks a corresponding real object. That is, he directly *takes* there to be a physical dagger externally present, without conceptualizing his inner experience in subjective terms. In such cases it is clear—to outsiders—that the locus of the relevant phenomenal qualities is, in some sense, in the subject's mind. They are wrongly interpreted by the subject as belonging to an external object.

Phenomenologically, deceptive hallucinations and veridical experiences are indiscriminable. Precisely the same phenomenon of projection takes place in the veridical case. In normal perception, the projection of inner states onto existing objects has the function of enabling the subject to form direct takings (perceptual beliefs) about the location of kinds in the world, takings that are sufficiently accurate to guide successful action. However, there need be no identity of the phenomenal colour quality of the inner experience and the external physical colour, so long as a suitable degree of isomorphism holds. So neither of the points that Johnston makes offers any basis for objecting to (detectable) spectrum inversion. What is lacking in Johnston's discussion is any serious treatment of the projectivist position with respect to colours, a view that does offer a plausible solution to the problems at issue here.

A related real-life case arising from variations in our subjective experience of colours gives rise to what I term 'the Shifted Spectrum' problem. There is now strong evidence that normal subjects differ slightly in their subjective experience of colour. In experiments on the determination of *unique hues*, it has been found that there is a significant amount of variation in the way that colours are perceived. There are complexities I shall ignore in outlining this phenomenon, but they do not, in any case, affect the main finding.

Colour researchers distinguish between the phenomenally simple hues—the unique hues, blue, green, yellow, and red—and (complex) hues that, considered from a subjective viewpoint, have a perceptually composite colour: thus purple is, in phenomenological terms, a mixture of red and blue; orange is seen to have a yellowish and a reddish component. In experiments, subjects are asked to identify the colours that they take to be the unique hues.

A subject will be asked, for example, to indicate which chip from a set of Munsell colour chips they perceive as completely blue, without any green or purple in it. The colour shade selected will correspond to the associated dominant wavelength. In such a manner it is possible, for each observer, to map each of the unique hues identified onto the visual part of the electromagnetic spectrum.

The surprising finding is that although subjects are self-consistent in their identification of unique hues over time, they do not all agree with each other on which colour shades are the unique hues. The variation is startlingly wide: the colour shade that some subjects identify as the unique blue is identified by other subjects as the unique green.[40]

So what is going on? One response is to appeal to cultural and other related factors, and to argue that the variation in hue allocation simply shows a difference in the way that subjects have learned the basic colour terms. The problem with this response is that, although it might explain minor variations and indeterminacy of the more complex binary hues (that subjects may not agree on what counts as a paradigm case of a purple hue, for example), it does not explain the fact that the unique hues are identified as having no other hue component.

Moreover, there are scientific reasons that can better explain the wide variation in response. When light from a narrow range of the spectrum impinges on the retina, all three types of cone in the eye will fire, although at different rates. A complex system of processing takes the input from the cones and ultimately produces the subjective experience of colour. There is, therefore, much room for physiological variation between observers, of the kind that will lead to different subjective experiences of the same objective properties. After all, at the extreme this is what happens in cases of colour blindness. The conclusion drawn by Kuehni (2004: 161) is:

> Most philosophers maintain a position of placing colours in objects. The finding of large individual repeatable variation in at least two of the four unique hues represents a serious obstacle to this position. It appears more likely that the brain/mind constructs images of the world rather than reconstructing them from nature.

I believe Kuehni is right on this issue. Subjects receiving the same input from an external physical colour source, in identical circumstances, appear to have different subjective colour experiences. Yet such differences in the subjective experience of colour do not, as far as we can tell, affect the abilities of subjects to deal successfully with the world. On a priori grounds, it is arguable that so long as subjects are able to exercise relational colour concepts, enabling them to discriminate between pairs of closely resembling shades, then they will not lose any practical abilities.

In an interesting paper, Michael Tye has defended the view that 'still there is a privileged class of Normal perceivers' who are accurate detectors of fine-grained hues. They happen—perhaps just through luck—to perceive the true colours of objects as they really are.[41] On the correlation view I favour, it is hard to make sense of such claims. There is *no* privileged class of normal visual perceivers who see things to be the colours that they really are. We have not evolved colour vision in order to accurately reflect monadic colour properties in objects, but to discriminate between objects in roughly the same category.[42]

[40] Unique hue variation is a well-established fact. For some discussion, see the introduction to Hardin's excellent (Hardin 1993).

[41] Tye (2006).

[42] It is of course still possible to account for *illusions* of colour by reference to a person's ability to detect and draw colour distinctions in agreement with those drawn by most observers in good conditions.

This ability helps someone to select the sweeter strawberries on a plant. Even Tye concedes that one main *present* function of the perception of differences in colour is to enable the fine discrimination between classes of objects with the same coarse-grained colour. The important point is that even if we could attach a meaning to the idea that the experiences of colour, for the lucky few, accurately reflected the properties of their environment, it remains the case that the phenomenon of unique hue variation demonstrates that the majority, who are supposed to have inaccurate experiences of colour, are still able to interact successfully with the world. As Tye is also forced to concede, we have no way of determining who belongs in the favoured minority of supposed accurate colour perceivers.[43]

These considerations about the actual and possible variations in our subjective awareness of colours all point to the same conclusion; the Independence Claim is vindicated. Differences in the awareness of phenomenal colour need not affect the ability of subjects to deal with the world—indeed, before careful experimentation many such differences pass unnoticed. But this is very much what we should expect on the Navigational Picture of perception. The precise nature of the phenomenal aspects of inner experiences is not important for the kind of knowledge that enables us to cope with the external world.

6.5.2 Sensory Substitution

A second line of thought that supports the Independence Claim arises from considerations relating to Sensory Substitution devices. The use of these devices presupposes a distinction between the sensations that subjects are immediately aware of in perceiving, and the objective features they detect, through perception, in the world. Those who start to employ them find that after a period of time there is a shift in their attention: whereas at first the awareness is mainly focused on their subjective sensations, after a while there is a transition. They start perceiving external objects in their surroundings directly. Although they are still in some sense aware of the sensations as a background to their consciousness of external objects, they no longer attend to them as such. It is still possible for subjects to switch their attention onto their inner sensations, but as they become more used to the devices, their perceptual focus is on outer things. This, again, is a form of projection: the sensations causally prompt the formation of conceptually rich perceptual experiences of the world.[44]

Such cases show clearly that navigation is possible without the immediate awareness of the external object interacted with, and lend further support to the independence claim. To object that sensory substitution devices have had only limited success, and that they only provide their users with a small amount of knowledge about their surroundings, is to miss the point. What they show is that subjects do not need to be immediately phenomenally aware of a subset of intrinsic properties of the

[43] See Tye (2007).

[44] For some discussion of the workings of sensory substitution mechanisms, see Lenay et al. (2003).

external physical object perceived, in order to have some degree of success in interactions with the world. Nor is it even necessary for there to be a precise correspondence, in all respects, between the phenomenal qualities immediately present and the external physical properties. All that we need in order to navigate about the world is some kind of isomorphism between the structure of inner experience and the structure of the physical world about us.[45]

6.5.3 *The Continuum Argument*

A rare and unfortunate visual condition, called achromatopsia, causes the victim to lose all awareness of colour in their vision. Typical subjects find it gradually harder to see the colours of things, although they still distinguish light and dark. They end up visually conscious of an achromatic world, only able to see various shades of grey.

It might be argued, in the spirit of the Confrontation Picture, that such cases only illustrate that, for any subject, there are restrictions on the range of objective properties that can be revealed in perception. Relatedly, there are species constraints with respect to perception: animals with only rudimentary vision may lack an awareness of the real colour of things, while humans lack a direct distal perception of electromagnetic phenomena, which certain fish perceive directly. These cases merely show some deficiency in the subject's perceptual system; they do not demonstrate that normal experiences are inner states, logically independent of the perceived world, as the Navigational Picture holds.

Yet these cases raise a difficulty for the Direct Realist conception of perceptual consciousness when explored further. Consider moving up the phylogenetic scale, from organisms that have only very rudimentary visual awareness, to higher animals such as primates and birds. Human beings are trichromates. We may be tempted to believe that normal humans, who have the complete set of three types of cone in the retina, see the full range of different colours. But other animals have different kinds of visual systems. Some see a greater range, into the ultraviolet part of the spectrum. Certain animals (including, it has been suggested, some human females) are tetrachromates, and—it is plausible to claim—experience hues unavailable to the rest of us. Pigeons are thought to have five different types of cone cells in the retina.

Now, it is important to appreciate the fact that there is no clear mapping of colours onto cone types. It is not the case that, as once assumed, one type of cone sees red, another blue, and so on. The opponent-pair system of colour vision works in a much more complex way. The vision of tetrachromates and pentochromates cannot map onto what we think of as normal human vision in anything like a straightforward way. Hence, it is unlikely that animals with more sophisticated vision simply see an

[45] It might be argued that in e.g. the Voice system, the subject is still immediately aware of some physical qualities, namely the sounds of the world. Even if this were true, it would not answer the main point. For the mapping of particular sounds to visual inputs is arbitrary. What the devices show is that we can *perceive* an external world feature F without F being immediately present in consciousness.

additional colour shade. It is perfectly possible that such animals see colours quite differently from the way we do, and that there is not even a partial overlap in the shades detectable by species with different kinds of retinas. If we think of the evolution, across different species, of a sensory system such as the eye, there seems to be a progression of possible kinds of colour experiences from the simple to the more complex and sophisticated. But this progression does not take the form of a smooth continuum, developing in a linear fashion, by a steady increase in the awareness of additional hues by different species. The way our vision compares with that of birds may be more like the way that the man with black, white, and grey vision compares with humans with colour vision. Very little in the achromatic sensory field is equivalent to the enormous range of phenomenal colours that normal humans make out. Equally, the colours that pigeons (and certain other birds) make out to be present in objects might well be of a very different nature to the range that we humans take to be present in objects. The claim is not that birds necessarily see more colours than we do, but that, on empirical grounds, it is highly probable that they experience objects as having a much richer set of colour properties than humans do, and that they can make out shades unavailable to human experience. There is certainly clear evidence that some non-human species can respond differentially to distinctions between patterns of wavelengths that human beings are unable to discriminate.

This presents a dilemma for the view that perception reveals the objective characteristics of the world immediately, through direct confrontation. If sight enables us to become aware of phenomenal colours, conceived of as qualities of the external physical world, then there are two main options: the first is to say that only the vision of normal human beings truly reveals the intrinsic colours really belonging to objects in the world. According to this first option, the visual systems of colour-blind subjects, *and also* of other creatures with greater powers of visual discrimination, are defective, and produce a constant stream of illusory experiences—even in cases where, in so far as their use of vision is concerned, they navigate around the world more successfully than we do. The second option is to claim that there is some other species—perhaps the pigeon, perhaps even some species not yet evolved, which can, or could, see the coloured world as it really is, while much of supposedly normal human colour experience is illusory, in the sense of not accurately reflecting the real colours that belong to physical objects. Neither option seems remotely plausible. Again, the appropriate conclusion to draw is that the role of perception is not to be explained in terms of confrontation and revelation, but in terms of successful interaction with the world. As Hardin has argued, the perception of colour has not evolved to represent the true properties of the environment, but to facilitate the functions of discriminating an object from its background, and of identifying and re-identifying objects.[46]

[46] See Hardin (2008), where arguments closely related to those adduced in the text are set out.

I believe that the three arguments set out above provide strong reasons for accepting the Independence Claim. For the purposes of successful interaction with the world in the navigational sense, what matters is the ability to locate, recognize, and discriminate objects, and to know how they will affect us. A suitable degree of isomorphism between the objects perceived and our inner experiences is sufficient for such activities. So long as we succeed in making beneficial use of objects, it does not matter whether or not perception provides an immediate awareness of the intrinsic sensible qualities belonging to external things.

On the view I am defending, navigation, in the sense explained, is the function central to our perceptual dealings with the world. But we also interact with the world in other ways. It is arguable that there exists an additional, distinctive, role for perception: we make use of perception in *examining*, and *inspecting* objects, in order to discover more about their precise nature. This raises some interesting matters about the more detailed ways in which perceptual experiences mesh with our actions, which I don't have space to deal with at the length they deserve. I shall confine myself to a general comment.

Analogous arguments to those considered above, in connection with the navigation function of perception, apply to its role in enabling us to examine objects: when I explore an object perceptually, turning it around and inspecting it closely, and so on, there are the same possibilities of spectrum inversion, and the like. Early chemical investigators made direct—and sometimes reckless—use of their senses in order to identify elements and compounds. But the central aim of this was to discriminate between different kinds of stuff, in order further to investigate their causal powers.[47] Experimenters required some practical means of identifying, and successfully re-identifying, different chemical kinds, in a consistent manner. All that an individual person requires for such recognitional purposes is an understanding of the stable, yet contingent, connections that hold between an objective kind and its subjective appearances. Again, the moral is that we don't have to assume that perceptual examination leads to the immediate awareness of the intrinsic properties of objects. In most cases what we are concerned with is how those objects will affect us, and affect each other: whether they will harm us by causing injury, or whether they can be put to practical use by way of providing food, tools, or shelter, and so on.

There is a further issue that connects with phenomenology of perception. There may be a deeper worry here about whether the Navigational Picture fully captures all there is to our awareness of objects and the kind of understanding of reality that we gain from our experience of the world. An objection might be made on the general grounds that the Navigational Picture suggests a conception of reality that is purely relational; the account offered is perhaps inadequate to explain our ordinary

[47] It is an interesting, and surely relevant, fact that Dalton, the founder of atomic theory and no mean experimenter himself, was colour blind.

common-sense idea that we deal with a world of substantial things, of physical objects that have intrinsic properties, in addition to their various relational properties.

Again, there is some truth in this objection, but it does not count against the Navigational Picture. Our understanding of the intrinsic nature of the kinds that make up our world operates at a number of different levels. Our grasp of objects comprehends more than an awareness of their spatial relations. In particular, our understanding of common-sense kinds is connected with their causal consequences, which include the ways they affect us through the senses. Part of what I grasp in knowing that a certain kind of stuff is, for example, common salt, is that it has a distinctive recognizable flavour. We gradually build up our ordinary knowledge about the kinds and inner natures of physical objects by investigating how they behave. It is arguable that our common-sense understanding of the intrinsic properties of objects, and of their material nature, is of a systematic nature, and has much in common with the way we form and justify scientific hypotheses.[48] We discover that an apple has nourishing properties, and grows under certain conditions, and is propagated by seed. At a deeper level, we discover through sophisticated experimentation that the intrinsic natures of kinds are connected with the properties of their micro-constituents. Gold turns out to have seventy-nine electrons in its atoms; the fact that gold looks yellow to most normally sighted humans should not be taken as revealing anything about its intrinsic nature, since, given the arguments above, the colour which it normally appears to have is a matter that is relative to perceivers and contexts, and does not directly reveal its essential constitution. Yet the fact that many kinds have a typical appearance is itself part of what we grasp in our common-sense appreciation of the nature of things.[49]

6.6 The Aesthetic Conception

There is one final picture of perception that I wish briefly to draw attention to, one which complements the Navigational Picture.

What I call 'the Aesthetic Picture' focuses on the sensuous, or sensational, aspect of experience—on the fact that perceptual experiences contain an essential phenomenal component, which distinguishes them from mere thoughts. Aside from its role in helping us to get about, perception can be appreciated as a process which produces

[48] As noted earlier, there is some scepticism about whether there exist intrinsic properties at the fundamental level: compare the discussion in Ladyman (1998), and the moderate structural realism argued for in Esfeld (2003) and Esfeld and Lam (2011). These points require more amplification and defence, for which I do not have space in the present chapter. I say more about them in my (Coates 2013).

[49] These arguments suggest that what it might be for a perceptual experience to be veridical or illusory is a complicated affair. Given the main argument of this chapter, one key aspect of veridicality is connected with the fact that a subject is able to determine spatial facts about the objects perceived directly, on the basis of experience. I leave more detailed discussion of this topic for a subsequent paper.

experiences that have aspects which we can contemplate and enjoy for what they are in themselves, in circumstances where neither revelation nor navigation matter.

I am thinking here of aesthetic experiences, or—since this notion is wide—of an important ingredient in much aesthetic experience, where the sensuous, non-cognitive, subjective nature of the experience is the primary focus of conscious attention. Aesthetic and related experiences in music and the visual arts certainly do have an important cognitive dimension; but there is, in addition, a way of responding to these artistic experiences by simply drinking them in, by enjoying what they are like at the phenomenal level, even when we are not trying to identify them or otherwise respond to them at a higher level.

The Aesthetic Picture is independent of, yet consistent with, the Navigational Picture outlined above. Perception, understood as involving navigational activity, is what enables me to find my way to an art gallery, a concert hall, or a restaurant. Looking at a painting, listening to some music, eating and drinking, and so on, will normally evoke some cognitive responses. I will exercise concepts relating to how the objective world is, or to how it is represented to be—I attend to the subtle manner in which a painting by Vermeer captures the faint shadows on a wall, I follow a fugal theme that keeps reappearing, I notice the different spices present in food, or the minerality in a wine, etc. I identify kinds, structures, and artistic creations. I respond by focusing in a cognitive manner on features that I perceive.

But such cognitive awareness arises against a background in which I am also immediately aware of a wide range of phenomenal qualities. Adopting a different conscious stance, the stance of introspection, I can reconceptualize my experiences, and focus my attention more directly upon the experiences themselves—or, more strictly, upon the sensuous, non-conceptual aspects of the experiences. In so doing, I can switch my attention away from the higher, cognitive aspects of my experience, and reflect upon, and attend to what the experience is like—I attend (by using concepts, of course) to the phenomenal qualities themselves. I immerse myself, and drink in the sounds, colours, or flavours immediately present in my experience.

But in adopting this second attitude, there is no reason to take the phenomenal qualities of which I am aware to belong out there in the world. I am simply focused upon what the subjective experience is like, in itself, *qua* experience. As far as *this* aspect of aesthetic experience is concerned, it would make no difference at all if I were hallucinating. In focusing upon the phenomenal aspect of my consciousness, I can disregard the intentional aspect of experience, and suspend any beliefs as to its veracity.

From the aesthetic standpoint, the idea that perception involves at its heart some kind of direct *revelation* of the external world again proves to be unnecessary. Reflection upon this aesthetic, or sensuous, dimension of perceptual experience supports the conclusion that nothing is lost from our intuitive understanding of what experiences are like, in themselves, if we regard them as inner states. What matters in perception, as far as the Aesthetic Picture is concerned, is, again, simply that the subject is aware of phenomenal qualities of some kind. What they belong to is irrelevant. These qualities *may* be, in some loose sense, isomorphic with the properties of the mind-independent objects perceived (they may, therefore, carry informational representational content about what is perceived). However, it is not necessary to claim that the subject is immediately aware of the intrinsic properties of those objects.

6.7 Conclusion

In this chapter I have explored some of the deeper motivations that underlie the competing accounts of perception put forward by Direct Realism and the Causal Theory of Perception. The main aim has been to show how a projectivist version of the Causal Theory makes sense, and does not entail a counter-intuitive analysis of experience. We can acquire perceptually based knowledge of the external physical world, while lacking an immediate awareness of some of the intrinsic properties of external things, such as their objective colours.

According to the Navigational Picture of perception, the central function of perception in our lives is to produce knowledge in a form that enables the perceiver to successfully interact with the world, so as to navigate around it, to examine it, and to make use of the objects in it. A further important aspect of perception consists in the fact that it involves phenomenal states, which the perceiver can focus upon for what they are in themselves, a feature that makes up one aspect of aesthetic enjoyment. In neither case do we need to claim that phenomenal qualities are located in the external world. These considerations support a projectivist view, according to which inner phenomenal states guide the concepts and categories we entertain directly about the external objects that we interact with.

It has been argued that a proper understanding of these roles that perception plays in our lives shows there are good reasons to uphold the Causal Theory. The rejection of Direct Realism does not imply paradoxical claims about the nature of experience. The Confrontation Picture of perception misleads us. Claims to the effect that the sensible qualities of external objects are immediately revealed in our perceptual experiences prove to be unnecessary.

Nothing is lost, according to the Navigational Picture of perception, if phenomenal colour qualities are viewed as located in the mind, and understood as belonging to inner states recruited to guide the perception of the external structural features of objects and the recognition of kinds. This is what projectivism and the Causal Theory of Perception assert. Moreover, nothing is gained by placing phenomenal qualities in the external world. As the metaphysical argument demonstrates, such a move fails to resolve the problem of explaining how the individual contents of our experiences are to be determined. Successful action does not require the revelation of the intrinsic sensible properties of external objects. The account of perception provided by the Causal Theory is adequate to explain our perceptually based dealings with the world.

It provides an obvious and straightforward answer to the problem of grounding individual content. The way is therefore open for a modified form of scientific realism, in which phenomenal qualities are properly understood as located in the mind/brain, and projected onto the world we interact with. However, the issue of their ultimate nature is a matter left entirely open by the arguments of this chapter.[50]

References

Allen, Keith (2011), 'Revelation and the Nature of Colour', in *Dialectica* 65/2: 153–76.

Armstrong, D. (1961), *Perception and the Physical World* (London: Routledge and Kegan Paul).

Block, N. (1990), 'Inverted Earth', in J. Tomberlin (ed.), *Philosophical Perspectives 4: Action Theory and Philosophy of Mind* (Atascadero, CA: Ridgeview), 53–79.

Byrne, A., and Hilbert, D. (2007), 'Colour Primitivism', in *Erkenntnis* 66/1: 73–105.

Campbell, J. (2002), *Reference and Consciousness* (Oxford: Clarendon Press).

Coates, P. (2007), *The Metaphysics of Perception* (London: Routledge).

Coates, P. (2009a), 'Perception, Imagination and Demonstrative Reference: A Sellarsian Account', in W. deVries (ed.) *Empiricism, Perceptual Knowledge, Normativity, and Realism* (Oxford: Oxford University Press), 63–100.

Coates, P. (2009b), 'The Multiple Contents of Experience: Representation and the Awareness of Phenomenal Qualities', in *Philosophical Topics* 37/1: 25–47.

Coates, P. (2013), 'Chess, Imagination, and Perceptual Understanding', in *Philosophy and Sport: Royal Institute of Philosophy Supplement* 73 (Cambridge: Cambridge University Press), 211–42.

Crane, T. (2011), 'The Problem of Perception', in Edward N. Alta (ed.), *The Stanford Encyclopedia of Philosophy* Spring, available at: <http://plato.stanford.edu/archives/spr2011/entries/perception-problem/>.

Drake, D. (ed.) (1920), *Essays in Critical Realism* (New York: Macmillan).

Egan, A. (2010), 'Projectivism without Error', in B. Nanay (ed.), *Perceiving the World* (Oxford: Oxford University Press), 68–96.

Esfeld, M. (2003), 'Do Relations Require Underlying Intrinsic Properties? A Physical Argument for a Metaphysics of Relations', in *Metaphysica: International Journal for Ontology and Metaphysics* 4: 5–25.

Esfeld, M., and Lam, V. (2011), 'Ontic Structural Realism as a Metaphysics of Objects' in Alisa and Peter Bokulich (eds), *Scientific Structuralism* (Dordrecht: Springer), Ch. 8.

Evans, G. (1982), *The Varieties of Reference* (Oxford: Oxford University Press).

Fish, W. (2009), *Perception, Hallucination and Illusion* (Oxford: Oxford University Press).

Grice, H. P. (1961), 'The Causal Theory of Perception', in *Supplementary Proceedings of the Aristotelian Society* 35: 121–52.

Hardin, C. (1993), *Color for Philosophers*, 2nd Edition (Indianapolis, IN/Cambridge: Hackett).

[50] Many thanks to Philip Goff, Trevor Levere, Paul Noordhof, Jonathan Salisbury, Paul Snowdon, and especially to Sam Coleman for discussion and helpful comments on earlier versions of this chapter.

Hardin, C. (2008), 'Color Qualities and the Physical World', in E. Wright (ed.), *The Case for Qualia* (Cambridge, MA: MIT Press), 143–54.

Hobson, K. (2013), 'In Defence of Relational Direct Realism', in *European Journal of Philosophy* 21/4: 550–74.

Jackson, F. (1998), *From Metaphysics to Ethics: A Defence of Conceptual Analysis* (Oxford: Clarendon Press).

Johnston, M. (1992), 'How to Speak of Colors', in *Philosophical Studies* 68: 221–63.

Johnston, M. (2004), 'The Obscure Object of Hallucination', in *Philosophical Studies* 120: 113–83.

Johnston, M. (2006), 'Better than Mere Knowledge? The Function of Sensory Awareness', in T. Gendler and J. Hawthorne (eds), *Perceptual Experience* (Oxford: Oxford University Press), 260–90.

Kind, A. (2003), 'What's So Transparent about Transparency?', in *Philosophical Studies* 115 (3): 225–44.

Kuehni, R. (2004), 'Variability in Unique Hue Selection: a Surprising Phenomenon', in *Color Research and Application* 29/2: 158–62.

Ladyman, J. (1998), 'What Is Structural Realism?', in *Studies in History and Philosophy of Modern Science* 29: 409–24.

Lambie, J., and Marcel, A. (2002), 'Consciousness and the Varieties of Emotion Experience: A Theoretical Framework', in *Psychological Review* 109/2: 219–59.

Langton, R. (1998), *Kantian Humility* (Oxford: Clarendon Press).

Lenay, C., Gapenne, O., Hanneton, S., Margue, C., and Genouelle, C. (2003), 'Sensory Substitution: Limits and Perspectives', in Y. Hatwell, A. Streri, and E. Gentaz (eds), *Touching for Knowing: Cognitive Psychology of Haptic Manual Perception* (Amsterdam and Philadelphia, PN: John Benjamins), 275–92.

Lewis, D. (2001), 'Redefining "Intrinsic"', in *Philosophy and Phenomenological Research* 58/2: 333–45.

Lewis, D. (2009), 'Ramseyan Humility', in David Braddon-Mitchell and Robert Nola (eds), *Conceptual Analysis and Philosophical Naturalism* (Cambridge, MA: MIT Press), 203–22.

Logue, H. (2011), 'Why Naive Realism?', in *Proceedings of the Aristotelian Society* 112/2: 211–37.

Lowe, J. (1995), *Locke on Human Understanding* (London: Routledge).

Lowe, J. (2008), 'Against Disjunctivism', in A. Haddock and F. Macpherson (eds), *Disjunctivism: Perception, Action, Knowledge* (Oxford: Oxford University Press), 95–111.

Macpherson, F., and Platchias, D. (2013), *Hallucination: Philosophy and Psychology* (Cambridge, MA: MIT Press).

Manford, M. and Andermann, F. (1998), 'Complex Visual Hallucinations', in *Brain* 121: 1819–40.

Martin, M. (2002), 'The Transparency of Experience', in *Mind and Language* 17/4: 376–425.

Martin, M. (2004), 'The Limits of Self-Awareness', in *Philosophical Studies* 120: 37–89.

Martin, M. (2006), 'On Being Alienated', in T. Gendler and J. Hawthorne (eds), *Perceptual Experience* (Oxford: Oxford University Press), 354–410.

Maxwell, G. (1970), 'Theories, Perception and Structural Realism', in R. Colodny (ed.), *The Nature and Function of Scientific Theories* (Pittsburgh, PN: University of Pittsburgh Press), 3–34.

Maxwell, G. (1972), 'Russell on Perception', in D. Pears (ed.), *Bertrand Russell: A Collection of Critical Essays* (New York: Anchor Books), 110–46.

McDowell, J. H. (1986), 'Singular Thought and the Extent of Inner Space', in P. Pettit and J. H. McDowell (eds), *Subject, Thought, and Context* (Oxford: Clarendon Press), 137–68.

McGinn, C. (1996), 'Another Look at Color', in *Journal of Philosophy* 93/11: 537–53.

Menzies, P. (2004), 'The Folk Theory of Colours and the Causes of Colour Experience', in I. Ravenscroft (ed.), *Minds, Worlds, and Conditionals: Essays in Honour of Frank Jackson* (Oxford: Oxford University Press), 141–60.

Millar, A. (1991), *Reasons and Experience* (Oxford: Clarendon Press).

Parker, A. (2003), *In the Blink of an Eye* (New York: Basic Books).

Peacocke, C. (1988), 'The Limits of Intelligibility: A Post-Verificationist Proposal', in *Philosophical Review* 97/4: 463–96.

Robinson, H. (1994), *Perception* (London: Routledge).

Sellars, W. (1967), *Science and Metaphysics* (London: Routledge and Kegan Paul).

Sellars, W. (1975), 'The Structure of Knowledge', in H. Casteñeda (ed.), *Action Knowledge and Reality* (Indianapolis, IN: Bobbs-Merrill), 295–347.

Sellars, W. (1982), 'Sensa or Sensings: Reflections on the Ontology of Perception', in *Philosophical Studies* 41: 83–111.

Siegel, S. (2008), 'The Epistemic Conception of Hallucination', in A. Haddock and F. Macpherson (eds), *Disjunctivism: Perception, Action, and Knowledge* (Oxford: Oxford University Press), 205–24.

Smith, A. D. (2002), *The Problem of Perception* (Cambridge, MA: Harvard University Press).

Snowdon, P. (1981), 'Perception, Vision and Causation', in *Proceedings of the Aristotelian Society* 81: 175–92.

Snowdon, P. (2005), 'The Formulation of Disjunctivism: A Response to Fish', in *Proceedings of the Aristotelian Society* 105: 129–41.

Strawson, G. (1989), '"Red" and Red', in *Synthese* 78/2: 193–232.

Travis, C. (2004), 'The Silence of the Senses', in *Mind* 113: 57–94.

Tye, M. (2000), *Consciousness, Color, and Content* (Cambridge, MA: Bradford/MIT Press), 165–6.

Tye, M. (2006), 'The Puzzle of True Blue', in *Analysis* 66/3: 173–8.

Tye, M. (2007), 'True Blue Redux', in *Analysis* 67/1: 92–3.

Tye, M. (2009), *Consciousness Revisited* (Cambridge, MA: MIT Press).

Valberg, J. (1992), *The Puzzle of Experience* (Oxford: Clarendon Press).

Weatherson, B., and Marshall, D. (2013), 'Intrinsic vs. Extrinsic Properties', in Edward N. Alta (ed.), *The Stanford Encyclopedia of Philosophy* Spring, available at: <http://plato.stanford.edu/archives/spr2013/entries/intrinsic-extrinsic/>.

Wright, W. (2003), 'Projectivist Representationalism and Color', in *Philosophical Psychology* 16/4: 515–29.

7

Real Direct Realism

Reflections on Perception

Galen Strawson

Philosophy is often a matter of finding a suitable context in which to say the obvious

(Murdoch 1964: 33)[1]

7.1 Introduction

I'm looking at a poppy in front of me in normal circumstances. Do I directly perceive the poppy? Common sense says yes, and I'm going to take it that common sense is right. There's no magic determinacy in the word 'direct', and its use in the philosophy of perception has caused horrible confusion, but this seems the best thing to say if we're going to use the word 'direct' at all when talking about perception. Certainly any perception of an object *x* involves a mental presentation or representation of *x*, as well as *x* itself. No mental (re)presentation, no perception. If anyone disagrees, the disagreement can only be a terminological matter of a kind that we must hope to be able to resolve. We don't, however, perceive the sensation-involving mental (re)presentation that must exist when we consciously perceive an object (for a qualification that has no place here, see Strawson 2015: §18). We perceive the object. We are, as some say, in 'direct perceptual contact' with the object.

I think it's relatively easy to state what a direct realist must hold if direct realism is true. The basic issues have been clear for a long time; they haven't been changed by advances in science. Descartes and Arnauld, perhaps, are the ones we should set our sights by, with some guidance from Reid. These philosophers' writings are open to different interpretations, but their shared belief that minds are immaterial certainly doesn't prevent them from articulating the sense in which perception of the world is

[1] When I cite a work I give the date of first publication, or occasionally the date of composition, while the page reference is to the edition listed in the bibliography.

direct. As Arnauld says, we can 'know material things... immediately, i.e. without there being any intermediary between our perceptions and the object' (1683: 77).

Conscious sensory perception is of course a causal process, involving states of the brain, as Descartes, Arnauld, and Reid all know. But this doesn't raise any problems for the claim that our perception of objects in the world may be said to be direct or immediate in the normal case.[2] The facts are relatively straightforward, when it comes to the core philosophical problems (as opposed to scientific problems) associated with a sensory modality like vision. When philosophers muddy things, it's usually enough to fall back on a lay-scientific understanding of light, reflection, and so on.

7.2 Direct Realism about Thought

I'm a direct realist about thought as well as perception. Just as we don't perceive mental representations of objects, but the objects themselves, so we don't think about mental representations of objects, but the objects themselves. I suspect that nearly all philosophers are direct realists when it comes to thought, however unreflectively, even when they're not direct realists when it comes to perception.

This point can be invoked to support direct realism in the case of perception. I think few would want to say that perceiving an object right in front of one puts a barrier between oneself and the object that doesn't exist when one thinks about that object! It's true that Descartes thinks that we can apprehend an object *clearly and distinctly* only when we think about it, and that we apprehend it only *confusedly* in perception. To say this, though, is certainly not to say that we aren't in direct mental contact with it in both cases.

7.3 A Caveat

I'll focus mainly on perception, and, conventionally, on vision. I'll assume that physicalism is true (by 'physicalism' I mean what one might call 'Hobbes-Russell-Feigl-Maxwell physicalism', physicalism that is truly realist—see pp. 218–19 below—about consciousness or experience), and that we inhabit a physical world more or less as we think we do. ('More or less as we think we do' is designed to rule out things like Berkeleian idealism while allowing for all the strangenesses of physics.) I'll start with a caveat, followed by some terminological preliminaries. Then I'll put down a sea anchor.

The caveat is this. The biggest mistake one can make, in starting out to give a theory of perception, is the mistake of thinking that one's theory has somehow to meet or answer scepticism about the external world. I think it's safe to say that any

[2] In section 7.9 I square Arnauld's fierce rejection of the idea that perception involves 'representative entities' with the claim that all perception involves mental representation.

philosopher of perception who starts out with this goal is going to go wrong—even if it's only a subsidiary goal.

More strongly: any theory whose terms permit the refutation of scepticism about the external world—either scepticism about its existence, or about our knowledge of its nature—is *ipso facto* refuted; for such scepticism is not refutable. To attempt to refute scepticism is to accord it too much force. To acknowledge that it is formally irrefutable, and then move on to other things, is to keep it in proportion. Whatever you do, don't ask direct realism to guarantee that we're in direct contact with objects in such a way that we can know that scepticism about the external world is false. Once the question of scepticism arises, direct realism takes a conditional form: *if*—given that—you're a real person in a real world more or less as you think you are, in the sense defined two paragraphs back, then the right or best thing to say is that you directly perceive objects; i.e. that direct realism is true. It certainly doesn't follow from this that you can know (or know you know) the nature of the objects that exist in your world. No realist theory of perception that has this consequence can be correct. More generally: direct realists don't need 'to offer a positive account of how beliefs about material objects are justified' (BonJour 2011: section 2.3). They don't have to engage with such epistemological issues. This is neither a requirement on a direct-realist approach, nor a necessary motive for one. Thinking otherwise has been a potent source of confusion.

Nor do direct realists need to endorse the view that what Mackie called 'colour-as-we-see-it' (Mackie 1976: 24) is, as St Augustine supposed, 'a quality that is spread out on the surface of bodies'.[3] This is fortunate, for although there's a clear sense in which there are hard facts about what colours things are (snow is white, blood is red), it's beyond reasonable doubt that colour-as-we-see-it isn't Augustinian.[4] Direct realism has no difficulty with this fact, for it allows, as any sensible theory of perception must, that perception is essentially a *transaction*, a transaction between perceiver and object perceived of such a kind that what is actually experienced in perception is a function both of the nature of the object and of the nature of the perceiver. It also allows, more particularly, that the same thing may possibly appear differently to—be experienced differently by—two different normal perceivers, in respect of colour, say, in the same lighting conditions, even while it remains true that both directly perceive the object and that both perceive the colour of the object, and that both agree in all their verbal colour judgements. Locke puts this point perfectly in 2.32.14–15 of his *Essay*. (It's independent of the issue between direct and indirect realism.)

[3] 'Une qualité répandue sur la surface des corps' (Malebranche c.1680–90: 6.68 characterizing Augustine's view; 1st ed: 'répandue dans les corps').

[4] I have nothing to say to those—'relationalists' or 'primitivists'—who doubt this rather beautiful fact, but I wish them well.

One of the perceivers may be Martian and the other human, but both may be human; it doesn't matter. The present point is that direct realism can't be expected to take on the burden of implying that perception gives us knowledge of the nature of external things 'as they are in themselves'. Direct perception is one thing; knowledge of the nature of the thing perceived is quite another.

One of the ironies of the view that colour is Augustinian is that it opens up the possibility that it is vanishingly unlikely, in the case of any individual, that he or she ever sees things as the colour they are, given that there is bound to be considerable interpersonal variation in colour-experience across human beings with normal colour-discrimination abilities. It also seems to have the consequence that we don't and can't actually know what colours things are. A thing that is Augustinian green might always produce red-experience in human beings with normal colour-discrimination abilities. More moderately, a thing that has specific Augustinian shade #1435 (say) might always produce colour-experience that is shifted a few degrees towards yellow (say) in human beings with normal colour-discrimination abilities.

Children are highly speculative creatures, and many of them spontaneously consider and take pleasure in (or worry about) the idea that other people may not perceive colours exactly as they do themselves—while realizing that they can never know whether this is so or not. Children quickly accept this possibility even as they persist in the view that 'colour-as-we-see-it' is 'a quality that is spread out on the surface of bodies'. There's obviously a tension in this position, given certain other natural assumptions, but it's hardly noxious in everyday life, and they're on the right track in their speculations about others, for it is (again) beyond all reasonable doubt that some—many—of those who make the same colour judgements don't experience colours in exactly the same way. Human beings vary strikingly with respect to the details of their possession of all common features that are objectively measurable; it would be astonishing if they didn't also vary with respect to common features that aren't objectively measurable. But this fact isn't grounds for an objection to any worthwhile version of direct realism. When my companions and I look at something and think that we may not be experiencing its colour in exactly the same way, this doesn't undermine our conviction that we're in direct perceptual contact with the object. Nor should it.

7.4 Real Realism about Experience

It makes perfectly good sense to talk of unconscious perception, unconscious awareness. The flexibility of the word 'conscious' allows us to say that one can be conscious of something of which one has no conscious awareness. One can also be said to be conscious of something *x* (subliminally) although one has no idea that this is so—so that one might even talk of unconscious consciousness of *x*. In this chapter, though, I'm going to restrict attention to paradigm cases of conscious perception, perceptions which essentially involve experiential qualitative character, experiential 'what-it's-like-ness', phenomenological character, which I'll simply call 'experience', for short.[5] Some, perhaps, think that bodily states (including 'enactive' states) can constitute perception without involving experience in the current sense, i.e. experiential (essentially mental) what-it's-like-ness. Such views are not my concern here.[6]

I'm a realist—a real realist—about experience. The pleonasm would be unnecessary if some philosophers hadn't claimed to be realists about experience while covertly denying its existence. Perhaps the best way to convey what it is to be a real realist about experience is to say that it's to take colour experience, or taste experience, or experience of pain, considered generally and just as such, i.e. just as subjective feeling, to be exactly what one took it to be—knew it to be in having it—before one did any philosophy: when one was six, for example, and was given food whose taste one didn't like, or asked a friend what something tasted like, or whether they liked the taste, or turned in the direction of a bright light with closed eyelids and experienced reddish-orange, and then covered one's eyes with one's hands and watched the reddish-orange dim to black; or wondered, as children often do at that age (vividly aware of the sense in which experience is essentially private), whether one's brother, sister, or friend saw colours exactly as one did oneself. Children of this age make many experiments with experience. They squeeze their eyeballs to see double, rub their closed eyes to 'see stars', block and unblock their ears, spin round until they're dizzy and then stop and watch the world swirling, fully aware that it's their experience, not the world, that is swirling. They're well aware that objects that have a constant colour appear to be different colours in different lights, that their faces and the faces of their friends look a different colour under a neon light in a bathroom mirror, and so on. They're fully competent with the general conception of experience that appreciation of these phenomena involves (the only conception of experience that concerns us at present) whether or not they can be said to possess this conception in any linguistically expressible form.

This is real realism about experience.[7] However many new and remarkable facts real realists about experience learn from scientists—facts about the neurophysiology of experience, or the 'filling-in' that characterizes visual experience, or 'change blindness', or 'inattentional blindness', or the complex and surprising mechanisms of taste experience[8]—their basic *general* understanding of what colour experience or

[5] This is the mass term use of 'experience'; adjective 'experiential'. I use 'phenomenological' rather than 'phenomenal', when speaking of the experiential-qualitative character of experience, because 'phenomenal' is for many strongly associated with sensory phenomenological character to the exclusion of cognitive phenomenological character. I take 'phenomenological' to be an essentially general word that covers all aspects of experiential qualitative character (see Bayne and Montague 2011).

[6] See e.g. Noë (2004).

[7] One might also characterize real realism about experience as the view of experience that is shared in all essentials by (to take a tiny sample) Block, Chalmers, Chomsky, Fodor, (early) Jackson, Kripke, Levine, Lockwood, McGinn, Nagel, Parfit, Quine, Searle—not to mention all philosophers prior to about 1915.

[8] See e.g. Grimes (1996), Simons and Levin (1997), Chun and Marois (2002), and Pessoa and de Weerd (2003).

pain experience (etc.) is remains exactly the same as it was before they did any philosophy. It remains, in other words, wholly correct, grounded in the fundamental respect in which to have experience is already to know what it is, however little one reflects about it. There is, to repeat, a fundamental respect in which *the having is the knowing*. This is because the knowing is just—just is—the having (it involves no 'introspection'). The having is all there is to the knowing, in this fundamental sense of 'know'; it's (non-discursive) knowledge 'by acquaintance'.[9]

The point can be extended—from general knowledge of what experience is to knowledge of the experiential character of particular experiences. It's not undercut by the fact that people may give sincere false reports of the character of their experience, or by evidence for the unreliability of introspection, for the following points remain untouched. (1) The experience is a real, concretely occurring process with a certain experiential-qualitative character. (2) Its experiential-qualitative character is—necessarily—the experiential character it has for the subject as it happens. (3) Its having the experiential-qualitative character it has for the subject as it happens constitutes the subject's knowing its experiential character in the present sense.

That said, it's worth adding that the present claim (that non-philosophers have a completely correct general understanding of what experience is) would remain untouched even if it could be shown that people can somehow be wrong in certain ways about the experiential-qualitative character of their current experience just in having it, rather than in some judgement they make about it.

There's no need to consider conceptual or propositional knowledge in this connection, but there's also no reason to deny that concept-exercising creatures may automatically come into possession of *concepts* of particular experiences and of particular kinds of experience as they have them, 'demonstrative' concepts whose content is given—fixed—simply by the character that those (kinds of) experience have for them as they have them, and which can as concepts feature as constituents of judgements and beliefs.[10] Plainly this doesn't give concept-exercising creatures any

[9] The view that the having is the knowing is now sometimes called *Revelation* (Johnston 1992: 223); it's close to the view Lewis calls the 'Identification Thesis', according to which 'anyone acquainted with a quale knows just which property it is' (Lewis 2001: 217). Using 'identify' in a rather unusual way, Lewis claims that common sense endorses the Identification Thesis: 'folk psychology says, I think, that we *identify* the qualia of our experiences. We know exactly what they are—and that in an uncommonly demanding and literal sense of "knowing what"' (Lewis 1995: 327). This seems correct, but Lewis thinks that physicalism requires one to reject the Identification Thesis: 'as a materialist', he writes, 'I reply predictably: the Identification Thesis is false' (Lewis 2001: 217). This, however, seems to be a mistake, a mistake about what materialism requires. It is perhaps the very big mistake (see the next section) of thinking that materialism is in tension with real realism about experience. (This said, I'm not sure what Lewis means by 'quale' or by 'knows just which property it is'.)

[10] One can allow that demonstrative concepts can carry infallibly known content into propositionally contentful thoughts, beliefs, and judgements, while continuing to maintain that fallibilism is sovereign as soon as one considers the semantic evaluation of such thoughts, beliefs, and judgements (their evaluation with respect to truth or falsity). Certainly one can agree with Hume that 'many of our ideas are so obscure, that 'tis almost impossible even for the mind, which forms them, to tell exactly their nature and composition' (Hume 1739–40: 1.2.3.1).

advantage over non-concept-exercising creatures when it comes to the knowing which is the having.

7.5 Real Physicalism

Real realism about experience is not only wholly compatible with physicalism; it's diagnostic of any serious or realistic physicalism. Some philosophers deny the existence of (real) experience, overtly or covertly, and call themselves 'physicalists', but the existence of the wholly concrete phenomenon of experience, as conceived of by real realism about experience, is a certainly known natural fact. It is therefore, for any remotely realistic physicalist, hence any *real* physicalist, as I'll say (defining 'real physicalist' by reference to 'realistic physicalist'), a wholly physical fact.

All physicalists, real or not, say that experiential states are physical states—neural states, in our terrestrial case. But when *real* physicalists say that experiential states are neural states, they don't mean anything like what some self-styled physicalists have seemed to mean by saying this. They don't mean that experiential states aren't really experiential states as conceived of by real realism about experience (six-year-old or pre-philosophy realism about experience), but are rather things whose whole nature can in principle be revealed by physics and neurophysiology. When *real* physicalists—Hobbes-Russell-Feigl-Maxwell physicalists, to choose a few names from a multitude—say that experiential states are neural states, they mean that experiential states considered specifically as such, i.e. considered as things whose nature as experiential is known to us by direct acquaintance (whether wholly or in part) simply in the having of experience, are wholly physical states.

It follows from their view that the intrinsic nature of the physical is fundamentally more than anything revealed by physics and neurophysiology. Real physicalists hold, as any realistic physicalist must, that experience wholly realistically conceived is as much a physical phenomenon as electricity. If you're not a real realist about experience, you can't really claim to hold that there's such a thing as conscious perception at all. This is because you deny the existence of something essential to the existence of conscious perception: experience.[11]

'If you focus on conscious perception in this way, you won't address the question of perception in full generality.' Any general theory of perception has to deal with the case of conscious perception, and the account I'm going to give generalizes to all cases of perception (see section 7.17).

Now for the sea anchor.

[11] Russell put the point strongly: 'we know *nothing* about the intrinsic quality of physical events except when these are mental events that we directly experience' (Russell 1956: 153, my emphasis); 'as regards the world in general, both physical and mental, *everything* that we know of its intrinsic character is derived from the mental side' (1927: 402, my emphasis). See also Feigl (1958, 1967), Maxwell (1978), Strawson (2003a).

7.6 The Sea Anchor: Representation

To be concerned with conscious perception, essentially experience-involving perception, is to be concerned with the relation between mind and reality, mind and world, as we loosely say. (It seems a safe remark, although we live in wild philosophical times.) And the first and fundamental fact about mind is that it only ever detects—makes contact with—anything in the world by representing it: no defensible conception of direct contact between mind and world can conflict with the fundamental fact that mind relates to reality by representing it. Mind has to represent reality in order to know about it in any way—in order to be in any sort of perceptual or cognitive contact with it. This is what mind does. This is the sea anchor. This is where we start from. If someone thinks there's a tension between direct realism and the view that the mind represents the world, they have a mistaken conception of what perceptual representation is.

One way to put things is as follows.

(1) For mind to *perceive* concrete phenomenon x in the world is necessarily for mind to *register* x in some way.

(2) For mind to *register* x in some way is for mind to *represent* x in some way.

So

(3) For mind to *perceive* x is for mind to *represent* x.

No one can object to (1), and I take (2) to state a necessary (trivial) condition of registration of x on the part of mind. I don't mean more by 'represent' than this. Conscious sensory perception of x obviously entails *some* sort of mental registration of x, and mental registration of x entails mental representation of x. Here we're not concerned just with representation, but with conscious perceptual representation, which also, of course, involves sensation, but the core notion is simply registering, mental registering, which needn't be conscious, or involve sensation. If you accept the idea that minds register things in perception, you already accept the idea that minds represent things in perception. Representation in this sense can be very primitive, but it is none the less a rock-solid necessary condition of perception—whatever is sufficient.[12]

One reason people have for being wary of the notion of representation can be expressed as follows: 'To suppose that a subject's perceiving x involves the subject's having a mental representation of x is to postulate something—the

[12] One can strengthen (2) into a biconditional stating a necessary and sufficient condition of mental registration, or indeed into an identity statement: mental registration is mental representation. I'm not concerned with currently popular theories called 'representationalism' or 'representationism', only with representation.

mental representation of *x*—existing in between the subject and *x* in such a way as to make the subject's perception of *x* indirect. And this is the classic indirect realist mistake.'

I agree that it's a mistake. A perception of an object must involve a mental representation of the object, but the representation doesn't get in the way. On the contrary. When a subject perceives an object, the subject's having a mental representation of an object is an essential part of what constitutes the subject's direct perceptual relation to the object. This is the key point in a sentence, and I'll repeat it in what follows (I think it had the status of a truism in the 1950s in the wave of direct realism that distinguished that decade). 'We see objects "directly" by representing them in visual experience' (McGinn 1983: 129).

Some, perhaps, worry about the 're-' of 'representation'. I could simply use 'presentation'. Certainly the 're-' carries no sense of something's being presented over again. As I use the word 'represent', the world's being *simply present* to one in thought or perception is its being represented in thought or perception, and necessarily so. It may also be present to one by being right next to one, but it's not present to one *in thought or perception* in any way at all unless and until it is in some way or other represented, registered, logged, in or by one's thought or perception. The sea-anchor fact about mind is that mind makes contact with and knows about things by representing them. It makes no contact with them whatever, of any sort whatever, unless it somehow represents them. That's the way mind is.

With that brief attempt at clarification, I'm going to continue to use the word 'representation'. Mental representation is mental presentation is mental registering. To hold that all perception involves representation isn't to be a 'representationalist' in the long-standard sense of this term.[13] It isn't, that is, to hold any sort of Lockean 'representative theory of perception', where a Lockean representative theory of perception is, essentially, a form of indirect realism.[14] There's a fundamental sense of representation in which all theorists must agree that all perception involves representation, however they classify themselves with respect to the directness of perception. The real issue between direct and indirect realism doesn't and can't lie here, however long philosophers fight over words.[15]

[13] See e.g. Mackie (1976: 37, 39, 41, 43, and passim), Woozley (1964: 33), Yolton (1984: 15, 102, 120).

[14] Nor is it to endorse representationalism in a recent confusingly different use of the term, the view that the phenomenological character of an experience is one and the same as its representational content, where its representational content is how it represents the world as being.

[15] I'm not going to consider the old question of whether or not some perception can or must be said to involve inference, and must therefore be indirect. It seems enough to say that not even the best possible theoretically motivated use of the notion of inference in the characterization of the causal process of perception could undercut the sense in which it's true to say that we directly perceive things in the world.

7.7 'Presentation'?

Some may find the word 'presentation' no better than the word 'representation'. They may think there's a tension between direct realism and the idea that the world is presented at all—that even 'presenting' gets between the mind and the world in such a way as to mischaracterize the directness of their relation.

To think this is to lack the sea anchor. One can show this as follows. Consider S, a human subject, and O, an object. They both exist in the world. Right now S does not perceive O. We can represent this as follows.

(4) S O

Now S perceives O. It's a standard case of conscious perception. All goes well.

What does it involve? Whatever it involves, it involves a connection, which we can draw as a line:

(5) S——————————O

What can we say about the line? First, that it represents a *causal interaction*. We may then add that O is *registered by or in S* in some way. No one, I think, will want to deny this, or deny that S changes in some way, and in particular—for this is a case of conscious perception—changes mentally in some way.

We can represent this change with a star as follows:

(6) S*——————————O

The mental change, *, is or involves the registration of O, *sc.* the representation of O. In the case we're considering now, S consciously perceives O, although S may not know what O is; it's a case of conscious, sensory perception. So the registration/representation, *, essentially involves experience, in particular sensory experience, whatever else it does or doesn't involve. No sensory experience, no conscious perception. This is bedrock—whatever one thinks it best to say about, say, animals who sense a coming earthquake.

Let the circle in the diagram below represent the totality of S's being as S perceives O, and let the star within the circle represent the registration-representation of O that was marked by a star in (6).

(7)

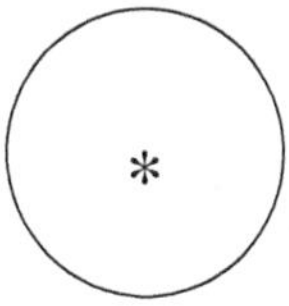

If S perceives O, consciously or not, there must be some such star in the circle. That's all that's meant by saying that all perception involves representation. This will be true even in the case of unconscious 'blindsight' perception, but we're now considering conscious perception, cases in which the existence of the star involves conscious sensory experience.

7.8 Three Fundamental Existents

One can say that there are three fundamental existents in question when it comes to perception: the subject of experience S, the representation R, and the object O. I choose the word 'existent' because it's maximally ontologically neutral. It doesn't entail that we have three separate objects, even if there's nothing wrong with saying that we do. It leaves open the possibility that one of the existents is correctly described as a property or aspect of another.

> 'Direct realists can't allow three things in this way, even if the word 'existent' is maximally ontologically neutral.'

They can, and they'd better. It's analytic that conscious perception involves registration/representation. Mind never makes contact with anything other than itself in any other way. This is what mind is; this is what it does.

> 'Why not adopt the "adverbial" idiom, and say that when Lucy sees a red triangle, she directly perceives the triangle, and is appeared to redly and triangularly?'

The adverbial idiom can be useful. Nothing I say about representation is incompatible with it. This seems to be another false—unnecessary—fight. For the physicalist adverbialist, the star in the circle marks the neural condition in virtue of which it's true to say that Lucy possesses the mental property of being appeared to redly and triangularly. Lucy and the red triangle are existents, so is the neural condition which is Lucy's having the mental property of being appeared to redly and triangularly. There are three relevant existents; there is no conflict of views.[16]

We can, then, think of the representation R as a property of the subject S. This leaves us with two objects, S and O, in the way direct realists prefer. That said, it's important that one can also think of R as an entity that is not a property (given a conventional metaphysical scheme of objects and properties), while remaining a direct realist. This is a crux, and I'll return to it in section 7.17.[17]

[16] The real physicalist knows that the neural condition essentially involves experiential qualitative character; some unreal physicalists deny this.

[17] Whatever the virtues of the adverbial view, it will still be true on any physicalist account that there is some state of the brain that can be correctly identified as that which constitutes the representation of the red triangle, and is an entity accessible to neural computational processes.

7.9 Arnauld

Arnauld, a staunch direct realist in the tradition of Descartes, passionately rejects Malebranche's idea that the process of perception involves 'representative entities' (*êtres représentatifs*). As Arnauld understands things, postulating representative entities commits one to indirect realism (it is in fact just a way of formulating indirect realism). I can, however, declare solidarity with Arnauld, in spite of the fact that he rejects the idea that perception involves 'representative entities'. Given the way I understand 'representation', Arnauld's 'representative entities' aren't representations! For representative entities in his sense are (by definition) mental entities that get in the way between subject and object in such a way that direct realism can't be true.[18]

Both Arnauld and Descartes acknowledge the existence of *states of the brain* that are caused by objects in the world affecting our sense organs, and that in turn cause our experiences of objects. But they don't take these states of the brain to be *mental representations*. (For one thing, they share an immaterialist conception of the mind given which physical states of the brain aren't mental items at all.) Nor are they, for Descartes and Arnauld, items of a sort that can be supposed to get between the subject and the object in such a way that we don't directly perceive objects, but only representations of objects.

I differ from Descartes and Arnauld in rejecting the immaterial mind, even as I agree with them, as a real physicalist, in being a real realist about experience. I also hold that some of the states of the brain involved in my perceiving the object are mental representations—conscious, sensation-involving mental representations—of the object. But I fully agree with Descartes and Arnauld that the states of the brain don't get in the way between me the subject and the object I perceive.

One of the nicest and wisest things about Arnauld is the way he tries to mediate between the indirect and direct realists, allowing that there are ways of taking some of the things indirect realists say given which they are acceptable (see e.g. Arnauld 1683: Ch. 6). One can't hope to get perception right unless one acknowledges this. It's true in the case of the crux mentioned at the end of 7.8, which I return to in section 7.17.

7.10 'Perception', 'Experience', 'Sensation', 'Representation'

'Perception', 'experience', 'sensation', and 'representation' all have plural-accepting count-noun uses as well as mass-term uses that have no plural. It's not that hard to use them harmoniously, but philosophers have understood them in considerably different ways, and moving from one to another can cause confusion. I think it's

[18] The term 'representative' is significantly different from 'representation', in a way I'll bring out in section 7.17.

worth noting this potential source of difficulty at this point, and writing down some of the relations between the words as used here.

I've restricted attention to *conscious* perception in this chapter, so a *perception* is necessarily an *experience*. It essentially involves *experience* in the real realist sense, and indeed *sensation*, and of course *mental representation*. So, too, the mental representation that is an essential part of a *conscious perception* is essentially experiential, essentially a matter of *experience*, at least in part. And its experiential character essentially involves sensation. It may well be that conscious perception can involve representation that has no experiential character in addition to representation that has experiential character; but it must always involve the latter.[19]

I need now to say something about 'externalism' and 'internalism'. But before that let me briefly explain what I mean by '(mental) content', since there's very little consensus about how this term is used. I'll continue to restrict attention to experience and to focus in particular on conscious perception—but not to the exclusion of conscious thought.

7.11 Content

I take the content of an experience to be: *everything that is experienced in the having of the experience*, everything that is experientially registered in any way, everything that the experience is an experience *of*, where 'of' is understood in the widest possible manner, and, in particular, in such a way that it covers everything that it is like to have the experience, experientially speaking, in addition to whatever objects the experience is an experience of.[20] When I look at a poppy, the experiential what-it's-like of my experience of the poppy is part of the overall content of my experience, just as much as the poppy is. It's not as if the content of my experience consists only of the poppy and its properties, while the experiential what-it's-like of my experience is 'just' the 'mode of presentation' (or some such) of the poppy and its properties, in

[19] It will almost always also involve cognitive experience, cognitive phenomenology (see e.g. Bayne and Montague 2011), but I'm leaving this point aside. Note that if there's any sense in which the unseen backsides of perceived objects are 'phenomenally present', as some like to say, then this is essentially partly a matter of cognitive phenomenology. Objection: 'unseen backsides may be present to the perceiver in so far as the perceiver has dispositions to act in certain ways'. Reply: they may perhaps be present in some sense, in this case, but not *phenomenally* present. That will require cognitive phenomenology, since phenomenal presence requires phenomenology by definition, and it's true by hypothesis that the backsides are not present by means of sense/feeling phenomenology. Objection: 'having dispositions to act in certain ways can affect or modulate or tone one's sense-feeling phenomenology in ways that render the backsides phenomenally present'. Reply: the toning must then amount to a form of cognitive phenomenology (it cannot be merely sensory phenomenology), if it's to constitute a respect in which the backsides of objects are phenomenally present.

[20] Compare Montague: 'the content of a perceptual experience is *whatever is given to one in having a particular perceptual experience*. It is whatever is given to consciousness, however this is further characterized. Since I take the phenomenological character of the experience to be part of what is given in the experience, it is part of the content of the experience' (Montague 2009: 497).

such a way that it's not correct to say that the experiential what-it's-like of my experience is part of the content of my experience. This restrictive 'externalist' conception of the content of perceptual states is well established in some philosophical circles, but it's profoundly unnatural. The experiential what-it's-like of my experience is, patently, *experiential content*; as is, also, the general mood-tone of my experience, the whole somatosensory background *continuo* that is part of my total experiential field as I look at the poppy.

Suppose, temporarily and for purposes of argument, that sensation isn't in itself intentional or representational in any way.[21] It doesn't follow that the existence of sensation doesn't essentially involve the existence of mental content. And of course it does. It involves 'sensory content'! It is sensory content! Sensory content doesn't have to be of or about anything in order to be mental content.[22] All experiential what-it's-like-ness is phenomenological content, hence mental content, independently of whether or not it can be said to be intentionally of anything. Consider a few of my philosophical 'Twins': my hallucinating 'Instant Twin', my 'Brain in a Vat Twin', and my 'Perfect Twin Earth Twin'.[23] Their three courses of experience and mine are very different, when it comes to the question what they're of or about, non-experientially speaking. In that sense our four courses of experience have quite different content. But there's a no less fundamental sense of content in which they have identical content, simply because they are by hypothesis identical in respect of experiential-qualitative character. They're all of exactly the same phenomenological-content *type*.

7.12 Internal and External Content

May we say that my Twins and I have different external content and identical internal content? Yes, for some purposes, but the distinction between internal and external content (or narrow and wide/broad content) isn't always clear.[24] This is partly because philosophers tend to think too much about trees and mountains and natural kinds like gold and tigers when characterizing external content, and not enough about other equally concrete, equally worldly items like pains, colour experiences, and conscious thoughts (either their own, or those of other people). We can, certainly, distinguish between the phenomenological and non-phenomenological

[21] Or at least that it is isn't intentional with respect to anything other than itself. I add the qualification for those who think, rightly, I believe, that sensation is always and necessarily intentional with respect to itself. See e.g. Brentano (1874), Montague (2009), Strawson (2015). For the view that experience isn't always intentionally related to itself even though it does always and necessarily comport awareness of itself, see e.g. Sartre (1943), Zahavi (1999).

[22] Even those who deny that it is always and necessarily of or about itself (see the preceding note) can agree.

[23] My Instant Twin has just popped into existence, a miraculous molecule-for-molecule copy of me. Perfect Twin Earth, unlike Classical Twin Earth, is qualitatively identical to Earth in every respect (the stuff they call 'water' on Perfect Twin Earth is H_2O, just as it is here).

[24] On this point see e.g. Segal (2008: 367), Strawson (2014).

elements of the content of a particular thought or perception, but this distinction doesn't line up neatly with the distinction between internal and external content.

In this situation of unclarity, I propose to define 'internal content' and 'external content' in a non-standard way as follows:

(8) the internal content of a conscious mental episode is its *concretely occurring phenomenological content.*

It's concretely occurring experiential what-it's-like-ness, considered just as such. The internal content of an experience is the total phenomenological being of the experience. My Twins and I resemble each other in having qualitatively identical internal content.

As for external content

(9) the external content of a mental episode is *all of its mental content that is not internal content as defined in (8).*

External content not only includes trees and hills; it also includes mental states, including phenomenological states. The internal content of a mental state or episode, i.e. its own concretely occurring phenomenological content, can feature as the external content of some other mental state or episode, because the latter state or episode can be of or about the former one. One can think about anything real. One can think about things outside one's light-cone, for one can think about the universe—everything that exists. A fortiori, one can think about concretely occurring phenomenological content, one's own or someone else's.[25]

My Twins' experiences are of the same internal-content-*type* as mine, but they are of course distinct as *tokens* of internal content. My currently occurring red-experience is or involves a clockable portion of internal phenomenological content, but it's also a token of a certain unclockable *type* of internal phenomenological content, and the type it is of is part of its *external* content, for that type isn't itself concretely occurring phenomenological content (some would say it's an abstract object, which is certainly something external to a mind, something that is not itself a mental item). When I think about my Twins' internal content, their internal content is part of the external content of my thought.

I take it, then, that there's both internal and external content as just defined, and that there's a lot more to external content than the things usually mentioned (mountains, trees, natural kinds). I've set out the distinction in order to say that as far as external content is concerned, I'm happy to agree with those who say that

[25] If all experience is 'self-intimating', if it essentially comports awareness of itself, as I believe, we face the intriguing question whether all internal content has itself as external content in some way. See Strawson (2014).

(10) one can't fully specify the content of an actual particular mental state like a thought about a poppy, or a perception of a poppy, without referring to the poppy itself.

I'm also happy to endorse a stronger formulation of this view, according to which

(11) the object of such a thought or perception (the poppy) is, quite literally, a constituent of that thought or perception.

Both (10) and (11) entail the essential 'object-dependence' of the perception, and they're wholly compatible with the view that there's also internal content, because the internal content of a conscious experience is (as remarked) simply its total occurrent phenomenological content. The character of this internal content can be fully characterized without any kind of reference to the poppy, because it is (*ex hypothesi*) identical to the character of the corresponding experiences of my Twins.[26]

7.13 No Entailment Relation between Direct Realism and Externalism

Some philosophers think there's an entailment relation between direct realism and externalism.[27] It seems, however, that this is a mistake. One can be a direct realist about perception, in holding that one's being in a certain mental state constitutes one's being in direct perceptual contact with an object, while denying externalism in the form of (10) and (11) or in any other form. One may for example hold that one's mental state takes one right up to the object, given the causal circumstances, delivering the object with no perceptual intermediary, even though the object doesn't have to be mentioned in specifying the core content of the mental state, and is not in any sense part of it. So, too, it seems that one can be an indirect realist about perception while being strongly externalist in accepting (10) and (11). On this view of things, the object needs to be mentioned in specifying the content of one's mental state, and is indeed part of it, considered as a whole, but it is so only via the mediation of another part of it.

[26] Conscious thoughts have phenomenological character—cognitive-phenomenological character—just as perceptions have sense/feeling phenomenological character (see Montague, this volume). That's why I'm using the cumbersome word 'phenomenological' rather than the word 'phenomenal' to characterize content. See note 5.

[27] Whether or not they also think that recognizing this entailment requires denying the existence of internal content.

7.14 No Entailment Relation between Direct Realism and Disjunctivism

Some philosophers think there's an entailment relation between direct realism and 'disjunctivism', which I take to be—hereby define as—the view that

> a veridical conscious perception *v* and a phenomenologically identical (hence subjectively indiscriminable) hallucination *h* are not in any fundamental respect states or episodes of the same mental or psychological type.

Let me call disjunctivism so defined 'disjunctivism*', for although this definition is—or was—standard, the meaning of the word appears to have changed over time.[28] Disjunctivism* is certainly false, given real realism about experience, which is certainly true, because it's certainly true that phenomenology is a matter of mentality, and that it is, as mental, of fundamental importance. It follows that the phenomenological character of a conscious mental episode like a perception is a fundamental feature of its overall mental/psychological character as a concrete existent. It follows in turn that there is a fundamental respect in which *v* and *h* are mental episodes of the same psychological type, simply in being phenomenologically identical. One may allow another fundamental respect in which *v* and *h* are of different psychological types, inasmuch as one is essentially and constitutively about an object, and so has a certain sort of external content, while the other isn't and doesn't, but this can't change the fact that there's a fundamental respect in which *v* and *h* are of the same psychological type.

Given that disjunctivism* is false, direct realists must hope that there's no entailment relation between direct realism and disjunctivism*. Fortunately, there isn't. One can be an unequivocal direct realist about perception, as I am, while fully acknowledging the fundamental, inescapable, common-sense respect in which *v* and *h* are mental episodes of the same psychological type. So, too, it seems possible to hold falsely that *v* and *h* aren't of the same psychological type in any fundamental respect (by taking similarity in respect of 'object-dependence' to be a necessary precondition of the correctness of any judgement of fundamental sameness of psychological type), while still insisting that perception is in some deep sense indirect, essentially mediated by a representation.

Direct realism may be what makes some find disjunctivism* attractive, and the two theses can no doubt be formulated in ways that entangle them in some constitutive way. But direct realism gives one no reason to favour disjunctivism* as understood here. Direct realists (philosophers of perception in general) should remember the caveat in section 7.3: they should never take their task to be the task of trying to defeat scepticism.[29]

[28] All names for implausible positions suffer this fate as they attempt to swallow cogent objections.

[29] Disjunctivism seems a good example of a theory that has no plausibility independently of the conclusion, already settled on, that it is engineered to produce.

7.15 Externalism Compatible with All-out Realism about Mental Representations

The next—simple—point is that acknowledging the existence of external mental content is wholly compatible with all-out (real) realism about mental representations. To say that an object or property *x* that one thinks about or perceives is and must be mentally represented by one, in order for one to think about it or perceive it at all, isn't to say or imply that *x* itself isn't part of the content of one's thought or perception, or that one isn't directly perceiving or thinking about *x*. On the contrary. *x* is part of the content of one's thought or perception precisely and only because it is mentally represented by one, and the fact that it is mentally represented by one is no bar to its being the case that one is directly perceiving or thinking about it, and not any representation of it. Depending on the details of the way in which one frames one's theory, the existence of the representation, caused as it is, is either what *constitutes* *x*'s being what one is thinking about or perceiving, or is at least a necessary part of what constitutes *x*'s being what one is thinking about or perceiving. This is philosophy of perception 101.[30]

7.16 Descartes's Direct Realist Externalism

I think Descartes puts it beautifully. Many present-day externalists say that the sun itself is literally a constituent of a thought or perception of the sun. Descartes says the same:

> the idea of the sun . . . is the thing [i.e. the sun] which is thought of . . . *the idea of the sun is the sun itself existing in the mind* . . . not of course . . . existing as it does in the heavens, but . . . in the way in which objects normally are in the mind.[31] (Descartes 1641: 2.75, my emphasis)

Obviously the sun doesn't exist in the mind in the way in which things exist in space. It exists in the mind in the way in which things exist in the mind—by being the object of its thought or perception—and hence by being mentally represented. What is neat—striking—about Descartes's formulation is the way it combines realism about the 'idea' or mental representation (necessary to any viable account of perception) with full-on externalism about the object of thought or perception (equally necessary

[30] Whether one takes the representation, caused as it is, to constitute all or part of the object's being part of the content of one's thought or perception depends on the richness of one's conception of a representation.

[31] As is well known, 'thought' is a general word for Descartes; it covers sensation, perception, and willing, as well as what we ordinarily think of as thought. Someone might contrive to misread 'the idea of the sun . . . is the thing which is thought of' in an indirect realist way, but the reading is ruled out by the immediately following words: 'the idea of the sun is the sun itself'. (Obviously this proposal is not compatible with a way of understanding what a subject of experience is that I favour in other contexts (see e.g. Strawson 2003b), according to which the subject is identical with the experience.)

to any viable account of perception) in a straightforwardly direct realist manner. We may say that the idea of the sun, the idea or mental representation of the sun, is the sun itself, in that the idea of the sun is the way in which the sun (the sun itself) exists in the mind as opposed to the way it exists in space, where it needs (as it were) more room.[32]

The idea or mental representation is not the sun itself in such a way that there can't be any idea or mental representation there at all in the case of a qualitatively identical hallucination. In the case of a hallucination, there's an idea or mental representation that is experientially indistinguishable from the idea or mental representation that is the sun in the case in which one sees the sun; but the idea or representation isn't, of course, the sun 'existing in the mind... in the way in which objects normally are in the mind'.[33]

Don't object that the idea of the sun can't be the sun itself because there's a causal (or representational) relation between the idea of the sun and the sun existing as it does in the heavens. Don't say that if this is really direct realism on Descartes's part, then (because of the inexorable nature of the law of identity, or Leibniz's Law) it must be a form of radical externalism that amounts at bottom to denying the existence of ideas or representations as distinctively mental items. Instead, listen to direct-realist wisdom as it finds powerful and delicate expression in Descartes's talk (however odd to us) of different ways in which concrete objects can exist, in the mind and in the extended world.[34] Note also that this way of putting things doesn't depend on Descartes's official dualism: it can be fully endorsed by real physicalists who take minds to be wholly physical entities while at the same time endorsing real realism about experience.

'It's no good. Descartes's way of putting things is hopelessly in tension with the idea that the existence of the representation consists in the subject's being in a certain experiential state that has a certain causal history. How (for one thing) can the sun itself be a state of the subject?'

[32] I omit Descartes's use of the word 'objective' in the quotation, because it is likely to mislead, given that he doesn't mean what we mean by the word. Once we have his definition of 'objective'—by 'the *objective reality of an idea*... I understand the entity or being of the thing represented by the idea, in so far as that entity is in the idea' (Descartes 1641:2.113–14) we can restore the word: 'the idea of the sun is the sun itself existing in the mind... not of course... as it does in the heavens, but objectively, i.e. in the way in which objects normally are in the mind'. This is object-dependent direct realism.

[33] The thought counterpart of a perceptual hallucination is a seeming thought about the sun on the part of my 'Instant Twin', who has just come into existence by cosmic chance and is having (cognitive) experience phenomenologically identical to mine as I now think consciously about the sun.

[34] Descartes allows that the existence of the sun as an idea in the mind is an 'extrinsic denomination' of the sun considered as existing in the heavens, and seeks to block the objection I've just mentioned as follows: 'If the question is "What is the idea of the sun?" and the answer is given that it is the thing that is being thought of, in so far as it is exists... in the mind [this is Descartes's own answer], no one will think that the idea is the sun itself, in so far as this extrinsic denomination is being applied to it' (Descartes 1641: 75).

The reply, I think, is that the sun itself, existing in the way in which things exist in minds, can *precisely* be a component of a state of the subject that has a certain causal history. That's precisely what's special about minds, and about the way in which objects can be in minds. Putting things in this way is a very nice way of expressing the essence of direct realism.[35]

There is of course a way of taking the claim that leads to confusion, but Arnauld can mitigate the difficulty:

> I take *perception* and *idea* to be the same thing. It must nevertheless be noted that, while this thing is single, it stands in a twofold relation, to the mind that it modifies and to the thing perceived in so far as this latter is objectively in the mind [see note 32], and the word 'perception' more directly refers to the former relation, the word 'idea' to the latter. Thus 'the *perception* of a square' has as its most direct meaning my mind perceiving the square, whereas 'the *idea* of a square' has as its most direct meaning the square [itself] in so far as it is *objectively* in my mind. (Arnauld 1683: 66)

The idea functions in such a way that the thing may be said to be literally a constituent of my thought or perception, when it is a physical object, for example.

Descartes and Arnauld allow a sense in which the representation can be identified with the object without falling down some Berkeleian rabbit-hole. The representation is the object, the real-world, spatially extended entity, existing in the mind in the way in which objects exist in minds. I do think this is a fine way of expressing the direct realist view (it may have scholastic antecedents), even if its attribution to Descartes and Arnauld is incorrect.[36] I am nevertheless going to continue to try to express direct realism without this identification.

7.17 Review

Consider a simple central case. Here I am, a standard-issue human being, looking at a poppy in normal conditions. We all know in broad outline what goes on in such a case. Photons impact on the poppy. Some are absorbed, some deflected. Some of those that are deflected impact on my retinas, where all sorts of amazingly complicated things go on. They pass through to my rods and cones and trigger electrical

[35] 'The whole philosophy of perception from Democritus' time downwards has been just one long wrangle over the paradox that what is evidently one reality should be in two places at once, both in outer space and in a person's mind' (James 1904: 11). But James's own 'radical empiricist' solution is hard to understand, and appears to be a form of idealism.

[36] The question whether this is Descartes's view is disputed (for a different view, see e.g. De Rosa (2010: 15–17); Van Cleve (2005)), and there are other potentially conflicting strands in Descartes's thought. Nor is it clear what Descartes would say about perceiving redness, on this account, for he holds that red-experience is a confused and obscure representation of what redness actually is in objects, and although he could certainly allow that red-experience is red itself existing in the mind in the way in which such properties normally exist in minds (given the way in which God has fashioned our minds), I don't know whether he would.

impulses in my optic nerve. Many more complicated things go on in my brain. I have a visual-sensation-involving experience with a certain highly complex phenomenological character. My having this experience is itself part of what goes on in my brain. The experience involves among other things a representation of the poppy; my representing the poppy is my perceiving the poppy. All this is completely straightforward. I'm describing something that is in one respect very simple, for all its extraordinary physical and neurophysiological complexity, a phenomenon that non-philosophers understand in general terms as well as—or better than—philosophers.[37]

All perception involves representation, so the defining claim of indirect realism can't be that all perception involves representation. What is it? No surprise. It's the claim that when one perceives an object, there is some palmary sense in which one directly perceives or makes direct mental contact with the mental representation of the object, not the object itself. This, just this, is the error—a conception of a subject, a representation, and an object which has the representation somehow interrupting the connection between the subject and the object. It conceives the representation as a *representative* of the object, as in a 'parliamentary representative'. The subject deals with the object's representative, not with the object itself. The subject perceives the representation, not the object itself.

To this direct realism simply replies that the subject doesn't perceive the representation. Rather, and again, the subject's being in the visual experiential state that constitutes its visually representing the object just is its seeing the object, given that the state is caused in the right kind of way for it to count as seeing.[38] In Descartes's dramatic terms, the mental representation, caused as it is, *is* the object; it may be said to be the object. It's the object itself existing in the mind in the way in which objects exist in minds, which is not the same way as the way in which they exist in space.

We can put the point in terms of experience. Indirect realism sets up a picture of a subject, an experience, and an object, and sees the experience as somehow interposed between the subject and the object. The response is the same: the experience is indeed an experience of the object, but it isn't located between the subject and object in such a way as to block the subject's direct perception of the object. Rather, the subject's having the experience (being in the neural state that constitutes its having the experience) is the subject's seeing the object. And one thing is certain: no experience, no seeing.

[37] See e.g. Gollisch and Meister (2010) and Da Silveira and Roska (2011) for an account of the extraordinary complexity of the processing that goes on in the retina alone.

[38] A visual experience of the object that is just like the visual experience of the object that the subject would have had given normal circumstances and normal operation of the visual system will not count as seeing the object if it is somehow deviantly caused by (say) the object's stimulating the olfactory nerves.

There is I think no more to say on this central issue. When I see a material object, the process is of course a causal process. The process is in this sense—and of course—causally mediated. But it is none the less direct—perceptually direct.

What happens in the case of unconscious perception? In this case there's no experience, and in particular no visual sensation. There is nevertheless, as in the case of conscious perception, a neural or bodily state or process that is one's registration/representation of the object. The difference is that this neural state or process is not an experiential one. Otherwise the cases are the same. One's being in the neural state is one's perceiving the object. And one thing is for sure: no neural or bodily representation, no perception, conscious or unconscious.[39]

So direct realists can perfectly well acknowledge three central existents, in the way proposed in section 7.8: the subject of experience S, the experience/representation E/R, or simply E,[40] and the object O. We can then ask about the relation between S, E, and O. Indirect realism is right to insist on E, but wrong inasmuch as it proposes that E stands between S and O in such a way that S perceives O only indirectly. Direct realism gets it right. E doesn't stand between S and O in this way. S doesn't see or perceive E. S has E, and S's having E is S's perceiving O. E is necessary, and given appropriate causation, sufficient for S's consciously perceiving O.

'To allow three existents is to steer close to the wind.' Not really. And even if it were, it would be worth it, because it brings us to the crux. We begin by allowing three *bona fide* existents, S, E, and O. Then we have various options. One is to say that E is a partly O-induced *property* of S, S's possession of which doesn't get in the way of, but on the contrary constitutes, S's perceiving O. On this account the three existents are two objects and one property (this is a version of the adverbial account described in section 7.8). But we can equally well continue to treat E as a kind of object rather than as a property. It is after all wholly constituted by components of the brain in a certain state of synergetic activation, and we can pick out this spatiotemporally located item, this brain synergy, as an object of thought and denote it by a name or noun just as comfortably as we denote S and O, without being in any way obliged to think of it as something that gets in between S and O in such a way as to support indirect realism. If you think of S as the whole organism, then E, conceived as an entity which is not a property, is a short-lived constituent of S (a pimple rather than a hand), and its being a constituent of S is S's perceiving O, or an essential part of S's perceiving O (depending on the richness of your conception of E). It's natural and proper to conceive of E in this way in some theoretical contexts; all one needs to

[39] If there is machine perception, then there is some state of the machine that can be rightly identified as the representation of the poppy. No one, perhaps, has fallen into the view that one can be in direct perceptual contact with an object when one has no conscious experience of it (perceiving it or being aware of it unconsciously or subliminally or peripherally) in a way in which one can't be in direct contact with it when one has a conscious experience of it, because the conscious image somehow gets in the way.

[40] Here I return to the case of conscious perception, and so put aside the more general 'R' (representation), which allows for unconscious perception, in favour of using 'E' (experience), which doesn't.

remember is that conceiving of it in this way doesn't create any pressure to think of it as something that gets in the way between S and O.[41]

This is the crux mentioned in section 7.8. Some philosophers may find it hard to accept, and I'm going to make things seem worse (to some) before trying to make them better: for just as there's nothing wrong with conceiving the experiential entity, the representation, as an object of some sort, so too one can think of it as a kind of causal intermediary between the subject and the object. Real direct realism can endorse the expression 'causal intermediary' and employ it without fear, for there is, after all, and of course, a causal process. There's no problem, because a causal intermediary isn't a perceptual intermediary, whether it's a synergy in the brain, a mental representation, a sensation, a state of the retina, or a photon. Whether it's a representation or a photon, it's part of the process—the causal process—of perception.

> 'I'm an indirect realist, and I find nothing to disagree with in your account of what you call "direct realism". So it can't really deserve the name "direct realism".'

Non sequitur. Everything is excellent.[42]

7.18 The Irrelevance of G. E. Moore

So I'm a direct realist. I'm a real direct realist, a direct realist who is clear on the point that all perception involves representation. Am I also a 'transparentist'? I doubt it. I accept one thesis endorsed by most of those who call themselves transparentists, but I reject the metaphor, which appears to be incompatible with direct realism.

The supposed *locus classicus* for the thesis of transparentism is G. E. Moore's difficult paper 'The Refutation of Idealism'. When we consider a 'sensation of blue', Moore says, and try to take the *consciousness* that is an 'element' of the sensation as an object of attention, the consciousness

> seems to escape us: it seems, if I may use a metaphor, to be transparent—we look through it and see nothing but the blue . . . the moment we try to fix our attention upon consciousness and to see *what*, distinctly, it is, it seems to vanish: it seems as if we had before us a mere emptiness. When we try to introspect the sensation of blue, all we can see is the blue: the other element [i.e. the consciousness as such] is as if it were diaphanous. (Moore 1903: 446, 450)

[41] I don't know whether this gets me into trouble with what one might call the new 'British school' of direct realists—philosophers like Brewer, Campbell, Martin, and Snowdon. In a full analysis of this matter it's necessary to grasp the respect in which the ontological distinction between objects and properties is metaphysically superficial, but there's no space to discuss this here (see e.g., Strawson 2008).

[42] Compare Coates's endorsement of 'critical' realism in this collection. It's not hard to understand why there has been so much disagreement about whether Reid is a direct realist or an indirect realist, for while there's an indisputable sense in which he has a right to be called a direct realist, he says many things of the following sort: 'In perception, whether original or acquired, there is something which may be called the sign, and something which is signified to us, or brought to our knowledge by that sign.' (Reid 1785: 2.11).

To say this is not, of course, to say that the consciousness element doesn't exist. Nor is it to say that it can't be detected, and Moore has no doubt that it can:

> Yet it *can* be distinguished if we look enough, and if we know that there is something to look for. My main object in this paragraph has been to try to make the reader *see* it; but I fear I shall have succeeded very ill. (Moore 1903: 450)

Why does Moore fear failure? Because he's trying to stamp out idealism, and he thinks that the principal reason why philosophers fall into idealism, at least in his time, is that *they fail to notice the element of consciousness in sensation because it's diaphanous*. His argument turns on the essential intentionality of contentful conscious experience, the intentionality that conscious experience necessarily has just in being contentful at all, and points up the sense in which almost all mental content, including e.g. blueness, must be thought of as something non-mental; from which it follows that idealism is false. The argument is complicated and ingenious, and in my opinion unsuccessful. But we needn't consider it because it has nothing to do with the present-day transparency debate in philosophy of perception. So we can set Moore aside.[43]

7.19 Sensation-Transparentism

We can turn instead to Reid and James. When we consider perception of things in the world, James says, we see

> how inveterate is our habit of not attending to sensations as subjective facts, but of simply using them as stepping-stones to pass over to the recognition of the realities whose presence they reveal.[44]

It's this—'sensations as subjective facts', in James's terms, sensations as subjective facts as contrasted with things like tables and chairs—that many have in mind when they talk about 'transparency': sensations or experiences thought of as subjective things that we look straight through, in some sense, when we have them, and so do not notice as such, when we perceive things in the world.[45]

[43] Moore's remarks appear to have been pressed into the service of views he would have utterly rejected, including even views which reject real realism about experience! On this see e.g. Kind (2003), Van Cleve (2005). Note also that he thinks that the blue that is all that one comes upon when one considers a sensation (because one fails to notice the element of consciousness), is an element of the sensation, and certainly not a property in the concrete external (physical) world.

[44] James (1890: 1.231). Compare the passage from Reid's *Inquiry* quoted in section 7.20, beginning 'The visible appearances . . .', which James later (1890: 1.241) quotes in part.

[45] See e.g. Tye (2000: 47), Hill (1991: 187). Both are cited by Van Cleve (2005).

This, as remarked, is not at all what interests Moore. He's not concerned with discerning the 'element' of sensation in our perception of things in the world. He's concerned with drawing attention to the element of *consciousness* in the 'mental fact' (Moore 1903) of *sensation*. This is because he thinks that failure to distinguish the bare element of consciousness from what the sensation is *of* (where this *of* may be wholly internalistically understood) is the fatal, primrose path to idealism. We have, however, put Moore aside, in order to consider the element of *sensation* in the phenomenon of *perception*, and the question whether *it*—sensation—is elusive or 'transparent', in the sense that all one seems to come upon in perception of the world is the *external object*, the something in the world (e.g. the colour blue conceived of as objectively there in the external world).

One might put this by saying that we're concerned with *sensation-transparentism* (not Moore's *consciousness-transparentism*). One might also call it *experience-transparentism*, or *representation-transparentism* (where the representation is assumed to be conscious), and I'll move freely between 'sensation', 'representation', and 'experience'. I'll continue to take 'experience' to denote experiential what-it's-like-ness, I'll temporarily take 'representation' to be effectively equivalent to 'sensation' or 'experience',[46] and I'll compress the three words into an acronym, *SRE*.

We're concerned, then, with SRE-transparentism. Is SRE-transparentism true? Is there any good sense in which the sensation or representation or experience that is essentially involved in and essentially constitutive of conscious perception is 'transparent' in ordinary everyday perception?

7.20 Reid on Transparency

There's certainly a sense in which SREs can be completely unnoticed by us. Thomas Reid puts the point well:

> the sensation of hardness may easily be had, by pressing one's hand against the table, and attending to the feeling that ensues, *setting aside, as much as possible, all thought of the table and its qualities*, or of any external thing. But it is one thing to have the sensation, and another, to attend to it, and make it a distinct object of reflection. The first is very easy; the last, in most cases, extremely difficult. We are so accustomed to use the sensation as a sign, and to pass immediately to the hardness signified, that, as far as appears, it was never made an object of thought, either by the vulgar or by philosophers; nor has it a name in any language. There is no sensation more distinct, or more frequent; yet it is never attended to, but passes through the mind instantaneously, and serves only to introduce, that quality in bodies, which, by a law of our constitution, it suggests. (Reid 1764: 5.2, 176; my emphasis)

[46] 'Experience', like 'representation', can denote something much richer than 'sensation'.

This is an excellent description of one of the fundamental 'transparency' phenomena.

Do Reid's remarks about the sensations of touch carry straight over to the case of vision? No, because there's a fundamental sense in which we are and must be fully aware of the experiential qualitative character of the sensation of blue when we look at the blue sky, lying peacefully on our backs—even though we're not thinking of the sensation as a sensation at all. This is obvious after a moment's reflection. It's enough to realize that, as we lie there looking at the sky, experiencing the qualitative character of the sensation of blue is what our seeing the blueness of the sky *is*![47]

It's a further point that we can if we wish take the sensation of blue as a specific object of attention. It requires some practice to be able to do this, in many everyday situations, as Reid remarks, but it's not that hard, at least in the case of colour experience. It's far harder in the case of the qualitative character of the sensation of hardness.

The case of vision is unlike the case of touch in another respect. Reid is well aware of this, too, and puts things differently in the case of vision. He doesn't talk of sensations, which are mental items, at all, but of 'visible appearances', which are on his account properties of objects. (They're the ways things look given one's relation to them when one sees them.) It's these visible appearances that we find it hard to attend to and 'make a distinct object of attention', in the case of vision, not our visual sensations:

> the visible appearances of objects are intended by nature only as signs or indications, and the mind passes instantly to the things signified, without making the least reflection upon the sign, or even perceiving that there is any such thing... The mind has acquired a confirmed and inveterate habit of inattention to them [the visible appearances]. For they no sooner appear than, quick as lightning, the thing signified succeeds and engrosses all our regard. They have no name in language; and although we are conscious of them when they pass through the mind, yet their passage is so quick and so familiar that it is absolutely unheeded.[48]
>
> (Reid 1764: 82 §6.3)

The phenomenon of unheededness is the same in the case of the sensations of touch and the visible appearances—

> that this is the case with regard to the sensations of touch, hath been shown in the last chapter; and it holds no less with regard to the visible appearances of objects (Reid 1764: 82 §6.3)

[47] The same general considerations apply in the case of taste, smell, and hearing (we are perhaps particularly inattentive to the experiential character of sounds-as-heard when they're spoken words we understand).

[48] He attributes to Berkeley the idea that 'the visible appearance of objects is a kind of language used by nature to inform us of their distance, magnitude, and figure'. In his later *Essays* he speaks more specifically of 'visible figure', magnitude, and so on, but the basic point is the same.

—but the unheeded items are of different sorts.

A few pages later Reid writes that

> the appearances of the same colour are so variable and changeable, according to the different modifications of the light, of the medium, and of the eye, that language could not afford names for them. And indeed they are so little interesting, that they are never attended to, but serve only as signs to introduce the things signified by them. Nor ought it to appear incredible, that appearances so frequent and familiar should have no names, nor be made objects of thought; since we have before shown, that this is true of many sensations of touch, which are no less frequent, nor less familiar.[49] (Reid 1764: 87 §6.4)

He's somewhat pessimistic about being understood on this point, except by painters:

> I cannot therefore entertain the hope of being intelligible to those readers who have not, by pains and practice, acquired the habit of distinguishing the appearance of objects to the eye, from the judgement which we form by sight of their colour, distance, magnitude, and figure. The only profession in life wherein it is necessary to make this distinction, is that of painting. (Reid 1764: 82 §6.3)

Nevertheless he makes the point clearly. Overall, he gives a brilliant account of the phenomena of unheededness or transparency. His (correct) view is not that we can't take the unheeded phenomena as objects of reflection, but that it's difficult to do so:

> it is indeed difficult, at first, to disjoin things in our attention which have always been conjoined, and to make that an object of reflection which never was before, but some pains and practice will overcome this difficulty in those who have got into the habit of reflecting on the operations of their own minds. (Reid 1785: 196 §2.16)

7.21 Is There Any Truth in Transparentism?

The general question remains. In what sense if any is the transparency thesis (the SRE-transparency thesis) true, in the case of vision? I'll address the matter without saying more about Reid, because he's not concerned with sensation-transparentism or SRE-transparentism in the case of vision, but rather with 'visible appearance'

[49] Reid notes (§6.2) Berkeley's analogous point about words and the ideas they stand for: 'No sooner do we hear the words of a familiar language pronounced in our ears, but the ideas corresponding thereto present themselves to our minds: in the very same instant the sound and the meaning enter the understanding: so closely are they united that it is not in our power to keep out the one, except we exclude the other also. We even act in all respects as if we heard the very thoughts themselves' (Berkeley 1707–10: §51).

transparentism.[50] That said, one can perform the Reidian exercise of focusing on the sensation one has when perceiving an object as much in the case of vision as in the case of touch. One can with 'some pains and practice' directly grasp it as a sensation.

One relatively easy way to do this is as follows. Suppose you're in a group of ten people looking at the blue sky. It occurs to you that you're probably not all having exactly the same colour experience, qualitatively speaking. You're surely right (it's beyond reasonable doubt, given human variation—see section 7.3). But that doesn't matter. What matters is that if you consider your colour sensation while involved in this reflection, you can easily apprehend it or experience it *as* a sensation—where this includes apprehending or experiencing the colour quality as a property of the sensation. Reflection on the nature of colour vision—on the fact that 'colour-as-we-see-it' is certainly not Augustinian colour, not 'a quality that is spread out on the surface of bodies' (see section 7.3)—can just as easily produce the same result. Everyone has this experience in Science 101.[51]

Consider as before three existents: the subject, the SRE, and the object. The subject is looking at the sky, which we may think of as an object for purposes of discussion, and having a sensation of blue, a blue-experience, in the real realist sense of 'experience'.[52] The sensation of blue is something fully concretely real. It's a state of the subject.[53] It's up for consideration as deserving the description 'transparent'. In what sense can it be said to be transparent? The best I can do is this: when I look at the blue sky, my natural sense is simply that I see the sky and the blueness of the sky. There is, to this extent, a *sense* in which I'm not aware of the sensation of blue (the point of the italics will become clear).

[50] Reid has less to say in detail on transparency in his later *Essays on the Intellectual Powers* than in his *Inquiry*, although he continues to stress the point that 'besides the sensations that are either agreeable or disagreeable, there is still a greater number that are indifferent [i.e. neither agreeable nor disagreeable]. To these we give so little attention that they have no name, and are immediately forgot as if they had never been; and it requires attention to the operations of our minds to be convinced of their existence' (Reid 1785: 274–5 §2.16).

[51] I return to this issue in the final section. Amy Kind helpfully distinguishes strong transparency, according to which 'it is *impossible* to attend directly to our experience; i.e., we cannot attend to our experience except by attending to the objects represented by that experience', from weak transparency, according to which 'it is *difficult* (but not impossible) to attend directly to our experience, i.e., we can most easily attend to our experience by attending to the objects represented by that experience' (Kind 2003: 230). I take it that Reid rejects strong transparentism in all its forms, and is a weak transparentist with respect to the sensations of touch. He doesn't in his *Inquiry* explicitly take up a transparentist position with regard to visual sensations, as remarked, but only with regard to 'visible appearances'. I think, though, that he would have agreed that it usually took some work to attend directly to visual sensations figured or conceived specifically as such.

[52] The blue-experience is not a blue experience, i.e. an experience that is blue (I hope no one will raise the objection that experiences are not coloured).

[53] For reasons given in section 7.17, the state—the SRE—can be legitimately thought of either as a property of the subject or as an entity (a brain synergy) that is not a property but a constituent part of the subject. Nothing hangs on this: in neither case does it get between the subject and the object in such a way as to cause difficulties for direct realism.

I think this is the only sense in which the SRE-transparency thesis is true, in the case of vision. And although it's fully concordant with (while not required by) direct realism, it needs immediate qualification. For there's also a fundamental sense, already remarked on, in which I am wholly and vividly aware of the sensation of blue, and must be, if it is to be true that I'm seeing the blueness of the sky. This is because my having the sensation of blue *is* my seeing the blueness of the sky, in the causal circumstances I'm in. No sensation, no seeing the blue of the sky! There is, furthermore, an utterly fundamental sense of 'sensation' and 'aware of' in which to have the sensation of blue at all is necessarily to be aware of it (a sense of 'aware of' given which a person's awareness of a mental state emphatically doesn't require its being taken as object of attention by another distinct mental state).[54]

Will it do to say that there's a sense in which I'm not aware of the sensation of blue *considered specifically as such*? There's a point to be made here, but the words 'considered specifically as such' aren't enough to make it. For although it's true that I don't in any express or attentive or (as the Phenomenologists say) *thetic* way consider or conceptualize the sensation specifically as a sensation (this is one natural way of reading the phrase 'considered specifically as such'), in my untrammelled looking at and deep appreciation of the colour of the sky (I don't do this any more than this wide-eyed six-month-old baby who is lying here beside me), there's another sense in which I am indeed fully aware of the sensation of blue considered specifically as such, simply in being aware of (simply in experiencing) the experiential qualitative character of the sensation!—as I must be, given that I am experiencing the blueness of the sky.[55]

7.22 Transparentism Incompatible with Direct Realism

So far we have the modest point that when one moves about the world perceiving this and that, one is often unaware of one's sensations in the following sense: one isn't aware of them in the way in which one would be aware of them if one were expressly or thetically conceiving or apprehending them as such, i.e. as sensations. I'll say that one is *C-aware* of a sensation if there is some sense in which one is aware of it

[54] The converse also holds: my being aware of the sensation of blue (in the sense of 'aware' which emphatically doesn't require one mental state taking another distinct mental state as object) *is* my having the sensation of blue. Note that this is fully compatible with Moore's correct assertion that 'to be aware of the sensation of blue... is to be aware of an awareness of blue; awareness being used, in both cases, in exactly the same sense' (Moore 1903: 449), although his concern here is somewhat different.

[55] Unnecessary note. This is not of course to say that what one might (roughly but clearly) call 'the sky's blue' and 'the sensation's blue' are the same. I take it that Galileo, Descartes, Locke, and Science 101 are right about this. The sky's blue is a light-reflection-and/or-absorption-and/or-emission property (or if you prefer, a disposition or power). The sensation's blue is something utterly different, a matter of 'colour-as-we-see-it'. Colour-as-we-see-it is, certainly, ostensibly a property of external objects. But it is for all that a strictly phenomenological property of experience, where phenomenological properties are wholly internalistically understood.

specifically as a sensation. The present point, then, is that one is often not expressly C-aware of one's sensations. This is compatible with the fact that one is also often aware of one's sensations, in one's most ordinary perceptual transactions with the world, not only in the sense noted above (the sense in which one must always be aware of them in order to be having any experience at all, and hence any conscious perceptual experience at all), but also in the C-awareness sense: the sense in which one is aware of one's sensations because one is in some manner conceiving of them or apprehending them specifically as such. This is obvious in the case of taste and smell—we almost always apprehend taste experiences and smell experiences specifically as sensations, when we have them, whatever else we do—and it's very often true in the case of touch and hearing. It's only in the case of vision, perhaps, that it seems that there is much less C-awareness.

I'll return to this point shortly. Then I'll consider the proposal that there's a respect in which one is *always* C-aware of one's sensation, a sense in which one always figures the sensation specifically as a sensation, albeit 'non-thetically'. For the moment, we have, again, the modest point that one is often unaware of one's (visual) sensations, in everyday unreflective experience, in the specific sense that one isn't *expressly* C-aware of them: one isn't conceiving of them or expressly figuring them specifically as sensations.

Are they then 'transparent'—at least in this case, and in this sense? This doesn't seem a good thing to say. The metaphors of 'transparency' or 'diaphanousness' seem unfortunate, because they carry the idea that we access the object *through* (*trans*-, *dia*-) the sensation, although we don't notice this, and the natural way to understand this is as follows. It's the idea that although our experience of an object is indeed *phenomenologically direct*, in the sense that we feel we are in direct contact with the object, it's *metaphysically indirect*, because one (the subject S) does in fact go *through* something else (the SRE) on one's way to the object (O). On this very natural understanding of 'transparentism', transparentism is incompatible with direct realism, because it requires the idea that the process of perception of an object does in fact metaphysically involve a passage through something—a sensation—even if we experience ourselves as directly in contact with the object.

One can put this by saying that transparentism splits into phenomenological transparentism and metaphysical transparentism, and that metaphysical transparentism must be false if direct realism is true, because it states that we see objects *through* SREs, even if phenomenological transparentism is true.[56]

Once again, this point doesn't bear on Moore's use of the term 'transparency'. He's concerned with the difficulty (but not impossibility) of taking *consciousness*

[56] One can allow—as one must—that perception is a causal process, without endorsing any metaphor of throughness. Note that the term 'phenomenological transparentism' isn't ideal either, because someone might perversely take it to suggest that there is some sort of *experience* of looking through something, albeit something transparent.

considered just as such, i.e. considered independently of what it is consciousness of, as the object of one's attention, when engaged in philosophically motivated examination of certain 'mental facts'—one's own occurrent sensations. So Moore is out of it—well out of it—so far as the present issue is concerned. The present doubt about the word 'transparentism' arises only when we put aside Moore's concern with consciousness-transparentism and turn to consider sensation-transparentism, SRE-transparentism, transparentism with respect to the SRE feature of the ordinary process of conscious perception of objects. This seems to be what most present-day *aficionados* of the term 'transparentism' have in mind.

7.23 Ceivism

I think that the notion of throughness (the 'trans-' or 'δια-' of 'transparent' and 'diaphanous') should be abandoned, for reasons just given. Once again, it's better to say simply that having the experience, in the causal circumstances one is in, *is* perceiving the object. On this account, there's *no* sense in which the subject sees the object *through* the experience, no sense in which the subject passes through something else to access the object. The throughness isn't just a bad metaphor, it's a mistake. The subject *has* the SRE, or is *in* the SRE state. In having the experience, in being in the sensation-involving representational state, the subject is in the state of seeing the object, given the causal circumstances: that is, the subject sees the object. The subject, being in the SRE state, 'directly' sees the object. There is in this fundamental sense nothing between the subject and the object.

Someone may think that throughness resurfaces in the 'per-' (through) of 'perception'. In reply one could propose the *per*-less noun 'ception' (verb 'ceive', pronounced 'seave'). According to direct realism, one doesn't perceive objects, one *ceives* objects ('ceives' derives from '*capere*', to take hold of). 'Ceivism' preserves the truth about directness that transparentism tries to express, while discarding the idea of throughness. It's 'anti-through-ism'. It honours the belief in the directness of perception that stems from the experience of the phenomenological directness of perception, while rejecting the non-phenomenological indirectness or 'throughness' of 'trans-' and 'dia-' and 'per-'. It does this without of course falsely suggesting that non-phenomenological (i.e. metaphysical) directness requires some sort of impossible non-causal immediacy.

Ceivism, then, is a straightforwardly metaphysical thesis. It states that the SRE that is the necessary representational element or 'moment' of any perception of an object is a property or part of the subject of such a kind that there is no defensible description of the process of perception according to which one perceives the object through a representation. It is therefore correct to say that one directly perceives—ceives—the object. Perception is ception.[57]

[57] If one knocks the 'S' for sensation and the 'E' for experience out of 'SRE' and reduces it to 'R' for representation, one can reformulate ceivism in a way that covers non-conscious perception (there are

7.24 Ceivism and Direct Realism

It now seems that the term 'direct realism' covers two distinct claims, one phenomenological, one metaphysical. *Phenomenological* direct realism is a view about the way we ordinarily experience the process of perception. *Metaphysical* direct realism is a view about the (best description of the) structure of the process of perception. Phenomenological direct realism records our experience of being in direct contact with the object in perception; as such it's fully compatible with the indirect realist idea that there's a sense in which we perceive objects through (possibly 'transparent') SREs. According to metaphysical direct realism, the correct description of the phenomenon or process of perception is, again, that it's a matter of direct contact between subject and object that isn't mediated through or by a representation in such a way that the contact must be said to be in some way indirect; although there must of course be a representation. Metaphysical direct realism is independent of any (phenomenological) view about how we *experience* ourselves as perceiving objects.

If this is right, the question about the relation between ceivism and direct realism splits in two. The first question is 'What is the relation between ceivism and *phenomenological* direct realism?' The answer is that neither implies the other. The fact that phenomenological direct realism is true is a contingent psychological fact about the standard case of human perceptual experience. It could possibly have been otherwise, compatibly with the truth of ceivism. It could not only have been the case that we were in perceiving objects always sharply or expressly C-aware, i.e. sharply aware of our (conscious) representations of objects conceived specifically as such, i.e. as representations; it could also have been the case that we naturally experienced ourselves (or that some other race of creatures experienced themselves) as making perceptual contact with objects only indirectly, and 'through', our (their) representations.

The second question is 'What is the relation between ceivism and *metaphysical* direct realism?' The answer, presumably, is that they're the same thing. It's plain that ceivism entails metaphysical direct realism (ceivism is 'anti-through-ism') and the only way to question the converse, i.e. whether metaphysical direct realism entails ceivism, is to raise a doubt about whether the case in which the SRE is thought of as some sort of *state* of the subject (whether because it is a property or a part of the subject) is really the only possible case in which it is correct to judge that metaphysical direct realism is true. I think it is—all other acceptable descriptions of the situation will in effect be equivalent. If so, ceivism is just a version of—another name for—metaphysical direct realism. But there's no need to insist on this (or to

non-conscious Rs, but no non-conscious Ss or Es): the R that is a necessary element of any perception of an object is a state of the perceiver of such a kind that there's no defensible description of the process of perception according to which in thought-experience the perceiver perceives the object through or indirectly by way of R.

commit oneself to the ontological ultimacy of the distinction between objects and their states). It's not as if we can't imagine how perception could be anything different. We can imagine all sorts of things. We can imagine creatures who really do have an inner theatre in their heads in which a homunculus subject of experience watches a representation of the world outside, so that it seems best to say that (metaphysical) indirect realism is true in their case even if phenomenological direct realism is also true, i.e. even if they experience themselves as in direct perceptual contact with objects (compare Mackie 1976: 44–6).

This, however, raises a doubt about the distinction between phenomenological and metaphysical direct realism. For all perception involves causal processes, and it now seems unclear what should guide our judgements about which causal processes count as metaphysically direct perception and which count as indirect. Why exactly are the creatures with the homunculi worse off than we are, in respect of metaphysical directness, given that they experience their perception as direct? Suppose there are creatures whose neuronal connections are ten times as long as ours, although their neural signals travel ten times as fast. Is their perception less direct, metaphysically speaking? What if my brain is located on another planet, connected by magically instantaneous radio links to my body on Earth in such a way that I have no idea that I am not all here, directly in front of the poppy?

I think these questions show that we cannot expect to come up with clear principles that allow us to say that causal process X is in fact metaphysically direct perception, ception, whereas causal process Y is metaphysically indirect perception. So perhaps metaphysical direct realism about perception is at bottom the same as phenomenological direct realism about perception. On this view, once we have the phenomenological facts about how creatures with a given perceptual system normally experience their perception, there is no further metaphysical issue about directness.

7.25 Awareness of Awareness

In this chapter I've tried to take back 'direct realism' as a name for a plausible view from those who have recently tried to co-opt it to name a suite of remarkably implausible views. I want to end by picking up two points I put aside in section 7.22. Many philosophers have claimed that when one perceives the world, there's an important sense in which one is unaware of the sensations that are a necessary part of one's perceiving the world. The question is whether and to what extent this is true. Once again I'll focus mainly on vision.

We have, first, the bedrock point that

(12) there's a fundamental sense in which we must be aware of the sensation, in ordinary everyday conscious perception, simply because having the sensation is an essential part of consciously perceiving the object, and having the sensation is also,

necessarily, being consciously aware of the sensation (though not in any reflective second-order fashion).[58]

This, however, is fully compatible with the idea that

(13) we are rarely expressly C-aware of the sensation, in ordinary everyday perception, i.e. we rarely conceive of it or expressly figure it as such, i.e. as sensation.

True. But this in turn is compatible with the idea that

(14) we are often C-aware of the sensation in some sense, in ordinary everyday perception, even if we're rarely expressly or thetically C-aware of it.

When we see a white table under a red light, for example, we're standardly aware of the respect in which our mental representation of it involves colour-experience of the sort we have when looking at pink things in ordinary light—even as it remains true to say that we see the table as white. To that extent we're genuinely C-aware of our sensation, in addition to being directly aware of the object. We're consciously aware of the straightforward respect in which the table looks pink (even though we may equally well say that it looks white, taking into account the red light), and that awareness already involves some awareness of the sensation as such, i.e. some C-awareness of the sensation, although this awareness may not be fully express or thetic. So, too, when we see ourselves in the mirror in the neon light of a bathroom, we're aware of the difference between the colour of our face as it appears in the mirror and the colour of our face as it appears in daylight. A paleface like myself thinks 'I'm not really that tanned'. So, too, when water feels cold to one hand and warm to another. Again we're directly C-aware of our sensation—however lightly, however non-thetically. And again this doesn't interfere with our being directly aware of the object. Focused attention may be single track; awareness isn't. 'Thought'—experience, awareness—'is quick'; and rich.[59]

Nor does C-awareness, awareness of one's sensations figured or apprehended as such, occur only in unusual cases. It's almost always present in the case of taste and smell, as already remarked, and commonly present in the case of experiencing texture by touch. In the case of hearing, it's standardly present when we hear a sound that we assume to be of constant volume grow louder as we get closer to its source or go round a corner, or in cases in which we hear a familiar sound we've heard more

[58] The case of touch is special, but it isn't an exception to (12) as stated.

[59] Hobbes (1651: 1.3). 'The mind thinks with extraordinary rapidity' (Darwin 1838: 544). 'How very quick the actions of the mind are performed... many of them... seem to require no time... seem to be crowded into an instant' (Locke, *Essay* 2.9.10). See also Strawson (1994: 18–21) ('An Account of Four Seconds of Thought').

clearly in other conditions. It's invariably present, I think, when we see objects dimly in dark conditions, and then experience being able to see better as our eyes adapt to the dark.

These kinds of things happen all the time. The human mind is, overall, tremendously aware of itself as mind, however dipping and fleeting this awareness can be (see Strawson 2009: 24–31). It's not just aware of the surrounding world; it's aware of its awareness of the world. And this is hardly surprising. Mind is in general aware of much of what is going on locally in the world, and its own awareness is itself part of what is going on locally in the world. Some philosophers picture us as fiercely locked to the outer world, typically unaware of our conscious mental processes as such.[60] They rebound from a fantasy they miscall 'Cartesianism', and consider dangerous, and fall into a greater falsehood—a view of human beings as absorbed in the world in such a way that they are

(15) standardly engaged only in thoughts that have to do with their immediate external surroundings

and

(16) rarely if ever C-aware: rarely if ever aware of their conscious mental processes apprehended as such.

The view is mistaken on both counts. As for (15), experimental results suggest that we're engaged in thoughts that have nothing directly to do with our immediate external surroundings a great deal of the time; probably most of the time (see e.g. Hurlburt et al. 1994). As for (16), I've already given reasons to doubt it, and it's arguable that it is in fact the opposite of the truth.

I like this passage from Gurwitsch:

> consciousness . . . is consciousness of an object on the one hand and an inner awareness of itself on the other hand. Being confronted with an object, I am at once conscious of this object and aware of my being conscious of it. This awareness in no way means reflection: to know that I am dealing with the object which, for instance, I am just perceiving, I need not experience a second act bearing upon the perception and making it its object. *In simply dealing with the object I am aware of this very dealing.* (Gurwitsch 1941: 330, my emphasis)

Gurwitsch's closing formulation—'In simply dealing with the object I am aware of this very dealing'—is better than his earlier one ('I am . . . aware of my being

[60] Locke supplies the correction: 'it is for want of reflection, that we are apt to think, that our senses show us nothing but material things. Every act of sensation, when duly considered, gives us an equal view of both parts of nature, the corporeal and spiritual' (1690: 2.23.15). The 'act of sensation' does this just in occurring.

conscious of [the object]'), given that the awareness of awareness in question doesn't require any express representation of oneself as the subject of the awareness.[61] The present point, though, is that even though there's a sense in which the subject isn't aware of himself as such, as mental subject, he is none the less aware of the perceptual dealing, the sensation-involving mental going-on, as such. And this is the normal case—the normal case of ordinary, situated, standardly alert, everyday perception. It's a routine point in the Phenomenological tradition. This C-awareness, this awareness of awareness, is standardly non-thetic, in Sartre's sense: it isn't in the focus of attention, but this doesn't mean that is isn't phenomenologically real. It's fully phenomenologically real.[62] It's part of the overall character of one's experience of the world as one sees the object, something that has to be mentioned in any attempt to give a full account of the overall character of one's experience. Experience is rich.[63]

7.26 Afterthought

I'm looking at my computer, and trying to attend explicitly or thetically to my visual experience of it as I do so. This is a Reidian exercise; it's not easy. I find, though, that I can do it. Do I perceive my computer only indirectly when I succeed? It's certainly not in the focus of my attention. I'm not capable of focusing my full attention simultaneously on my visual experience of my computer, considered specifically as such, and my computer. It is, however, a separate question whether I then perceive my computer only indirectly.

The answer, I think, is No. I perceive my computer directly as before. Even though I'm paying attention to my visual experience of my computer considered specifically as such, I have no sense that it's *getting in the way* of my experience of the computer, in such a way that I perceive the computer only through it, or indirectly. I'm attending to the visual experience, but the computer is also wholly present to me. It seems to be no more true that I perceive the computer only indirectly in this case

[61] This, in fact, is the principal ('non-egological', Sartrean) point of the paper from which this quotation is taken: 'the subject in his dealing with the object, aware as he is of this dealing, is nevertheless in no way aware of his ego, much less of his ego's involvement in his dealing' (Gurwitsch 1941: 327).

[62] It would be superficial to think that the claim about C-awareness is obviously false in the case in which one is (for example) watching an exciting film.

[63] C-awareness as characterized here is not the same as the basic awareness of awareness that is constitutive of the very existence of experience, according to the self-intimation thesis mentioned in section 7.21. If the self-intimation thesis is correct, as I think it is, then all animal experience necessarily involves basic awareness of awareness, but we needn't suppose that it involves C-awareness. I'm not certain that Gurwitsch is talking only about (non-thetic) C-awareness, as opposed to basic awareness of awareness, in this passage, but the present suggestion, in any case, is that much adult human conscious perception does involve some C-awareness in addition to necessarily involving basic awareness of awareness. We needn't decide the issue, however, for the present point is simply that the possibility and common occurrence of C-awareness is entirely compatible with the truth of direct realism. (If it weren't, direct realism would be false.)

than it's true that I perceive an object only indirectly if it's on the periphery of my awareness. Peripherality doesn't in itself compromise directness, and the same goes for lack of 'theticity'.

Suppose someone who concentrates on his visual experience of the computer comes to feel that he's perceiving the computer through the visual experience, or indirectly. I think this might happen. But I'm not inclined to say that he would then be right. When we consider individual cases of perceptual experience, rather than perceptual systems, as in section 7.24, I think we can legitimately distinguish metaphysical from phenomenological direct realism, and say that metaphysical direct realism continues to hold (because one's perceptual system is of such a kind that one standardly experiences oneself as directly perceiving objects), even if phenomenological direct realism fails in this particular case. I'd be inclined to classify any such sense of indirectness of perception as an illusion produced by focusing.

Proust has a striking description of looking at the world while absorbed in reading as a child (perhaps he paused and looked up, perhaps not): 'when I saw an external object, my awareness that I was seeing it would remain between me and it, enclosing it inside a thin mental border that prevented me from ever directly touching its substance'.[64] One can have a similar experience of detachment when listening intently to the radio, or a talk, and the causation can run the other way (one's experience of detachment makes one aware of one's awareness, rather than one's awareness of one's awareness causing an experience of detachment). Another way to become aware of one's awareness while continuing to experience oneself as (and to be) in direct perceptual contact with external objects, has already been mentioned: it's enough to look at something and wonder whether others are seeing its colours as one is oneself.

When one begins the Reidian exercise, the shift of attention from the computer to the visual experience of it requires a studied reconceptualization of what one is experiencing. In time it becomes easier. When I look across the room at some bright clothes, I find I can take the visual sensation as object of attention more easily, disengaging by means of a relatively effortless version of what one has to strive to do in order to see shapes in 'magic-eye' pictures. Written words are different again. When one reads fluently and understands what one is reading, one seems to take almost no notice of the words considered as visual entities. For some, shifting attention to the visual experience of the words may be harder than shifting attention to the visual experience of the computer, as the meaning of the words hijacks attention and interferes with one's seeing them just as black and white marks. Perhaps painters can flip more effortlessly.[65]

[64] 'Quand je voyais un objet extérieur, la conscience que je le voyais restait entre moi et lui, le bordait d'un mince liséré spirituel qui m'empêchait de jamais toucher directement sa matière' (Proust 1913: 1.83).

[65] I'd like to thank Ned Block, Brian Garrett, Amy Kind, Michelle Montague, Nini Praetorius, François Récanati, and Alison Simmons for their comments. I also learnt from audiences at the Université de Fribourg, the Danish Society for Philosophy and Psychology in Copenhagen, the Institut Jean Nicod in Paris, and the Australian National University in Canberra.

References

Arnauld, A. (1683/1990), *On True and False Ideas*, translated with an introduction by Stephen Gaukroger (Manchester: Manchester University Press).

Bayne, T., and Montague, M. (2011), *Cognitive Phenomenology* (Oxford: Oxford University Press).

Berkeley, G. (1707–10/1975), *Philosophical Commentaries* in M. R. Ayers (ed.), *Philosophical Works* (London: Dent).

BonJour, L. (2011), 'Epistemological Problems of Perception', in Edward N. Zalta (ed.), *The Stanford Encyclopedia of Philosophy*, at <http://plato.stanford.edu/archives/sum2011/entries/perception-episprob/>.

Brentano, F. (1874/1995), *Psychology from an Empirical Standpoint*, introduction by Peter Simons, translated by A. C. Rancurello, D. B. Terrell, and L. McAlister (London: Routledge).

Chun M. M., and Marois, R. (2002), 'The Dark Side of Visual Attention', in *Current Opinion in Neurobiology* 12: 184–9.

Da Silveira, R., and Roska, B. (2011), 'Cell Types, Circuits, Computation', in *Current Opinion in Neurobiology* 21: 664–71.

Darwin, C. (1838/1987), 'Notebook M', in *Charles Darwin's Notebooks, 1836–44*, ed. P. Barrett et al. (Cambridge: Cambridge University Press).

De Rosa, R. (2010), *Descartes and the Puzzle of Sensory Representation* (Oxford: Oxford University Press).

Descartes, R. (1641/1985), *Meditations* and *Objections and Replies*, in *The Philosophical Writings of Descartes*, Volume 2, translated by J. Cottingham, Robert Stoothoff, and Dugald Murdoch (Cambridge: Cambridge University Press).

Feigl, H. (1958), 'The "Mental" and the "Physical"', in *Concepts, Theories, and the Mind-Body Problem* (Minneapolis, MN: University of Minnesota Press).

Feigl, H. (1967), 'Postscript', in *The 'Mental' and the 'Physical'* (Minneapolis, MN: University of Minnesota Press).

Gollisch, T., and Meister, M. (2010), 'Eye Smarter than Scientists Believed: Neural Computations in Circuits of the Retina', in *Neuron* 65: 150–64.

Grimes, J. (1996), 'On the Failure to Detect Changes in Scenes across Saccades', in K. Akins (ed.), *Perception (Vancouver Studies in Cognitive Science)* (New York: Oxford University Press), 89–110.

Gurwitsch, A. (1941), 'A Non-Egological Conception of Consciousness', in *Philosophy and Phenomenological Research* 1: 325–38.

Hill, C. (1991), *Sensations* (Cambridge: Cambridge University Press).

Hobbes, T. (1651/1996), *Leviathan*, ed. Richard Tuck (Cambridge: Cambridge University Press).

Hume, D. (1739–40/2000), *A Treatise of Human Nature*, edited by D. F. Norton and M. Norton (Oxford: Clarendon Press).

Hurlburt, R., Happé, F., and Frith, U. (1994), 'Sampling the Form of Inner Experience in Three Adults with Asperger Syndrome', in *Psychological Medicine* 24: 385–95.

James, W. (1890/1950), *The Principles of Psychology*, Volume 1 (New York: Dover).

James, W. (1904/1912), 'Does Consciousness Exist?', in W. James, *Essays in Radical Empiricism* (London: Longmans, Green and Co).

Johnston, M. (1992), 'How to Speak of Colors', in *Philosophical Studies* 68: 221–63.

Kind, A. (2003), 'What's So Transparent about Transparency?', in *Philosophical Studies* 115: 225–44.

Lewis, D. (1995/1999), 'Should a Materialist Believe in Qualia?', in D. Lewis, *Papers in Metaphysics and Epistemology* (Cambridge: Cambridge University Press).

Lewis, D. (2001/2009), 'Ramseyan Humility' in D. Braddon-Mitchell and R. Nola (eds), *Conceptual Analysis and Philosophical Naturalism* (Cambridge, MA: MIT Press), 203–22.

Locke, J. (1690/1975), *An Essay Concerning Human Understanding*, edited by P. H. Nidditch (Oxford: Clarendon Press).

Mackie, J. L. (1976), *Problems from Locke* (Oxford: Oxford University Press).

Malebranche, N. (c.1680–90), *Oeuvres complètes, tomes 6 et 7. Recueil de toutes les réponses à M. Arnauld* (Paris: Vrin).

Maxwell, G. (1978), 'Rigid Designators and Mind-Brain Identity', in C. Wade Savage (ed.), *Perception and Cognition: Issues in the Foundations of Psychology* (Minneapolis, MN: University of Minnesota Press), 365–403.

McGinn, C. (1983), *The Subjective View: Secondary Qualities and Indexical Thoughts* (Oxford: Clarendon Press).

Montague, M. (2009), 'Perceptual Experience', in A. Beckermann, B. McLaughlin, and S. Walter (eds), *Oxford Handbook of the Philosophy of Mind* (Oxford: Oxford University Press).

Moore, G. E. (1903), 'The Refutation of Idealism', in *Mind* 12: 433–53.

Murdoch, I. (1964/1970), 'The Idea of Perfection', in *The Sovereignty of Good* (London: Routledge and Kegan Paul).

Noë, A. (2004), *Action in Perception* (Cambridge, MA: MIT Press).

Pessoa, L., and de Weerd, P. (eds) (2003), *Filling-in: From Perceptual Completion to Cortical Reorganization* (New York: Oxford University Press).

Proust, M. (1913/1987), *Du côté de chez Swann: A la recherche du temps perdu I* (Paris: Pléiade).

Proust, M. (1913/2002), *In Search of Lost Time: The Way by Swann's*, trans. Lydia Davis (London: Penguin).

Reid, T. (1764/2000), *An Inquiry into the Human Mind*, ed. D. Brookes (Edinburgh: Edinburgh University Press).

Reid, T. (1785/2002), *Essays on the Intellectual Powers of Man*, ed. D. Brookes (Edinburgh: Edinburgh University Press).

Russell, B. (1927/1992), *The Analysis of Matter* (London: Routledge).

Russell, B. (1956), 'Mind and Matter', in B. Russell, *Portraits from Memory* (Nottingham: Spokesman), 145–56.

Sartre, J.-P. (1943/1969), *L'Être et le néant* (Being and Nothingness), translated by H. Barnes (London: Methuen).

Segal, G. (2008), 'Narrow Content', in A. Beckermann, B. McLaughlin, and S. Walter (eds), *Oxford Handbook in the Philosophy of Mind* (Oxford: Oxford University Press).

Simons, D. J., and Levin, D. T. (1997), 'Change Blindness', in *Trends in Cognitive Science* 1: 261–7.

Strawson, G. (1994), *Mental Reality* (Cambridge, MA: MIT Press).

Strawson, G. (2003a/2008), 'Real Materialism' in L. Antony and N. Hornstein (eds), *Chomsky and His Critics* (Oxford: Blackwell), 49–88, and in G. Strawson, *Real Materialism and Other Essays* (Oxford: Oxford University Press).

Strawson, G. (2003b/2008), 'What Is the Relation between an Experience, the Subject of the Experience, and the Content of the Experience?', in G. Strawson, *Real Materialism and Other Essays* (Oxford: Oxford University Press).

Strawson, G. (2008), 'The Identity of the Categorical and the Dispositional', in *Analysis* 68/4: 271–82.

Strawson, G. (2009), *Selves: An Essay in Revisionary Metaphysics* (Oxford: Oxford University Press).

Strawson, G. (2014), 'Internal and External Content', at <http://www.academia.edu/11942205/Internal_and_external_content>.

Strawson, G. (2015), 'Self-Intimation', in *Phenomenology and the Cognitive Sciences* 4: 1–31.

Tye, M. (2000), *Consciousness, Color, and Content* (Cambridge, MA: MIT Press).

Van Cleve, J. (2005), 'Troubles for Radical Transparency', at <http://www-rcf.usc.edu/~vancleve/>.

Woozley, A. D. (1964), 'Introduction', in John Locke, *An Essay Concerning Human Understanding*, ed. A. D. Woozley (London: Collins).

Yolton, J. (1984), *Perceptual Acquaintance from Descartes to Reid* (Minneapolis, MN: University of Minnesota Press).

Zahavi, D. (1999), *Self-Awareness and Alterity: A Phenomenological Investigation* (Evanston, IL: Northwestern University Press).

SECTION III

The Kinds and Character of Phenomenal Qualities

8

A New Argument for Realism from Perceptual Content

E. J. Lowe

8.1

Why, if at all, should we be *realists* about the 'external world' of common-sense ontology? I am prompted to raise once more this thorny age-old question by some interesting recent work of Athanassios Raftopoulos. In his excellent and thought-provoking book *Cognition and Perception* (Raftopoulos 2009), Raftopoulos suggests that realism—as opposed to various types of constructivism, conventionalism, and relativism—can be defended only if it can be argued that perception includes some species of *nonconceptual content* which serves to 'individuate' objects in the perceiver's environment and thereby fix the reference of perceptual demonstratives in a manner which does not rely on the perceiver's repertoire of concepts (including, above all, his or her *sortal* concepts). And he argues at length that just such a species of nonconceptual content can indeed be attributed to perception and exploited in an argument for realism. However, I think it may be questioned both whether (1) realism can be defended *only* in this way and also, more fundamentally, whether (2) it really *can* be defended in this way. In this connection, I shall raise some doubts in the present chapter concerning the adequacy of Raftopoulos's conception of 'object individuation', as this notion is applied to perceptual processes. In particular, there seems to me to be some confusion, or at least a questionable degree of idiosyncrasy, in Raftopoulos's use of the terms 'object' and 'individuation', and likewise in his related use of the terms 'sortal' and 'identification'. I shall argue that the perceptual mechanisms appealed to by Raftopoulos cannot in fact serve to single out environmental objects uniquely and that our perceptual systems *must* be able to exploit sortal distinctions of a very broad kind in order to achieve this task. But I shall also argue that, even if the perceptual individuation of objects relies in this way upon the deployment of at least *some* sortal 'concepts', this need pose no special threat to realism, since it is perfectly possible and indeed very plausible to maintain that the relevant sortals are ones that are, for evolutionary reasons, both 'innate' and well-attuned to real distinctions in nature. Consequently, they need not and should not be seen as 'floating free' of such distinctions or as being empirically and metaphysically 'ungrounded', in any sense that could give comfort to the antirealist.

In addition to all this, however, I shall further contend that Raftopoulos's response to antirealism is ultimately question-begging and circular, failing to tackle antirealism at its real philosophical roots. This is because Raftopoulos formulates and defends his account of the nonconceptual content of perception in terms which just *presume* the truth of current empirical scientific theories in neurophysiology and neuropsychology and thus in terms which are already presumptively *realist*. If one is to argue non-question-beggingly *from* nonconceptual perceptual content *to* realism, then, I believe, one needs to be able to identify a species of nonconceptual content to be found in perception which is (1) introspectively accessible by the perceiver and (2) suited by its intrinsic character to constitute inductively good evidence for the existence of an 'external world' conforming in its broad nature and structure to the realist's conception of such a world. The final task of this chapter will be to sketch and defend precisely such an account of the nonconceptual content of perception. It will be seen that nonconceptual content of the required kind differs markedly from the type of nonconceptual content appealed to by Raftopoulos and yet is perfectly consistent with the latter (or something close to it), so that we need not maintain that perception can include the former only at the expense of *excluding* the latter. In effect, my claim will be that Raftopoulos has not delved *deep enough* into the structure of nonconceptual content to find a *level* of such content that is suited to the task of combating the antirealist in terms which do not implicitly beg the question against such a philosopher.

Before beginning my detailed critique of Raftopoulos's position, however, I want to quote two important passages from his book which encapsulate key features of his approach and main line of argument. First, a claim—with which I have considerable sympathy—concerning the relationship between perception and our knowledge of the external world:

> [T]o make any claims whatsoever about the externalia, one must argue *from* perceptual states *to* the external world. (Raftopoulos 2009: 341)

Second, Raftopoulos's own summary of his main line of argument:

> Here is my argument for a restricted form of realism:
>
> (i) To get in contact with the world through vision, one must break the circle of representations.
>
> (ii) To break that circle... at least some visual states must have nonconceptual *representational* content.
>
> (iii) There is a part of visual processing... that induces in us states with nonconceptual representational content.

(iv) The nonconceptual content has features that we consciously perceive as of properties of objects . . .
(v) Our interactions with the world on the basis of this content are largely successful.
(vi) In order for [this to be the case], a subset of the [nonconceptual content] must present correctly some of the real properties of the external objects. (Raftopoulos 2009: 342)

8.2

Raftopoulos, as I have already indicated, has as one of his main aims the defence of a moderate form of realism—one that is opposed to the antirealisms inspired by various versions of constructivism, conventionalism, and relativism, of the kinds that have pervaded much thinking in the philosophy of science and metaphysics during the last fifty years or so. He seems to think, and perhaps rightly so, that a common root in all of these antirealist positions is a conviction that all perception—and, more specifically, all perceptual *content*—is thoroughly and inextricably infused with *concepts* or *interpretations* or *descriptions*. One finds this idea, for instance, in Wilfrid Sellars's (1963) rejection of what he called 'the myth of the given', in N. R. Hanson's (1958) insistence that all observation is 'theory-laden', and in Thomas Kuhn's (1962) talk about scientific 'paradigms' and 'normal science'. Raftopoulos accordingly considers that realism can be defended only if it can be shown that perception includes some kind of *nonconceptual* content, which serves to 'individuate' objects in the perceiver's environment in advance of the perceiver's deployment of *concepts* or *descriptions* of any type to *characterize* or *classify* those objects. This would be a kind of content which thereby serves to *fix the reference of perceptual demonstratives*—'this' and 'that', as used by the perceiver to pick out such objects, whether in speech or merely in thought—in a way that does not rely on the perceiver's idiosyncratic stock or repertoire of classificatory concepts. For the latter, by implication, are all regarded as being suspect, from an antirealist point of view, on account of their supposed cultural or historical relativity and consequent lack of permanence and universality—a suspicion that Raftopoulos himself seems to share at least in some measure. In this fashion, then, Raftopoulos hopes to marshal evidence against the antirealist in favour of at least a *modest* species of realism, according to which we human subjects are not *radically* mistaken about the real nature of the 'external world', to the extent, at any rate, that our basic referential apparatus in everyday talk and thought succeeds in latching on to particular things which do genuinely exist as distinct and intersubjectively accessible constituents of mind-independent reality.

Let me now begin my evaluation of Raftopoulos's views by saying that I agree with him that perception includes a distinctive kind of nonconceptual content—indeed, like him, I think that there is more than one kind of such content—but that I disagree with him about certain aspects of this content and also disagree with him about how, precisely, considerations concerning such content can be marshalled in favour of realism. And here I should emphasize immediately that all of my own philosophical sympathies lie entirely on the side of realism. Now, with regard to the question of realism, I want to say, in the first place, that I am *not* convinced that realism can be defended *only* by appealing to some notion of nonconceptual content. But, also, I do not consider that Raftopoulos in fact focuses on the *right kind* of nonconceptual content for the purposes of an argument from perceptual content to realism, nor indeed that the kind of *argument* from such content that Raftopoulos deploys is one that will *or should* make any impression upon, much less satisfy, his antirealist opponents—who are, I consider, entitled to regard his style of argument as being fundamentally question-begging and circular.

However, before I come more specifically to the question of realism, I want to register some doubts about Raftopoulos's account of 'object individuation' in perception. To begin with, I think that Raftopoulos is somewhat confused—or, at least, *confusing*—about both 'objects' and 'individuation'. Indeed, I think that he is also confused or confusing about what *he* calls 'identification' and 'sortals'. Most importantly, I do not believe that the perceptual mechanisms that he appeals to in his account of the nonconceptual content of perception can in fact serve to single out environmental objects *uniquely* and in *that* sense 'individuate' them. However, it seems that by 'individuation' Raftopoulos himself *doesn't* really mean individuation in this sense: rather, he means something like *discrimination*, as I shall soon explain. Moreover, by 'identification' he means something like *classification* and, more specifically, classification under a *sortal* concept or description. (As we shall shortly see, these uses of the terms 'individuation' and 'identification' are non-standard ones, at least in the philosophical community.) So, the overall picture that Raftopoulos seems to be offering us is something like the following one. Even before our sortal concepts are brought to bear upon the contents of perception, our perceptual mechanisms serve to 'parse' the environment around us into discriminably distinct 'objects', thus 'individuating' those objects for us and enabling us, for instance, to *track* them as they move. Only when our higher-level cognitive capacities are brought to bear on these perceptual contents do we 'identify' any of those objects, that is, *classify* them, whether explicitly or only implicitly, as belonging to this or that *sort* or *kind* of object—as it might be, as being a *table*, a *cat*, or a *tree*. And then Raftopoulos's point is that, while the latter process of 'identification' is conceptually infused or theory-laden and hence subject to antirealist anxieties about the intersubjective variability of different 'conceptual schemes', the initial process of object 'individuation', being nonconceptual, is *not* vulnerable to such anxieties and consequently serves to provide an intersubjectively *invariant* domain of reference for perceptual demonstratives, thereby securing the truth of at least a moderate form of realism concerning the 'external world'. All human subjects, it may thus be supposed, at least 'parse' their perceived environment into the same basic 'objects', ensuring a limit to the amount of possible disagreement between them regarding the constituents and structure of 'external reality'. It won't be a case, then, of 'anything goes', depending on one's conceptual scheme, regarding the nature of the 'external world', rendering that world effectively noumenal, in a Kantian sense.

Let me revert at this point to some matters of terminology. I prefer to use the term 'individuation', at least as it applies to an activity of perceivers or of their cognitive mechanisms, to mean—and in this regard I believe that I am just following current mainstream philosophical practice—the *singling out of an object as the particular individual thing that it is*: not just a *discrimination of its boundaries* (see Lowe 2007). A simple example will show what I mean by this distinction. If we have before us a certain *cat*—say, Tibbles—then Tibbles will at this moment be composed of a certain discrete hunk of feline tissue: and, of course, Tibbles and that hunk of feline tissue will *share their spatial boundaries*. If, say, Tibbles is black and is sitting in front of a white screen, then a normally sighted person will certainly be able to *discriminate* Tibbles from his surroundings, because Tibbles's spatial boundary will be sharply delineated by the colour-contrast between his blackness and the whiteness of the screen. But to *discriminate* Tibbles in this sense is not at all the same as *individuating* him in the standard sense of the term 'individuate', since Tibbles and the hunk of feline tissue composing him have the *same* boundaries and yet are different individual objects. 'Discrimination', then, does not mean the same as 'individuation' in the standard philosophical sense of the latter term. However, the perceptual mechanisms to which Raftopoulos appeals in his account of nonconceptual content can only secure the *discrimination* of environmental objects, not their *individuation* in the standard sense—a fact which is unfortunately obscured by Raftopoulos's non-standard use of the term 'individuation' to mean, in effect, mere discrimination. (According to Raftopoulos, 'When one perceives a scene, the first thing one usually does is parse it in[to] discrete objects, *thereby individuating them*' (2009: 90, emphasis added).) For Raftopoulos's usage will naturally suggest to many of his philosophical readers that the perceptual mechanisms to which he appeals in his account of nonconceptual content really can serve genuinely to *individuate* environmental objects, when in fact they can do no such thing.

Next, there is the question of the appropriate use of the term 'object'. Here, I suggest, we should insist that something counts as an 'object' only if it has *determinate identity*—that is, only if there is a fact of the matter as to *which* object it is (see Lowe 1998: 28–57 and Lowe 2007). And, again, in this I am just following standard philosophical practice, I believe. Both Tibbles and the hunk of feline tissue composing him—call it *H*—are objects in this sense. But, most importantly, they are clearly *different* objects, since Tibbles can, in time, come to be composed of a *different* hunk of feline tissue, owing to metabolic processes that Tibbles necessarily undergoes in virtue of being a living organism and, more specifically, an *animal*. Now, a subject of perception can individuate—*single out uniquely*—a particular object only if he or she can *identify* it, in the sense of *tell which object it is* and thereby *tell it apart from other objects*. This, of course, is not *Raftopoulos*'s use of the term 'identify' since, for Raftopoulos, to 'identify' an object is just to *classify* it as being of this or that *sort* or *kind* and hence to apply a certain *sortal concept* to the object or to judge it to fall under a certain such concept. (According to Raftopoulos (2009: 113), the term 'object identification', as he uses it, 'attempts to convey the notion of an object… as falling under a certain description'.) But, again, I find his terminology here confusing and certainly out of line with common practice in *philosophical* discussion, however things might be in other disciplines such as, perhaps, cognitive science or sociology. The upshot, however, is this. Because Raftopoulos means *classify sortally* by 'identify' and thinks that such classification operates only *subsequently* to the 'individuation' of objects—by which he really means only their *discrimination*—he never really gets to grips with the question of how a subject can acquire and exercise an ability to *tell which object an object is*: that is, to *identify* objects, in my philosophically more familiar sense of 'identify', which links 'identification' to an object's individual *identity*, rather than to its general *sort* or *kind*. *Discrimination* of an object does not serve to identify it in this sense, since, for example, Tibbles and the hunk of feline tissue *H* are discriminated *together* by our nonconceptual perceptual mechanisms, as the latter are characterized by Raftopoulos, because Tibbles and *H* have *the same spatial boundaries*. But, given that these mechanisms cannot *identify* objects, in my sense of 'identify', they don't provide our higher-level classificatory concepts with items that are even *suitable* to be assigned to this or that *sort* or *kind*. They don't serve to pick out *objects with determinate identities*, prior to any sortal characterization of them, to which sortal classifications can then be applied. And yet this is what Raftopoulos's readers, owing to his misleading choice of terminology, may well be tempted to *suppose* that those mechanisms can do and, indeed, what he himself may well suppose them to be capable of.

Moreover, it seems that an account like Raftopoulos's can never explain what we now *need* to explain—namely, how a subject can acquire and exercise an ability to *tell which object an object is and tell it apart from others*—for the following simple reason. Identifying an object—in my sense of being able to tell *which* object it is—only makes sense relative to an appropriate *classification* of that object as belonging to a certain broad *sort* or *kind*, because the identity-*criteria* of individual objects are clearly sortal-relative. For instance, the criterion of identity governing *Tibbles* is that of a *living organism* and differs fundamentally from that governing *H*, which is that of a *hunk of matter*. A living organism can, for instance, survive—that is, *preserve its identity through*—a change of its material parts, whereas a hunk of matter cannot. Hence, only a subject possessing at least an implicit grasp of this criterial difference can be in a position to *identify* Tibbles, in my sense of 'identify', that is, tell *which* object Tibbles is: for this at least requires the subject to be able to tell, for instance, that Tibbles is distinct from *H*, in the sense of *know that Tibbles and H are not one and the same object*—even though Tibbles and *H* presently coincide spatially and so share the same spatial boundaries, rendering them *perceptually indiscriminable* at the present moment.

Now, Raftopoulos might urge at this point that what I have just said concerning identification renders me vulnerable to the attacks of antirealists, because I am committing myself to the claim that a subject cannot 'individuate' perceptible objects in the environment independently of deploying his or her repertoire of *sortal concepts*, thus making all perceptual content—or, at least, all perceptual content of a relevant kind—irredeemably 'theory-laden' and hence open to cultural and historical variation and instability. But, in the first place, I don't see why the concession that certain sortal concepts play the role in question, even if it has to be made, renders anyone who makes it automatically vulnerable to antirealist attacks of this sort. Even granted that perceptual demonstratives, on the view I am now proposing, would rely on the deployment of sortal concepts of certain very broad kinds—such as the concepts of 'living organism' and 'hunk of matter'—I see no reason why a realist cannot plausibly claim that the sortal concepts in question, at least in a primitive form, are *innate* components of human cognitive and perceptual systems, being built into those systems in the course of human cognitive evolution and shaped by evolutionary processes in such a way that they are *attuned to real distinctions in nature.* Just because they are 'conceptual' resources, we needn't conclude that they are therefore completely arbitrary or are mere products of cultural or linguistic history. Indeed, when Raftopoulos himself talks of the 'objects' which, according to him, the human perceptual system succeeds in 'individuating' nonconceptually, it turns out that what he has in mind are something like so-called *Spelke-objects*, which are *topologically connected, possess spatial boundaries, are 'rigid', and can move continuously as cohesive wholes* (see Spelke 1990 and Raftopoulos 2009: 100–5). But these seem to be, to all intents and purposes, pretty close to what I meant earlier by *hunks of matter* (certainly, it is the latter that most nearly satisfy the characterization just given in terms of connectedness, boundedness, rigidity, and the ability to undergo cohesive continuous movement). However, Raftopoulos seems to be labouring under the misconception—which, to be fair, is quite common, especially amongst cognitive scientists and psychologists—that when we use the term 'object' to mean something like *this* we are *not* deploying a *sortal* concept and hence that an 'object' in this sense is something that can be singled out prior to *any* classification of it as belonging to a certain sort or kind. That is simply not so, however, and this is a point whose importance is such that it deserves further elaboration.

It would be quite wrong to suppose that we can single out a particular *object* in the foregoing sense and then only *later* assign it to any one of indefinitely many different sorts or kinds, such as 'cat' or 'toy' or 'ornament'. For an 'object' in this sense—a 'Spelke-object' or 'hunk of matter'—is *already* conceived as something of a certain sort or kind, albeit a very *broad* kind, governed by a criterion of identity which is in fact *incompatible* with, for example, the criterion of identity governing any *cat*. (The very fact that 'objects' in this sense are said to *move* implies that there must be some principle constraining their identity both at a time and over time, since movement requires the *same* object to be in *different* places at *different* times—a crucial point that I shall return to later.) A hunk of matter is not something that can be classified as *being* a cat, for no hunk of matter can be *identical* with a cat. The reason is simple and we have already pointed it out: a cat, being a living organism, can preserve its identity through changes which *cannot be survived* by a hunk of matter, and indeed *vice versa.* And the same reasoning applies to a *Spelke-object*, if indeed that differs significantly from a hunk of matter: a *Spelke-object* cannot *be*—that is, *be identical with*—a cat or other living organism. It can at most *coincide* for a period of time with a cat, sharing its spatial boundaries for a while with the latter. So 'object', in the sense implicitly understood by Raftopoulos, is *itself* a sortal term, *not* a term which can find application *prior to any sortal classification whatever* of the items encountered in perception. Of course, I do not recommend this use of the term 'object' myself, precisely because it is so misleading. In my own usage, 'object' is what David Wiggins (1980; 2001) calls a *dummy* sortal, carrying with it no commitment to any particular criterion of identity for the items to which it applies. But, for reasons already made plain, one cannot *identify* or *individuate* (in *my* senses of these terms) anything as an 'object' in this sense, precisely because it is so indiscriminate in its application. The term 'object' as used by *Raftopoulos*, however, is far from being so indiscriminate. As I say, it seems to be pretty much what is meant by a 'Spelke-object' and fairly close to what I mean by a 'hunk of matter'. And *neither* of the latter terms is unconstrained in its application by considerations to do with *identity at and over time*—the sort of constraints that are standardly captured by the *criterion* of identity governing the application of a *sortal* term. Indeed, a sortal term, in the broadest sense, precisely *is* a general classificatory term whose use is constrained by a specific criterion of identity governing the items to which it applies. That is how the expression 'sortal term', originally coined by John Locke, was recruited into the current philosophical literature by philosophers such as P. F. Strawson (1959) and David Wiggins (1980), so to use it in any other way would be seriously misleading.

It turns out, then, that *Raftopoulos himself* is, very probably, actually committed to something like the position that I am proposing, whereby our pre-reflective perceptual mechanisms not only *discriminate* objects in our environment but also (in my sense) *individuate* at least some of them, as individual instances or exemplars of a certain broadly defined *sort* or *kind*, namely, as something very like individual 'hunks of matter' or (if this is anyhow significantly different) 'Spelke-objects'. It is then a moot point whether these perceptual mechanisms exhibit an application only of this *one* general sortal classification, with its associated criterion of identity, in their pre-reflective 'segmenting' of the perceived environment into discrete objects moving through space and time, or whether, for instance, they *also* apply a sortal classification roughly corresponding to the concept of a *living organism*, with its very different associated criterion of identity. Certainly, there is strong empirical evidence that even very young infants are sensitive, in their instinctive perceptual responses, to the distinction between things that are 'alive' and things that are not, but that is not enough to show that their sensitivity in this respect includes a sensitivity to relevant differences between the *identity-conditions* of living and non-living things, as is reflected, for example, in the different criteria of identity governing *living organisms* and *hunks of matter*, or in the different criteria of identity governing *living organisms* and *material artefacts* (for instance, between the criterion governing *cats* and that governing *toy* cats). But let me emphasize once again the very important point that *any* theorist who maintains that our pre-reflective perceptual mechanisms can somehow pick out items in our environment and *track them as they move* must be committed to acknowledging that those mechanisms somehow embody a sensitivity to the synchronic and diachronic *identity-conditions* of the items in question and thereby must be, effectively, *classifying* those items sortally, since precisely what it *means* for an item to fall under a certain sortal characterization, however broad, is for it to comply with a certain criterion of identity both at a time and over time. Theorists, including Raftopoulos, who think that items can be 'picked out' and 'tracked' *independently of any sortal characterization of them whatever* betray, I believe, a seriously distorted understanding of what 'sortal' classification really involves. It first and foremost involves a proper sensitivity to an item's distinctive *identity-conditions*, as captured by the criterion of identity governing it. It is quite false, however, to think that a 'sortal' term in this sense has to be something nearly as specific as, for example, 'cat' or 'table' or 'tree'. It can be quite as general as 'object', in the somewhat misleading sense in which this term is used by Raftopoulos, for even in this sense it is necessarily associated with the satisfaction of certain identity-conditions both *at* a time and *over* time, given that it is being used to denote items capable of *moving through space and time.*

8.3

Now, I said earlier that, in my view, Raftopoulos's strategy for defending realism isn't either (1) the only available one or even (2) an entirely satisfactory one. As I have just indicated, I think that one can defend realism by appealing to the *innateness* of certain 'sortal' concepts, at least *as* successfully as one can by deploying Raftopoulos's strategy (which isn't, of course, to say that *either* strategy is fully satisfactory). Secondly, however, I do think that Raftopoulos is right to contend, as he does, that the only way to defend realism compellingly against the sort of antirealists that he has in mind is to argue *from* perceptual content *to* realism, not least because their scepticism arises from doubts about the reliability of perception as a guide to mind-independent truth. I am also happy to acknowledge, indeed, that it is only the *nonconceptual* content of perception that should ultimately be appealed to for this purpose (although not because I share the antirealists' scepticism about the universality and stability of human concepts quite generally). However, my immediate objection to Raftopoulos's own attempt to implement an argument for realism of this type is—as mentioned earlier—that his version is at bottom just question-begging and circular. This is because Raftopoulos openly and deliberately appeals to *scientific* evidence drawn from empirical work by neurophysiologists and neuropsychologists in support of his claims that perception has the type of nonconceptual content that he attributes to it. However, this is just to assume the *truth* of the scientific theories that such evidence relies on—it is to assume, not least, that *brains* exist, that they are composed largely of *neurons*, and that our perception is a product of *brain-processes* involving the interaction of neurons stimulated by *physical events* (events such as the emission of *photons*) occurring in our external environment and affecting our *sensory organs* (such as our *retinal surfaces*). But these are all *realist* assumptions of a quite specific kind, all of which are thoroughly 'theory-laden' and so subject to the antirealists' sceptical concerns.

To argue at all compellingly against the antirealist, we need to be able to appeal to features of the nonconceptual content of perception which can be identified wholly *introspectively*, without any appeal to antecedently assumed empirical scientific theories. Now, is the kind of nonconceptual content described and appealed to by Raftopoulos of a suitable type for this dialectical purpose? I think *not*. For even if it could be contended (as Raftopoulos himself does not contend) that it is purely *introspectively* ascertainable that perception has nonconceptual content of this kind, this is supposed to be content which is still *representational*, even though not *conceptual*, in character. It is supposed, more specifically, to be content which represents the *physical environment* of the subject as being a certain way, namely, as being articulated into three-dimensional objects situated *outside* the subject and capable of undergoing movement with respect to the subject. But an antirealist—such as, to take a classic historical example, *Berkeley*—can easily claim that the mere fact that our perceptual states *represent* to us the existence of such an external, three-dimensional environment in which we ourselves are located gives us no good reason to suppose that such an environment really *does* exist. In short, we have yet to be persuaded of the *veridicality* of any such representational content, notwithstanding its supposedly 'nonconceptual' character. Why—the antirealist may ask—couldn't extramental reality (if indeed there is any) be *utterly unlike* the 'external world' as the nonconceptual content of our perception *represents* it to be? Why shouldn't it be the case that extramental reality—*God*, perhaps—equips us with this kind of representation *not* because it is in any way *veridical*, but just because it is somehow conducive to our wellbeing or our survival for us to *take* extramental reality to be like this?

In this context, then, the crucial step (v) in Raftopoulos's own summary of his argument, cited earlier in section 8.1, has very little dialectical force against his antirealist opponents. Step (v), recall, was this: 'Our interactions with the world on the basis of this [nonconceptual representational] content are largely successful' (Raftopoulos 2009: 342). But, as I have just indicated, a sufficiently sophisticated antirealist, such as Berkeley, can readily contend that 'success' in our projects is perfectly consistent with the radical non-veridicality of the representational contents of our perceptions because, say, the *real* source of our perceptions is a benevolent deity who has our wellbeing in mind in conferring upon our perceptions contents of precisely this 'illusory' kind.

8.4

Fortunately for realism, there is, I believe, a solution to the foregoing difficulty, but it is one which involves delving down much deeper into the introspectively accessible nonconceptual content of perception, to a level not recognized by Raftopoulos (nor, to be fair, by most present-day philosophers of perception, given their hostility to anything that is suggestive of 'sense data'). I can only very roughly sketch this solution here, which begins as follows. And, for ease of exposition, I shall focus exclusively on the case of *visual* perception, as indeed Raftopoulos himself largely does. Very well, then: as I have argued elsewhere, there is, I believe, a component or level of nonconceptual visual content that is *topologically* two-dimensional and *metrically* spherical (or fairly close to spherical). That is to say, the visual field of a normally sighted human subject is at any given moment articulated into *regions*, often differentiated by phenomenal colour differences, and these regions individually and collectively exhibit a *two-dimensional topology* and a *spherical geometry* (see Lowe 1986). For simplicity, I concentrate on the case of *monocular* vision, since the stereoscopic effects of binocular vision, while not affecting the topological structure of the visual field, in the sense of rendering it anything other than two-dimensional, are of course significant for depth-perception and certainly give the perceiver an *impression* of three-dimensionality, even though the visual field itself is not *extended* in three dimensions.

I shall deal, rather briefly, with the topological point first, the details of which I have set out previously (Lowe 1986). The following is a simple theorem in the topology of two-dimensional surfaces. Given any two separate points, *A* and *B*, in such a surface, it is always possible to draw a closed line or *loop*, *L*, around *A*—this loop being confined to the surface in question—such that any line (likewise confined to the surface) connecting *A* to *B* must intersect the loop *L*. Figure 8.1 illustrates this fact.

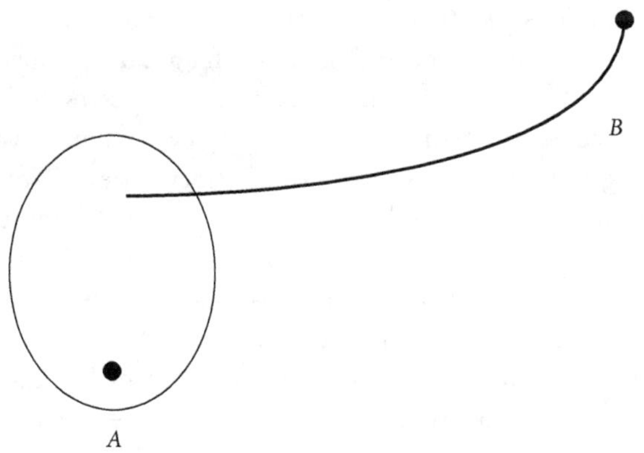

Figure 8.1

Now, to see how this theorem is exemplified by the visual field of a normally sighted person, consider any two 'points' in that field: for instance, suppose that one is looking at a distant hillside on which two houses *appear* as two small coloured 'dots', *A* and *B*, separated from one another. Then it will always be possible to take a thin piece of coloured wire bent into the shape of a loop, *L*, and position it so that it *appears* to encircle *A*, in such a fashion that any other thin piece of coloured wire, positioned so as to *appear* to connect *A* to *B*, must *appear* to intersect the loop *L*.

Since the word 'appear' is multiply ambiguous, it is vitally important, of course, that we recognize the intended sense of 'appear', as I am using it in the foregoing example. This is sometimes called the 'phenomenal' sense of 'appear'—although the expression 'phenomenal', being a philosophical term of art and hence subject to dispute itself, is not altogether helpful in this context. The relevant sense is, I think, best brought out by means of further examples. A good example for this purpose, I consider, is the following one, which draws on the phenomenon of 'size constancy' in visual perception. If one holds one's two thumbs together in front of one, and then gradually moves one of them further away, all the while fixing one's gaze on the two thumbs, the more distant thumb will *not* appear to get 'smaller' as one moves it progressively further away. However, if one repeats this exercise while directing one's gaze *not* at the two thumbs, but rather at a point a few degrees of arc above or below them, then the more distant thumb *will* indeed appear to get increasingly 'smaller' as one moves it further away: the 'size constancy' phenomenon that manifests itself in the first version of the procedure entirely vanishes in the second version, and indeed in a very striking fashion. Now, the sense in which the more distant thumb *appears smaller* than the nearer thumb in the second version of the procedure is the sense of 'appear' that I am applying in my description of the experiment with the two distant houses and the two pieces of wire. In the latter experiment there is, of course, a perfectly good sense in which the two wires may *not* 'appear' to intersect, since one of them may 'appear', in *this* sense, to be in front of the other. Similarly, in *this* sense of 'appear', the second piece of wire may not 'appear' to connect the two houses, since it may not 'appear', in *this* sense, to touch either of them—nor, in *this* sense of 'appear', may the two houses 'appear' as dots. *This* sense of 'appear' is sometimes called the 'epistemic' sense—although, again, the terminology here, being technical, is not as helpful as it might be. Setting terminology aside, however, I simply want to point out that we are dealing, in such examples, with two distinct senses of 'appear'—the sense in which, for instance, the two thumbs *do* 'appear' to remain the same in size and the sense in which they *do not*—and that it is the *second* sense that I am appealing to in my argument concerning the topology of the visual field: a sense of 'appear' that I am happy to call the *phenomenal* sense, now that we have managed to pin it down. The thesis is that *visual appearances*, in the *relevant* sense of 'appearance', are two-dimensional. And the hillside example with the two houses seems to confirm this thesis quite compellingly. So I shall pass on from the *topology* of the visual field to its *geometry*.

Now, when I say that the visual field is *metrically spherical*, or exhibits the metrical characteristics of a spherical geometry, what I mean is that topologically distinct regions of the visual field—typically distinguishable by their phenomenal colours, which serve to mark out their boundaries—possess visual *shapes* whose properties typically conform to the principles of just such a geometry. Here, however, we have to consider the visual field not merely as it is *at a moment*, but rather as it *evolves* over a continuous period of time—a period whose duration may be relatively short, such as a few seconds, or considerably longer than this. Another simple, self-performable visual experiment illustrates this important fact about the visual field. This experiment may be conducted as follows.

Take a thin piece of coloured wire bent into the shape of an equilateral Euclidean triangle and view this, to begin with, in a small central region of one's visual field (by holding it at a suitable distance away from one's eye). Next, gradually bring the wire triangle progressively closer towards the centre of one's eye. It will then be observed that the phenomenal character of one's visual field changes in the following way: a progressively larger *triangular* region of that field, outlined by the phenomenal colour of the wire, will be presented to view, in such a fashion that the sum of the *internal angles* of this triangular region progressively increases beyond 180 degrees to a theoretical maximum of almost 360 degrees (attainable only when one's eye is actually *inside* the wire triangle). Since the *actual* experiment is a little tricky to perform in practice—owing to the need to utilize the periphery of one's visual field in order to generate the strongest effect—it may be helpful to reinforce its lesson with the aid of a simple but compelling *thought experiment*, as follows. Suppose that, instead of having at most 180-degree vision, one had *360-degree* vision, enabling one to see the visual scene all around oneself in a single view, without needing to turn one's head in any direction. And suppose that one were approaching, in a straight line, an archway constructed from three iron rods in the form of an equilateral Euclidean triangle. While one was at a considerable distance from the archway, it would appear—in the phenomenal sense of 'appear'—as a small, almost Euclidean, equilateral triangle lying in one's direction of travel. However, imagine how it must appear as one gets very near to and actually *passes through* the archway. Clearly, at that point the archway must appear as *encircling* one in every direction, with no apparent 'corners'. Its phenomenal appearance will gradually have been transformed from that of a small, almost Euclidean triangle whose internal angles sum to approximately 180 degrees, via a continuous series of ever larger spherical triangles, until finally it takes the form of a 'great circle' of a sphere, which is the limiting case of a spherical triangle. As one then proceeds through and away from the archway, it will present the appearance of a reverse sequence of ever diminishing spherical triangles in the direction opposite to one's direction of travel until, once again, it has the appearance of a small almost Euclidean triangle, but now 'behind' instead of 'ahead' of one.

Now, this experimental exercise, both in its original and in its thought-experiment form, just serves to illustrate an almost ubiquitous phenomenal feature of normal human visual perception, alluded to earlier: namely, the fact that the visual field is almost always articulated into chromatically differentiated spatial regions whose typical evolution over time conforms, in the foregoing manner, to the metrical principles of a spherical geometry. There are, of course, various exceptions to this—for example, in conditions of complete darkness, or when the subject is viewing a uniformly coloured surface, such as a white wall, in very close proximity to it. For present purposes, I am ignoring also more complex situations in which—speaking in 'realist' mode—we would say that objects in our environment are themselves undergoing changes of size or shape, unlike the presumed situation in the case of the 'archway' thought-experiment. If there were *never* stability of size or shape in environmental objects, then, it seems clear, our visual appearances would be practically useless to us as guides to the structure of our environment, and experiments of the kind that I am describing would be impossible to perform. However, the fact that we very frequently *do* find them possible and indeed quite easy to perform provides, I believe, significant testimony in favour of external world realism, as I am about to explain.

There is, of course, a very obvious *physiological* explanation for the almost ubiquitous phenomenal feature of normal human visual perception just described. This is that each region of the visual field corresponds to a geometrically similar region of the subject's *retina*, which is an approximately (hemi)spherical surface and thus one that possesses an approximately spherical geometry. For example, in the case of the wire triangle, as it is brought progressively closer to the eye, an increasingly large *spherically triangular region of the retina* is stimulated by light rays from the wire incident upon the retinal surface. Now, of course, this *physiological* explanation is not something that we can assume to be correct in a debate with a thoroughgoing antirealist, for whom the truth of the physiological claims involved in that explanation are still entirely open to question. Nonetheless, *the phenomenological fact itself*, for which this physiological explanation has been offered, is unassailable, since it is ascertainable by introspection alone in the manner just described. Bear in mind here that while the *instructions for performing the experiment* are couched in physical terms, the *phenomenal character* of the visual experience thus generated does not call upon any such terms for its proper description. And this is why this kind of phenomenological fact is suitable for recruitment in an argument in defence of realism, since it begs no relevant question against the antirealist. Precisely *how* it may be recruited for this purpose we shall now proceed to see.

What can be established introspectively, in the foregoing manner—supplemented if need be by many other self-performable experiments of a similar kind—is that the phenomenal content of visual experience possesses formal spatial features in virtue of which it is true to say that the visual field has, *geometrically speaking*, the properties of a central 'projection' of a three-dimensional Euclidean space upon a two-dimensional spherical surface. Being a 'projection' in this sense is a purely *formal* relational property of a spatial manifold of any kind. It is in this sense, for instance, that we can say that Mercator's geographical 'projection' of the Earth's surface in an atlas is a 'projection' of a spherical surface upon a flat one (or, more accurately, a cylindrical one). In the case of the visual field, we have a *central* projection of a three-dimensional Euclidean space upon a spherical surface, meaning that the 'lines of projection' go from points in the Euclidean space to a point at the *centre* of the (notional) sphere whose surface is the surface of projection. Incidentally, this fact about the visual field was recognized long ago by Thomas Reid in his 'geometry of visibles', so I am saying nothing fundamentally new here. It explains, amongst other things, why it is that the cloudless night sky appears to us as a *dome*, giving rise to the traditional description of the starry heavens as a celestial *sphere*. But it is vital to recognize that a two-dimensional spatial manifold can have all the *formal properties* of a 'central projection' of this kind without there needing to *be* any three-dimensional spatial manifold of which it really *is* such a 'projection', much less for the two-dimensional manifold actually to be *embedded* in such a three-dimensional one. Hence, in describing the visual field in this way we are not simply *assuming* the existence of any 'external' three-dimensional space of any kind, such as *physical* space. Nonetheless, given that this formal characteristic of the visual field is so pervasive, constant, and consistent, we are entitled to assume that it is not just accidental and hence that it calls for some kind of *causal explanation*. And now we are in position to propose, as a case of 'inference to the best (or simplest) explanation', that it is reasonable to *infer*, as a *cause* of this pervasive and stable geometrical characteristic of the visual field, *the actual existence* of a *real* three-dimensional Euclidean spatial manifold and indeed a *real* 'projective' mechanism, in the form of something akin to light rays, incident upon a *real* (hemi)spherical sensory surface, akin to the retina—in short, an 'external' world possessing the basic structure and form that realism traditionally assigns to it and in which we as perceiving subjects are *located* and *embodied*.

Of course, this is not to imply that human subjects acquire a belief in such an external world *by inference* from the spatial properties of their visual fields—neither by any conscious process of inference nor by any unconscious or 'subpersonal' one executed by the visual systems in their brains. We are not concerned here with the *acquisition* of belief in an external world, only with its *justification*. Obviously, too, there are in principle alternative possible 'explanations' for the relevant spatial properties of the visual field other than the 'realist' one which posits a real three-dimensional Euclidean space 'external' to the subject. For instance, taking a lead from Descartes or Berkeley, it is possible to suppose that God or an 'evil demon' has just decided, for good or ill, to *give us* visual experiences which present us with a visual field possessing precisely the projective properties that have just been described, thus making it *seem to us as if* we inhabit a real three-dimensional Euclidean space. (For, clearly, the projective properties in question are intimately involved in its *seeming to us* that we do inhabit such a space, even if our belief that we do is not generated by any kind of inference from those properties to the existence of such a space.) But it seems evident that any such alternative 'explanation', while *conceivable*, is really just *parasitic* upon the preferred realist explanation of the relevant phenomenological facts. The alternative hypotheses are all just ones which claim that the 'true' explanation *mimics* the effects of the realist explanation, without providing any detailed account of *how* these effects are supposed to be produced. And that, at least in part, is why the realist explanation is indeed the *best* and *simplest* explanation, even if it is not the *only possible* explanation. The phenomenological facts in question, then, give us *good but not conclusive* reason to be realists—and this, really, is the best that one can ever hope to achieve in a debate with any confirmed antirealist.

Why, it may be asked, can't the antirealist reply to me just as I envisaged him replying to the realist who merely invoked the (nonconceptual) *representational* content of visual experience—by urging, for instance, that some deity has simply determined, perhaps for the sake of our wellbeing, to confer upon us visual perceptions which have the systematic projective geometrical features that I have just described? My answer is that by advancing from the representational to the formal *geometrical* content of visual experience we open up a possible form of *explanation* of the phenomenal character of our visual experience which is much more powerful than anything that can be offered by the realist who confines his or her attention purely to the representational content of visual experience. For now we can invoke the hypothesis of a three-dimensional Euclidean space incorporating a suitable projective mechanism to explain why our visual experience takes the form it does—and do this *without* appealing, in a way that would be blatantly question-begging, to any presumed scientific facts concerning our physiology. The hypothesis in question requires only *a priori mathematical concepts* for its coherent formulation. The merely representational realist, by contrast, cannot, without appeal to physical concepts and theories, formulate any substantive explanation of the visual phenomena, but is reduced in effect to saying that the representational content of our visual experiences is best 'explained' by the putative fact that it is caused by environmental objects whose properties are broadly what our visual experience *represents* them as being. But this sort of 'explanation' is very thin indeed and consequently presents little challenge to a determined antirealist. By contrast, the sort of explanation that I am offering on behalf of realism is both simple and powerful, serving to explain *in detail* why the course of our visual experience proceeds as it typically does.

8.5

I have urged that we *can* formulate an argument *from* perceptual content *to* realism which does not beg any question against the antirealist by assuming the truth of any theory couched in terms of objects and properties supposedly belonging to an extramental 'external world'. But, as we have seen, in order to construct such an argument we need to be able to identify *introspectively* certain aspects of the nonconceptual content of perception which are not only nonconceptual but also *non-representational* in character, unlike the kind of nonconceptual content appealed to by Raftopoulos, which is not only representational but also, supposedly, not immediately accessible to phenomenal consciousness but attributable to perception only with the support of empirical scientific theory. I have also tried to show that introspectively accessible nonconceptual content of the required sort *can* be found, in the form of the characteristic projective geometrical features of the visual field, which provide good evidence for the truth of a moderate form of realism, according to which we really do inhabit an 'extramental' three-dimensional space occupied by persisting objects possessing relatively stable spatial structures—a space that is Euclidean in form, at least at the scale at which our sensory engagement with it takes place.

As it stands, this argument for realism is just a rough preliminary sketch which needs to be filled out in many ways to make it as compelling as it could be. But it is at least indicative of the *kind* of task that needs to be undertaken, I believe, if one is to engage the antirealist on terms which are not implicitly question-begging and circular, in any attempt to argue *from* perceptual content *to* realism. Some may now conclude that such a task *cannot* be successful and give up the debate with the antirealist altogether. Others will try to persuade us that antirealism can be challenged effectively in some quite different way, such as by insisting that only a thoroughgoing 'externalist' account of perceptual content is even intelligible—a claim which, for my own part, I find not merely implausible but questionably even coherent. Interesting and bold though Raftopoulos's attempted argument for realism is, however, I feel that it falls between two stools—that of a properly *non-question-begging* argument from perceptual content to realism on the one hand, and that of a putative defence of realism which rejects altogether the idea that what is either possible or needed, in order to defeat the antirealist, is an argument *from* perceptual content *to* realism.

References

Hanson, N. R. (1958), *Patterns of Discovery* (Cambridge: Cambridge University Press).

Kuhn, T. S. (1962), *The Structure of Scientific Revolutions* (Chicago, IL: University of Chicago Press).

Lowe, E. J. (1986), 'The Topology of Visual Appearance', in *Erkenntnis* 25: 271–4.

Lowe, E. J. (1998), *The Possibility of Metaphysics: Substance, Identity, and Time* (Oxford: Clarendon Press).

Lowe, E. J. (2007), 'Sortals and the Individuation of Objects', in *Mind and Language* 22: 514–33.

Raftopoulos, A. (2009), *Cognition and Perception: How Do Psychology and Neural Science Inform Philosophy?* (Cambridge, MA: MIT Press).

Sellars, W. (1963), *Science, Perception and Reality* (London: Routledge and Kegan Paul).

Spelke, E. S. (1990), 'Principles of Object Perception', in *Cognitive Science* 14: 29–56.

Strawson, P. F. (1959), *Individuals: An Essay in Descriptive Metaphysics* (London: Methuen).

Wiggins, D. (1980), *Sameness and Substance* (Oxford: Blackwell).

Wiggins, D. (2001), *Sameness and Substance Renewed* (Cambridge: Cambridge University Press).

9

Can We Really See a Million Colours?

David Papineau

9.1 Introduction

It is widely assumed that human beings are capable of well over a million different conscious visual responses to coloured surfaces.

The evidence for this is the psychometric data on 'just noticeable colour differences'. When two coloured surfaces are presented simultaneously and adjacently, normal human beings can detect very fine differences. They are capable of consciously registering colour differences between well over a million differently coloured sample surfaces, varying in hue, brightness, and saturation.[1]

It might seem natural to infer from this that we humans must have a repertoire of more than a million conscious responses to coloured surfaces. After all, when we are presented with a pair of adjacent surfaces, surely our consciously registering a *difference in colour* must derive from our first having *one* colour response to the left-hand side surface, and *another* colour response to the right-hand surface, and thence registering that there is a difference.

However, this assumption, which I shall call the 'orthodox view', is not mandatory. In this chapter I shall offer an alternative account of the discrimination data. On this alternative view, detection of colour differences is a gestalt phenomenon: we can often consciously see straight off that two adjacent surfaces are different in colour without first consciously having two different responses to each surface.

This alternative view is consistent with our being capable of far fewer than a million conscious colour responses when we are presented with colour samples on their own. Perhaps we have a limited number of such non-comparative conscious colour responses. If the detection of colour differences between adjacent surfaces

[1] Pointer and Attridge (1998), McCamy (1998). It is relevant to what follows that the ability to discern simultaneous colour differences between non-juxtaposed surfaces falls off rapidly with increasing spatial separation (Sivic 1997: 163).

does not derive from prior non-comparative responses to each surface, there is no need to posit a million such responses to account for the discrimination data.

The alternative view fits well with the fact that humans perform very poorly on same/different tasks when colour samples are presented successively rather than simultaneously. When two coloured surfaces are presented at separate times, the number of different surfaces that can reliably be judged to be the same or different by most observers is of the order of a few dozen, even under ideal conditions (Hamwi and Landis 1955).

Orthodoxy attributes this poor performance in the diachronic successive matching task to some kind of memory limitation. On the orthodox view, subjects are capable of distinct conscious responses to a great many more than a few dozen different coloured surfaces; so their inability to make reliable same/different responses to more than a few dozen successively presented surfaces must be due to some sort of failure to retain knowledge of their earlier response until the later presentation.

But, on my alternative view, we don't necessarily have to attribute the poor performance in the successive matching task to memory deficiency. Perhaps most humans are capable of no more than a few dozen conscious responses to coloured surfaces presented singly in the first place, and the reason that they aren't reliably attuned to finer distinctions in the successive same/different task isn't that they can't hold the relevant fine-grained information in memory, but simply that they didn't have it in the first place.

However, this is more than I need, or indeed want, to say. The main burden of my alternative view is that we have *far fewer* conscious colour responses to surfaces presented singly than the million plus assumed by orthodoxy. It would be an extra claim to equate this number with the few dozen categories over which subjects can perform reliably in the successive same/different tasks. Maybe subjects do have significantly more than a few dozen available conscious responses to surfaces presented singly, but fail to manifest these in the successive matching tasks because of difficulties in retaining the relevant information in memory.[2]

As will become clear in what follows, my alternative view makes it a matter of internal cognitive architecture how many different conscious colour responses humans can make to surfaces presented singly. The number of such responses depends on the organization of the brain, and is not something that can easily be ascertained from psychometric or even introspective data.

[2] This diagnosis receives prima facie support from evidence that performance in colour memory tasks is enhanced if the subjects have names for the colours involved (Roberson et al. 2005). Of course this evidence does not *prove* that the limited performance is due to memory constraints—the names may matter, not because they help subjects to remember colours, but because they shape the single-colour responses which subjects are capable of in the first place (cf. Roberson et al. 2004, Winawer et al. 2007). It is consistent with my alternative view that subjects' single-colour responses cannot outstrip the colour categorizations made by their culture and reflected in their colour vocabulary. But, again, this is more than I need or want to argue here. For a survey of relevant recent data in this hotly debated area see Regier and Kay (2009).

We should also bear in mind that the range of such responses is very likely to vary from individual to individual. It will be entirely consistent with my alternative view that variations in culture, training, and natural endowment should make a significant difference to the repertoire of non-comparative colour responses available to different individuals. Maybe some individuals are indeed only capable of a few dozen such responses, while others—painters or interior decorators, say—are capable of many hundreds.

For both these reasons, it would make no sense for me to offer any definite number for the number of colour responses humans in general are capable of. Still, having made these points, it will sometimes be useful to have a number to play with, and so I shall on occasion assume that there are a hundred single-colour responses available to humans. But this will be for illustrative purposes only, and should not be taken to deny that the real number will depend on details of brain structure, and moreover will vary across individuals.

More generally, in what follows I shall be offering an alternative to the orthodox account of the structure of colour perception. However, this alternative will be something of a speculative simplification. No doubt a full understanding of colour perception will show it to be more complicated than I portray it here. The physiology of colour vision is by no means fully understood, and future findings are sure to add to our understanding of the structure of conscious colour vision.

However, the primary purpose in this chapter is not to establish a precise positive account of conscious colour vision, but to cast doubt on orthodoxy. For this purpose, it will be convenient to formulate a simple alternative, and to show that the existing evidence favours it over orthodoxy. But it should be borne in mind that variations on this alternative would be equally well-supported by that existing evidence, and could well be favoured by future evidence.

One final preliminary. My focus in all that follows will be on phenomenal properties. That is, I shall be concerned with the range of *ways it can consciously be* for an individual in colour vision. In this respect, I shall have a narrower focus than much other philosophical work on colour vision, in that I shall aim to bracket off questions about the ontology of colour. I shall be exclusively concerned with the range of *conscious mental states* involved in colour vision, and not with the range of *properties of surfaces* that such states might be tracking.[3]

[3] Peter Mandik's 'Color-Consciousness Conceptualism' (2012) appeals to a distinction between non-comparative and comparative colour perceptions that is close to that defended in this chapter. But his primary focus is on the representational contents of the perceptions rather than their qualitative nature, and it is not clear to me whether he ends up endorsing my thesis that humans are capable of far fewer than a million colour responses to surfaces presented singly. Mandik acknowledges David Rosenthal's important earlier discussion of non-comparative and comparative colour concepts (Rosenthal 2005: 188–9). But Rosenthal too seems not to deny that humans are capable of a million-plus 'mental colours'. The relation between Rosenthal's and Mandik's positions and my own is complicated by the fact that Rosenthal, and I suspect Mandik too, will not count the million-plus responses as *conscious* if they are not individually conceptualized, whereas I am not assuming any kind of higher-order approach to consciousness. Still, even

Moreover, I shall aim to remain as neutral as possible about the nature of conscious phenomenal properties. As it happens, I think that conscious vision is designed to represent features of the external environment, and so will on occasion talk about conscious colour perception in representational terms; I also think that conscious phenomenal colour properties are to be identified with 'syntactic' features of the vehicles of such representation, rather than with the abstract representational contents of those vehicles. However, I do not think that the main points in what follows depend on these commitments. Those who have other views about the nature of the phenomenal properties should be able to transpose my arguments into their own theoretical frameworks.

9.2 Two Kinds of State

On the view I propose, our conscious colour experience is the joint product of two different kinds of perceptual state.

The first kind of state arises in response to single surfaces, and is designed to categorize the surface as of a certain colour. Here I hypothesize that the visual system is capable of something like 100 different colour responses. I shall refer to perceptual states of this kind as 'categorical'. We can think of them of corresponding to ordinary colour terms, such as pink, orange, purple, navy blue, olive green, and so on.[4]

The second kind of perceptual state arises when the visual system is presented simultaneously with two coloured surfaces side-by-side. This kind of state will convey information about the *relation* between the two surfaces. The simplest version of such a perceptual state would simply indicate whether the two samples are the *same* or *different* in colour. But it is consistent with my view that such states should also indicate the relative locations of the two samples in various colour dimensions: thus they might indicate which sample is *more* red than the other, and similarly for *more* yellow, more *saturated*, and *brighter*.[5] I shall refer to states of this kind as 'relational'.

if we put this difference to one side, I deny, where they seem to accept, that our sensory systems generate a million-plus single-colour responses, whether or not we count these responses as conscious.

[4] A central piece of evidence for the now widely-accepted 'opponent-process' account of colour perception (Hurvich and Jameson 1957) is the ability of subjects reliably to estimate the *proportion* of red/green or blue/yellow in any spectral colour (Werner and Wooten 1979). This quantitative ability may seem in tension with my hypothesis of a limited range of categorial single-colour responses. However, this tension is only apparent. The subjects' estimates are by no means so precise as to entail that they are capable of more than a few dozen distinct categorial colour responses. And my view can perfectly well allow that these categorial responses depend on the activity of opponent channels in ways that can to some degree be recovered by introspective reflection.

[5] This particular set of dimensions is suggested by the opponent-process theory. But my view is not committed to this theory, and could equally well accommodate different dimensions of colour relations, and also more specific qualitative comparative judgements (for example: much redder/redder/same redness). I shall return to the issue of dimensions of colour relations towards the end of section 9.6.

The crucial point for my purposes is that the visual system should be able to issue in a relational judgement that two adjacent samples viewed simultaneously *differ* even in cases where the two surfaces produce the *same* categorical colour response. That is, the two surfaces both elicit the same version of the first kind of categorical state—they both strike the viewer as *orange*, say—but nevertheless elicit a relational state that indicates a colour *difference* between the two samples.

If the relational state simply conveyed symmetrical same/different information, then this would imply that in such a case the conscious experience of the viewer would be essentially the same with respect to the two adjacent surfaces: the viewer would see the left-hand sample as *orange* and as *different* from the right-hand sample, and similarly see the right-hand sample as *orange* and as *different* from the left-hand sample.

But if the relational states also convey information about which sample is more red/yellow/saturated/bright, then the situation need not be so symmetrical. The viewer may not only judge relationally that two oranges are different, but also that the left-hand sample is more *red* than the other, and similarly for the other dimensions. To this extent, the observer's conscious experience of the two samples will be different: one will be seen as more red, say, and the other correspondingly as less red.

Still, my view does have this striking consequence: looking at orange_{23} next to orange_{24} can be just like looking at orange_{27} next to orange_{28}. (I am here using 'orange_{23}', 'orange_{24}', and so on to refer to the surface properties of samples that are just noticeably different in colour when presented side-by-side.) In both cases—orange_{23} next to orange_{24}, and orange_{27} next to orange_{28}—the viewer would have the categorical information that the two adjacent surfaces are both orange, plus relational information to the effect that the left-hand sample is more/less red/yellow/saturated/bright than the other. If our conscious awareness is the product of the two states conveying this information, as I am supposing, then our conscious awareness of the two pairs will be just the same.

This is in striking contrast to orthodoxy. On the orthodox view, orange_{23} next to orange_{24} must look different to orange_{27} next to orange_{28}. For orthodoxy takes our awareness of colour differences to derive from our awareness of the individual colour of each sample, which implies that each orange_{k} must produce a different colour response on its own, and thus that different pairs of such surfaces will do so too.

Here is a way of conveying my view of colour perception. Imagine that a friend is looking at two side-by-side samples that are invisible to you. Your friend *tells* you, say, that the samples are both orange, and that the left-hand sample is more red, less yellow, less saturated, and more bright than the right-hand sample. I say that the information that your friend has provided exhausts the information that you would get even if you were looking at the samples yourself.

9.3 The Debate about Non-Conceptual Content

Many readers will have been introduced to questions about the range of colour responses available to humans in connection with the debate about 'non-conceptual content'. While this debate is not my focus in this chapter, it may be helpful to explain what my view implies about it.

The debate about non-conceptual content concerns the representational powers of perception. Can perception represent facts that cannot be conceptualized by the perceiving subject?

To keep things simple, let me assume that representational contents are 'Russellian', depending on the object and properties represented, and not on their modes of presentation. Now assume that some subject perceptually represents that some *a is F*. Must the subject possess concepts that refer to *a* and to *F*? The conceptualists say 'yes', the non-conceptualists 'no'. (To bring out the possibility of non-conceptual representation, imagine that some insect represents that the leaf in front of it is edible, say, in a way that does not require that it can refer to that leaf, or to the property of edibility, in other representational contexts.)

One of the most familiar arguments for non-conceptual representation appeals to the 'fineness of grain' of colour perception. The idea is that the psychometrical data on just noticeable differences show that we are capable of visually representing over a million different colours. But it seems highly implausible to suppose that we have over a million colour concepts. (If we can conceptualize all those colours, how come we are so hopeless at retaining visual information about colours over time?) So conscious vision can represent properties for which we have no concepts (Evans 1982, Peacocke 1992).

Nearly all the literature on this argument accepts that the discrimination data do show that we can visually represent a million different colours. The debate has focused rather on whether or not we have a corresponding range of colour *concepts*.

Conceptualists have responded to the 'fineness of grain' argument by appealing to 'demonstrative' colour concepts. The idea is that such 'demonstrative' colour concepts can be formed when a specific colour sample is in view, and can be expressed by the phrase 'that colour'. Since there is nothing to stop us forming concepts like these for all the million-plus colours we can represent, so the conceptualists argue, there is no reason to suppose that our representational powers outrun our conceptual repertoire (McDowell 1994, Brewer 1999).

Non-conceptualists have objected that these putative demonstrative concepts do not really qualify as concepts. A minimum requirement for the possession of concepts, they argue, is that such possession subserves the retention of information over time. But subjects are typically unable to retain information about fine-grained colours they saw a moment ago. So we should not credit them with any corresponding concepts (Raffman 1995, Kelly 2001).

One possibility open to conceptualists at this point is to respond that their opponents are setting the standards for concept possession too high, and that there are good reasons for crediting us with fine-grained demonstrative concepts despite their failure to allow information retention (Brewer 2005, Chuard 2006).

However, the position I am defending in this chapter allows a quite different defence of conceptualism, one that does not call for any dilution of standards for concept possession. This is because my view rejects the assumption that gets this whole debate off the ground, namely, the assumption that humans are able visually to represent a million different colours. On my view, we can only represent a hundred-odd categorial colour properties in the first place (as well as being able to represent that two surfaces seen side-by-side differ from each other in certain dimensions). So there is no need to posit a million concepts to render all representation conceptual. A hundred or so will do (plus a few concepts to represent two adjacent surfaces being relationally different in certain dimensions).

Put it like this. My view agrees with conventional non-conceptualists that we have a highly limited number of colour concepts. But, from my perspective, this is quite enough to render all colour representation conceptual, since we don't represent any more than a highly limited number of colours to start with.[6]

9.4 Pictures and Features

Some readers may be feeling that this would be a fine way to defend conceptualism, if my view were true—but that as yet I have offered no earthly reason to suppose it is true. Moreover, they may well feel that the orthodox theory of a million different conscious colour responses is far more in line with obvious facts than my outlandish suggestion that we are only capable of a hundred responses or so.

In this section I shall aim to cast doubt on the idea that the orthodox view is forced on us by any obvious facts. In subsequent sections I shall offer further positive considerations in favour of my alternative view.

If conscious vision worked in a pixel-like pictorial manner, by first consciously determining the local qualities of each minimal region in the visual field, and only thence inferring the properties of larger regions, then I agree that the orthodox view of colour perception would follow. However, it is highly doubtful that conscious vision does work in this pictorial manner.

Note that the issue is not whether viewing a real scene produces the same kind of conscious response as looking at a picture. This is of course trivially true, given that pictures (at least traditional representational pictures) are *designed* to produce the same kind of conscious visual reactions as normal scenes. Rather the question is whether our conscious awareness of an overall scene is metaphysically determined by our prior conscious awareness of each minimal region of the field, in the way that the

[6] For a more detailed defence of conceptualism along very similar lines, see Mandik (2012).

large-scale visible properties of a picture are arguably metaphysically determined by the visible properties of each of its minimal regions.

While it might seem natural to suppose that conscious vision works in this pictorial way, this doesn't fit what the brain does. Perhaps the information registered by the retina at any time can be considered to comprise a kind of pictorial representation of what is seen (though it will be both fleeting and highly degraded outside the central foveal region). But I take it that this retinal state is certainly not conscious. And all later stages of visual processing work in a highly non-pictorial manner. Far from trying to identify local properties of minimal regions, different processes strive to discern spatiotemporally non-local features, such as orientations, shapes, motions, and colours, prior to 'binding' together features that are co-instantiated in the same objects. The processes that discern these features progressively discard much of the information that provides input for their analysis. The whole point of these processes is to sift through noisy, multifarious, and often equivocal inputs and reach a verdict on, say, the orientation of some edge or the shape of some surface. They will then transmit this verdict to other parts of the brain, but not the basis on which they reached it.

Now, it is a matter of some controversy, to put it mildly, exactly which brain states correspond to the phenomenal properties that constitute *conscious* vision. But, whatever the precise answer to this question, there is no immediate reason to suppose that there is a range of such possible conscious states corresponding to all the million-plus surface colour properties that are just noticeably different. It is an interesting question whether the *inputs* to the processes giving rise to conscious colour states contain enough information to identify all these different surface properties. But, even if they do, it does not follow that the conscious *outputs* of these processes include distinct states for each of these million-plus surface properties.

On my view, there is one cognitive process that categorizes single surfaces into one of a hundred-odd kinds, and another that discerns a limited range of relations between adjacent surfaces. While both will use fine-grained wavelength information as input, this information will have been discarded before they produce their outputs. So on my view conscious visual perception will not be capable of anything like a million potential responses to coloured surfaces.

Of course, I have not yet given any definite argument that there *isn't* a cognitive process capable of producing such fine-grained conscious colour outputs. Such arguments will come in a moment. This section's purpose, remember, is only to show that there is nothing in the basic workings of visual perception to *force* us to recognize such a mechanism.

Does not introspection show us directly that conscious vision works pictorially? When we reflect on the nature of our visual experience, can't we just *see* that each minimal area of the visual field plays its part in determining the character of the whole? Well, no doubt introspection shows us that each minimal area of the visual field has a range of definite properties. But I see no reason to accept that it shows us that these properties are determined in a bottom-up way, with conscious vision first fixing the local qualities of minimal regions, and then allowing this to determine the conscious properties of the whole.

We should ask ourselves—what would it seem like if vision worked in a gestalt manner, with many relational non-local features, such as shapes and motions and colour differences, entering directly into conscious perception, independently of any conscious registration of local qualities that might determine them? I say that things would then seem to us just as conscious vision actually does. There is nothing in introspection itself to show us that conscious vision works in a bottom-up pictorial way. (Indeed, if you ask me, the idea that conscious vision works pictorially derives from confused reflection on the physical nature of pictures, rather than from any deliverances of introspection.)

While we are on introspection, it is worth remarking that there are two oft-remarked features of introspectible visual experience that fit rather better with my view than orthodoxy.

The first is the subjective *categoricality* of colour perception. When we look at a picture of some region of colour space, we do not experience a continuous variation in the relevant dimensions, as we do when we are noting the loudness and pitch of noises, say, or the warmth and hardness of surfaces. Rather, we see a set of distinct colour regions (orange, yellow, green, turquoise, . . .), divided by fairly definite boundaries. This argues that the conscious brain is placing viewed surfaces into a limited number of discrete categories, rather than locating them at some position along a continuous spectrum.

The second relevant feature is our ability simultaneously to see adjacent regions of some variably illuminated surface as of the *same* categorial colour yet as *differing* in colour (Cohen 2008). From an orthodox point of view, this can seem puzzling. When we see the whole surface as having the same colour, it's not just that we judge the different regions to be different shades of some determinable colour—different shades of red, say. Rather we see the whole surface to be just one determinate colour, one specific shade of red (our colour perception shows us that we'd need only one kind of paint to produce a surface like that). But how can this be part of our visual experience, on the orthodox view, if we simultaneously see different regions of that surface to be different colours?

However, from my alternative point of view this phenomenon is just what we should expect. The different regions of the surface are being categorized as the same colour (courtesy of the process that makes such categorial judgements), while at the same time adjacent regions are being experienced as different in colour (courtesy of the process that detects relational colour differences).

9.5 Functions of Colour Perception

It will be helpful to think about the *functions* that colour perception is designed to serve. We can distinguish two basic such functions.

First, there is the classification and re-identification of objects. Is that a robin? Is this cherry ripe enough to eat? Is that John's dog? Is this my scarf?

This first function could be served perfectly well by a repertoire of about a hundred colour categories. Anything more would seem like overkill. After all, the different instances of a given natural type—such as different robins or different ripe cherries—are likely to vary in more fine-grained chromatic respects. And even a given object—such as John's dog or my scarf—will vary in colour over time. For purposes of classification and re-identification, a million different colour categories would seem quite unnecessary, and indeed liable to lead to distinctions that are positively counter-productive.

The second function is the discernment of three-dimensional physical form. One of the primary functions of human vision is to construct a representation of the medium-sized physical objects in our environment, including their sizes, shapes, orientations, relative positions, and so on. The brain uses many clues to do this, but crucial first steps are the identification of the visible edges which mark the boundaries of objects in the visual field.

The standard assumption is that the visual brain identifies these features by detecting loci which mark light *intensity* differences—that is, lines where the light intensity on one side is different from that on the other. But, as we shall see in the next section, it also uses loci of chromatic *wavelength* differences. From a functional perspective this is unsurprising, given that loci of chromatic differences are often better guides to the presence of edges than intensity differences alone. This is because they are not generated by mere shadows in the way that intensity differences are: the light from either side of the line produced by a shadow will necessarily vary in intensity, but will generally not vary in wavelength. This point is all the more significant if we consider our evolutionary history. As Israel Abramov has observed in this connection, 'primates developed in an arboreal environment, which is characterized by a bewildering and random array of leaves and shadows' (Abramov 1997: 110).

Edge-detection will benefit from a very fine-grained sensitivity to wavelength differences, even if categorial colour classification does not. Any consistent locus of discontinuity in the wavelength of reflected light is likely to indicate an edge, however small. The edge-detecting function will thus be served by the maximal sensitivity that the eye and brain can manage. There is no overkill in detecting the most precise colour *differences*, even if we have no use for fine-grained *absolute* colour classifications.

Functional considerations thus give us every reason to suppose that there are two distinguishable colour-related processes in the visual brain. One will be concerned to categorize single surfaces into a hundred-odd kinds, as an aid to the classification and re-identification of objects. The other will be concerned to detect colour relations between adjacent regions of the visual field, in the service of the discernment of three-dimensional visual form.

We might model the first process as a kind of neural net with a hundred-odd output nodes. When it is presented with any surface, one of these output nodes will be activated.

We can expect this 'surface classifier', as I shall call it henceforth, to manifest 'colour constancy'. That is, it will be able to judge surfaces as retaining the same colour even across a wide range of changes of illumination. Such changes of illumination can radically alter the amounts of different wavelengths of light that surfaces transmit to the eye. But such changes of illumination will of course not alter the surface properties of the objects with those surfaces. Given its function, the surface classifier will thus need to factor out the optical differences caused by changes in illumination, and instead track surface properties that are invariant with respect to such changes.

The second kind of process might be modelled as comparing the light received from adjacent regions in the visual field in various dimensions, and subtracting the relevant quantities from each other. It will note whether the answer is positive, negative, or zero, but will throw away the absolute values of these quantities, since these absolute values are irrelevant to its function of discerning three-dimensional form. It will register fine-grained differences between surfaces even when these differences are too small to make any difference to the verdicts of the surface classifier.

Note how the outputs of this 'difference detector', as I shall call it, will also be insensitive to changes of illumination. Such changes will affect the absolute values of the optical quantities the detector is comparing, but in general will leave the relative values unchanged. This insensitivity is as it should be, given that changes in illumination do not normally signal changes in three-dimensional form.

In my view, our conscious colour experience is the joint product of the outputs of these two different processes. In the first place, we experience surfaces as having one of a hundred-odd colours. But alongside this we also experience adjacent regions of the visual field as differing in colour, even in cases where the two regions prompt the same response from the colour classifier.

9.6 Mechanisms and Dissociations

The existence of two distinguishable colour mechanisms is amply confirmed by what is known of the neurophysiology of colour vision.

It is widely accepted that chromatic wavelength information is carried to the primary visual cortex by the lateral geniculate nucleus by two kinds of cells. There are the L/M cells that are stimulated by long-wavelength L cones and inhibited by medium-wavelength M cones (or vice versa)—these are standardly called red/green opponent cells. And then there are the S/(L+M) cells that are stimulated by short-wavelength S cones and inhibited by the sum of L and M cone signals (or vice versa)—these are standardly called yellow/blue opponent cells (Abramov 1997: 101–5, Shapley and Hawken 2011: 704).

It is also widely supposed that these two types of cells bear some relation to the opponent 'red-green' and 'yellow-blue channels' posited by the 'opponent-process theory of colour vision'. According to this theory, experienced categorial hues are determined by the levels of activation of two such opponent channels: that is, we can think of such hues as points in a two-dimensional space whose axes are the activation levels of these two channels. This theory thus offers a nice explanation of why we can have hues that strike us as a mixture of red and blue or yellow, or green and blue or yellow, but none which seem a mixture of red and green, or of blue and yellow.

How exactly the two kinds of chromatic cells in the lateral geniculate nucleus might relate to the two posited channels of the opponent process theory is not a straightforward matter (Hardin 1993: 54–8, Abramov 1997: 107). However that may be, though, it is clear that the determination of experienced categorial hues is not the *only* upshot of the chromatic information carried to the visual cortex by the L/M and S/(L+M) cells.

Many of the cells in the primary visual cortex are '*double-opponent*' cells. These are cells that fire when they get contrasting inputs from opponent cells which themselves respond to different but adjacent regions of the visual field. For example, we might have a cell that is excited when L/M inputs responsive to one region of the visual field are opposite in sign to L/M inputs from an adjacent region.

Cells of this kind are designed to detect *spatial changes* in optical properties. They fire when adjacent regions of the visual field produce *differing* optical responses. Many such double-opponent cells are also *orientation-selective*. They fire only when the locus of optical discontinuity lies in a specific direction. The function of these double-opponent cells is clearly to serve the recovery of three-dimensional form, by helping to identify whether edges are present in some region, and determining their orientation when they are (Shapley and Hawken 2011: 704).[7]

Until relatively recently it was supposed that the detection of form depended predominantly on achromatic information about spatial discontinuities in light intensity. However, it is now clear that the double-opponent cells in V1 that subserve the recovery of three-dimensional form are generally just as responsive to chromatic information as to achromatic information (Shapley and Hawken 2011: 707). This is unsurprising, given the point made in the last section about the importance of chromatic discontinuities for identifying edges in an environment containing shadows.

[7] If these cells are specifically sensitive to *spatial* variation, then they will be unable to account for any ability to detect fine-grained colour differences in samples displayed in immediate *temporal succession*. However, it seems likely the mechanisms underlying the perception of *motion* involve cells that are sensitive to *temporal* variation in *chromatic* information (Shapley and Hawken 2011: 703–4). If so, this would explain an ability to detect fine-grained temporal colour changes across short time intervals.

It is sometimes said that double-opponent chromatic cells provide the basis for *colour constancy* computations (Kentridge et al. 2003, Heywood and Kentridge 2003). But this can be a bit confusing. Certainly these cells can detect whether or not transmitted wavelength *alters* from one spatial region to another, and to this extent can sometimes detect that a certain area is *uniform* with respect to wavelength properties. And this can then inform a visual verdict that the relevant area is part of a single surface with a uniform surface colour property. Moreover, none of this processing is going to be affected by variation in background illumination, since double-opponent chromatic cells, like double-opponent cells in general, are sensitive to *differences* in optical properties between different regions, and not to the absolute value of these properties.

But, for just this reason, double-opponent chromatic cells on their own are no good for computing *which* uniform colour a surface has. The information they convey can help to determine that a given area is all one colour, but it does not determine what that colour is. The information about absolute wavelengths that is needed to identify categorial colour has been discarded by the time we get to the outputs of double-opponent chromatic cells. These cells can convey that one region is 'more red' than an adjacent region, say, but this information is consistent with the two regions having a wide range of categorial colours. Double-opponent cells are thus designed to identify colour changes, so to speak, not the colours themselves. So they provide a basis for colour constancy only in the sense that they help discern the three-dimensional form which is an essential precondition for the attribution of uniform colours to surfaces. They do not determine those colours themselves.

I thus take the double-opponent cells in the primary visual cortex to be part of the *difference-detecting* mechanism postulated in the last section. They inform a process that eventually issues in conscious judgements as to whether adjacent regions differ or coincide in colour, possibly augmented by judgements as to the relative positions of the surfaces in a few colour dimensions, such as red-green, yellow-blue, or bright-dark. This process does not reach any conclusion about the categorial colours of surfaces.

What now about the other mechanism postulated in the last section, the 'surface classifier'? Well, the location of a 'colour centre' in the human brain has been a topic of intense debate over the past few decades. In the 1970s Semir Zeki showed that cells in area V4 in the monkey brain responded reliably to surface colours across changes in illumination, and to this extent seemed to be operating as a surface classifier.[8] Subsequent work has sought to identify an analogue of V4 in humans, but specific suggestions have proved highly controversial. In any case, it is not clear that V4 is dedicated specifically to colour rather than form, even in monkeys.[9] Moreover, there is evidence that certain areas yet further forward in the human brain ('VO-1' and

[8] Zeki (1978). [9] Shapley and Hawken (2011: 713).

'VO-2') are highly activated by coloured stimuli.[10] A recent survey article on colour vision suggests that 'perhaps VO-1 is a memory bank of colours that is compared with incoming color signals from V1' as an aid to object recognition using 'association of current input from the world with prior experience'.[11]

In any case, it is clear that at some point the human brain issues in categorical colour responses that are unaffected by changes in illumination. As I said right at the beginning, the precise range of such responses is not a matter to be decided behaviourally or introspectively, but will depend on facts of cognitive architecture. But we have seen no reason at all to posit anything like a million such possible responses, and reflection on their function argues that the range of such responses will be far more limited in number.

If I am right that there are two distinguishable cognitive mechanisms that make use of chromatic signals, then we should expect to find dissociations in injured subjects who possess one mechanism but not the other. And this is exactly what we do find.

Let me first consider the possibility of the difference detector without the surface classifier. Precisely this dissociation is arguably found in patients with the condition called 'cerebral achromotopsia'. These are subjects who have suffered damage to the occipital ventral cortex near to the areas that have been conjectured to comprise the 'colour centre', and as a result have lost the ability to see hues.[12] They report that everything is black and white and grey. Even so, they can easily detect boundaries between surfaces that differ only in transmitted wavelength and not in brightness.[13] The natural explanation for this condition is that these subjects still possess the difference-detecting mechanism even though they have lost the surface classifier.

An interesting question which arises at this point is whether achromatopsics like this will still be capable of conscious judgements to the effect that one surface is more red, say, than another. The survival of some such ability might seem to be an implication of my argument so far. Even though the achromatopsics deny seeing hues, I am supposing that their chromatic difference detector is intact, and I have posited that this difference detector does not just issue in judgements that adjacent surfaces are chromatically *different*, but also pronounces on the relative location of the surfaces in various dimensions, including red-green and yellow-blue. The achromatopsics may not experience these differences as normal hue experiences of greater redness or yellowness, but this does not mean that they cannot display their sensitivity to them in other ways.

I do not know the answer to this question, nor whether there are any relevant empirical data.[14] I suspect it would not be easy to test for the relevant abilities. Many

[10] Brewer et al. (2005). [11] Shapley and Hawken (2011: 714).
[12] Zeki (1990). [13] Heywood et al. (1998).
[14] Achromatopsics standardly fail the Farnsworth-Munsell 100-hue test which requires the chromatic ordering of coloured chips (Heywood and Kentridge 2003: 488). But this failure is arguably attributable to

patients reported as suffering from cerebral achromatopsia have only partial loss of hue vision, and in addition many of them have various other cognitive deficiencies.[15] In practice it could prove difficult to be sure which aspects of their performance on various tasks are due to which deficiencies.

In any case, there is no reason to be strongly committed to the specific suggestions I have made so far about the dimensions of comparative chromatic judgements issuing from the difference detector. For this mechanism to pronounce on which of two surfaces is redder, or yellower, or even brighter, there would need to be a clear division between double opponent cells in V1 that responded to the relevant channels of optical information, such as red-green, yellow-blue, or bright-dark. However, it is not clear that the relevant double opponent cells are specialized in this way. Rather, many of them seem to take in information from a mix of these channels (Shapley and Hawken 2011: 706–8). If the V1 double-opponent cells do not display the relevant specialization, then the difference detector cannot be informing subjects about those specific dimensions of difference, and so must be making other qualitative comparisons, if it is making such comparisons at all.

Let me now turn to the possibility of the converse dissociation, the surface classifier without the difference detector. Given the difference detector's importance for form vision, subjects who lack it will be unable to discern three-dimensional form. (There is no serious possibility of subjects who have lost the chromatic difference detector still being able to discern form by means of brightness information alone. Even if, contrary to the doubts expressed in the last paragraph, there are indeed double-opponent cells in V1 that are specialized for achromatic information, their spatial proximity to chromatic double opponent cells makes it likely that they will also be compromised by any lesions that incapacitate the latter.) The loss of form vision means that such subjects will be unable to perform colour constancy computations, since these rest on a prior identification of surfaces to which to assign uniform colours. Even so, a range of patients have been reported in whom the loss of form vision is combined with the retention of conscious hue experience.[16] As we would expect, these patients cannot separate changes in background illumination from genuine changes in the colour of surfaces, and so experience the former as shifts in hue. The natural way to account for these patients is to suppose that their surface classifier is still operating, in that it is producing categorial colour responses when fed wavelength information, even in the absence of the fine-grained chromatic difference-detection needed to discern form.[17]

their loss of categorial hue responses, and does not necessarily show that they are incapable of any pairwise chromatic comparisons.

[15] Davidoff (1997: 119–22), Shapley and Hawken (2011: 714).

[16] Heywood and Kentridge (2003: 494).

[17] Certain cases of colour anomia, a condition where the ability to name colours is impaired, might also seem to indicate the presence of the difference detector without the surface classifier. In one thoroughly studied such case, the patient retained hue vision, and was normal in many colour tasks, but performed

9.7 The Intransitivity of Indiscriminability

Further support for my alternative account of colour perception comes from reflection on the apparent intransitivity of colour indiscriminability. From the point of view of orthodoxy, this intransitivity is extremely puzzling. My alternative account makes it much easier to understand.

In this section I shall explain the phenomenon and the puzzles it poses for orthodoxy. In section 9.8 I shall show how my alternative point of view helps resolve these puzzles.

Consider a sequence of gradually varying colour samples where successive samples are below the threshold of a just-noticeable difference, but where the first and last are noticeably different. That is, $sample_1$ is indiscriminable from $sample_2$ when viewed side-by-side, and $sample_2$ similarly indiscriminable from $sample_3$, . . . and $sample_{k-1}$ is similarly indiscriminable from $sample_k$, yet $sample_1$ and $sample_k$ *are* discriminable when they are viewed side-by-side.

There is no doubt that it is possible to construct real examples of such sequences. However, if we assume the orthodox account of colour perception, they are very puzzling. On the orthodox account, a judgement that two samples viewed side-by-side are the same colour derives from the identity of the viewer's responses to each side: the awareness of sameness is a consequence, as we might put it, of 'the look of the left-hand side' being the same as 'the look of the right-hand side'. However, if this is what is going on, then it ought not to be possible to get sequences where the indiscriminability does not transmit from beginning to end. If the look of the first sample is the same as the look of the second, and the look of the second the same as that of the third, and so on, then can the look of the first possibly be different from that of the last? Identity is a transitive relation, and this seems to leave no room for the looks of the first and last not to be the same.[18]

I shall be concerned in the rest of this chapter with this very specific paradox about 'colour looks'. It is worth distinguishing it from the more general phenomenon of sorites paradoxes. A sorites paradox arises whenever the first of a sequence of slightly differing objects $o_1, \ldots o_k$ satisfies some predicate 'P', and the last does not, yet there is

oddly when asked to sort a range of colour chips from across the spectrum in 'whichever way he saw fit'. Where normal subjects would uncomplicatedly put the chips into around eight groups corresponding roughly to colour terms like red, yellow, brown, green, blue, purple, and so on, this subject produced unusual groupings. His strategy was to pick up two chips and compare them to each other, placing them in the same group if they struck him as maximally similar (Roberson et al. 1999). The combination of these pairwise comparisons with the inability to form normal groupings might seem to call for explanation in terms of the difference detector without the surface classifier. However, given that this subject retained hue experience, and didn't report that everything looked black and white and grey, I am disinclined to suppose that he had lost the surface classifier, the outputs of which I am taking to constitute hue experience. Rather I would suggest that the subject's naming deficiency prevented him from grouping his conscious categorial colour responses into larger similarity classes in the way that normal subjects do.

[18] A number of writers have argued on these grounds that the very idea of definite phenomenal properties is incoherent (Armstrong 1968, Dummett 1975).

a plausible tolerance principle of the form: *if* o_n *is P, then* o_{n+1} *is P*. In general, consistency in the face of such sorites sequences requires the rejection of the relevant tolerance principle; different theories of vagueness thus all agree in holding that certain instances of the relevant principles are not definitely true. But no corresponding move seems to be available with the 'looks' paradox generated by the orthodox view of colour discrimination. For this paradox does not depend on a tolerance principle, but on the simpler 'identity assumption' that:

(I) sample_n and $\text{sample}_{\text{n+1}}$ are visually indiscriminable if and only if the type of visual response produced by sample_n is the *same* as that produced by $\text{sample}_{\text{n+1}}$.

Note that the same sequences that generate our 'looks' paradox may well also generate a range of more familiar sorites paradoxes. Thus suppose that our sequence of samples takes us from a definitely red sample to a definitely orange one. Then ordinary sorites issues will be raised by the application of the predicates 'red' and 'looks red' to this sequence of samples, and also by the application of predicates like 'experience as of red' to the sequence of visual responses to the samples. I have nothing special to say about these sorites paradoxes. My concern, to repeat, is not with these paradoxes, but with the more specific 'colour looks' paradox generated by the orthodox view of colour discrimination and the *identity* assumption it is committed to. (Note how the latter paradox will arise even if our sequence of samples remains *within* the definite oranges, or within any other nameable or conceptualizable colour category which might generate sorites problems, as long as the first sample is side-by-side distinguishable from the last. Our problem is not to do with transitions between categories, but with the way colour discrimination is assumed by orthodoxy to depend on identities and differences between 'looks'.)[19]

There are two main lines of response to the 'colour looks' paradox in the literature, which I shall call the 'standard line' and the 'minority line'.

The standard line accepts that the indiscriminablity of colour samples is indeed intransitive, and resolves the paradox by modifying the identity principle (I).[20] It continues to endorse one half of this principle—if two samples are discriminable, they must produce different conscious visual responses—but denies the other half, and holds that in some cases two samples can be indiscriminable even they do *not* produce the same conscious visual response. The idea here is that, as we move along the sequence, the conscious responses produced by at least one pair of adjacent samples must differ, in order to account for the difference in responses produced by the first and last samples. But this will be a difference in conscious responses that will

[19] Rosanna Keefe (2011) emphasizes how specific solutions to the 'looks paradox' do not necessarily help with more general problems raised by vagueness.

[20] Goodman (1951), Wright (1975), Williamson (2000).

not be reflected in the visual discriminability of the relevant pair of samples, since it is given that all adjacent pairs are visually indiscriminable.

The difficulty facing this line is obvious. In what sense can two samples have different conscious 'looks' if they are visually indiscriminable? Surely their indiscriminability means that they consciously look the same. The idea that these samples produce different conscious responses seems of dubious coherence. If the responses are *consciously* different, how can the subject be unaware of this?[21]

The minority line insists that genuine indiscriminability of conscious looks must indeed be transitive (after all, it is a matter of identity), and instead aims to deal with the paradox by denying that there are any genuine empirical sequences manifesting such intransitivity of indiscriminability.[22] Adherents of this line allow that there are of course sequences of physical *samples* that are sequentially pairwise indistinguishable even though the first and last are distinguishable. But they deny that such sequences generate an intransitive sequence of indistinguishable 'looks', on the grounds that the same *sample* need not generate the same '*look*' in different contexts. In particular, they suppose that at least one sample_k will generate one 'look' when compared with sample_{n-1}, but a different 'look' when compared with sample_{n+1}. This can then account for the difference in the 'looks' produced by sample_1 and sample_k, quite consistently with the transitivity of the identity of 'looks': since we aren't guaranteed a sequence of identity of 'looks' as we go along the sequence of samples, there is no reason why the 'look' produced by the first and last sample should be the same.

Now, there are certainly many cases where the conscious colour response produced by some surface varies with context, as a wide range of contrast and adaptation effects testify. However, from the point of view of orthodoxy, it is not so obvious why this general phenomenon of context-dependence should apply here. The particular suggestion at hand is that some sample_n will shift appearance so as to look the same as sample_{n-1} in one comparison, and the same as sample_{n+1} in another. But why should this happen? If sample_n is *capable* of looking different from sample_{n-1} in certain contexts (for example when it is compared with sample_{n+1}), then surely we would expect it to display this potential difference when it is actually juxtaposed to sample_{n-1}. Putting surfaces next to each other should surely make it easier to detect colour differences, not harder.

As we shall see in the next section, there is a sense in which I am happy to agree with the minority view about the effect of such juxtapositions on certain categorial classifications. However, my explanation of this phenomenon will hinge crucially on my non-orthodox view of the mechanisms of colour perception. Without such

[21] See Graff (2001) for a sustained argument that orthodoxy is committed to the transitivity of indiscriminability.

[22] Raffman (2000), Graff (2001).

attention to mechanisms, it seems ad hoc to suggest that juxtaposition will make surfaces seem similar, rather than highlight their differences.

9.8 Intransitivity Resolved

The account of colour perception offered in this chapter makes the apparent intransitivity of colour indiscriminability much easier to understand.

Note first that, on my account, the notion of 'indiscriminability' as applied to pairs of colour samples is ambiguous. On the one hand, it can mean that there is no 'difference' response when they are viewed side-by-side. On the other, it can mean that they are placed in the same colour category when viewed successively.

So let us distinguish between two samples being $\text{indiscriminable}_{\text{side-by-side}}$ and their being $\text{indiscriminable}_{\text{singly}}$. Two samples are $\text{indiscriminable}_{\text{side-by-side}}$ if the viewer can detect no difference when they are juxtaposed. Two samples are indiscrimina-$\text{ble}_{\text{singly}}$ if they produce the same colour classification when each viewed on their own.

First consider $\text{indiscriminability}_{\text{singly}}$. It seems clear that this must be transitive. After all, if a whole sequence of colour samples each produces the same categorial colour response when viewed singly, then so in particular must the first and the last.

But there is nothing at all problematic about this, since there is no reason to suppose that there are any empirical sequences that manifest intransitivity of indis-$\text{criminability}_{\text{singly}}$. Such a sequence would be one where sample_1 produced the same categorial response as sample_2 when they were viewed successively, and sample_2 similarly the same categorial response as sample_3, and so on . . . yet the last sample produced a different categorial response to the first sample. But there are not going to be any such sequences.

To make it clear why, suppose that the first sample produces the categorial response *orange* and the last the categorial response *yellow*. Well, then there must be some point along the sequence where the viewer's categorial colour classifier switches from *orange* to *yellow*. It must switch somewhere, and that is where it does.[23] So it won't be the case that every pair of successors as we go along the sequence will be $\text{indiscriminable}_{\text{singly}}$. For some n, sample_n will produce one categorial colour response, but sample_{n+1} a different categorial response.

Now consider $\text{indiscriminability}_{\text{side-by-side}}$. Now there will certainly be empirical sequences of samples that manifest the intransitivity of $\text{indiscriminability}_{\text{side-by-side}}$—just manufacture a sequence of samples whose successive pairwise differences along some dimension of colour variation are below the threshold of 'just noticeability', but make the sequence long enough that the first and last will be noticeably different.

However, no paradox is generated by this intransitivity. We can simply accept that $\text{indiscriminability}_{\text{side-by-side}}$ is indeed intransitive. That is simply how

[23] The precise point at which the surface classifier switches may be affected by a number of factors, such as the order in which the samples are presented. This will not matter to any of the arguments that follow.

these side-by-side comparisons work—differences that are too small to see can add up, so to speak, to a visible difference.

This no longer generates any paradox because my gestalt view denies principle (I) and so does not allow the indiscriminable$_{\text{side-by-side}}$ relation to impose a transitive equivalence relation on the samples.

The point is clearest in connection with an intransitive colour sequence all of whose members lie within some one colour category, say *orange*. The successive orange pairs are not noticeably different, but the first and last are. If the indiscriminability$_{\text{side-by-side}}$ of the successive samples implied a sameness of 'looks', and the discriminability$_{\text{side-by-side}}$ of the first and last a difference in 'looks', then we would face the apparent paradox discussed in the previous section. But on my gestalt view there is no such implication. Judgements of sameness$_{\text{side-by-side}}$ and difference$_{\text{side-by-side}}$ are neat gestalt judgements, not derived from comparisons of prior 'looks' responses to each sample. In particular, there is no inference from the difference$_{\text{side-by-side}}$ of the first and last sample to their having different 'looks' when viewed singly. Indeed, these two samples, along with all the others, will actually share the only response evoked when they are viewed on their own, namely, the categorial response *orange*.

Still, what about the case where we move from one category into another via a series of indiscriminable$_{\text{side-by-side}}$ comparisons—from the oranges into the yellows, say?

Now it is *given* that the look$_{\text{singly}}$ of the first sample is different from the look$_{\text{singly}}$ of the last. The first is *orange* and the last is *yellow*. And this means, as above, that there must come a point, as we move along the sequence of samples, that some sample$_n$ will be *orange* and the next sample$_{n+1}$ will be *yellow*. Yet at the same time it is given that this same pair are indiscriminable$_{\text{side-by-side}}$—like all the successive pairs, their difference is below the threshold of just-noticeability.

This might seem very odd, but from my perspective it is still not paradoxical.

On the orthodox view, remember, judgements of discriminability$_{\text{side-by-side}}$ are taken to derive from the difference or identity of the 'look' of each sample. And this leaves orthodoxy with no obvious way of explaining how the relevant samples can possibly be indiscriminable$_{\text{side-by-side}}$ when the 'look' of one is *orange* and the 'look' of the next is *yellow*.

But from my perspective I can simply point out that the indiscriminability$_{\text{side-by-side}}$ of these two samples, on the one hand, and their separate 'looks', on the other, are products of two *separate mechanisms*, the difference detector and the surface classifier, respectively. The surface classifier will put the samples in two different boxes if they are presented separately (it has to switch somewhere and this is where it does); while the difference detector will register the two samples as indiscriminable (because it is triggered by chromatic differences between adjacent samples and this difference is below its threshold).

This might be curious, but it is clearly not incoherent.

In one respect, my position is similar to the majority view that denies transitivity by rejecting half of the principle (I). That view, remember, upheld the intransitivity of indiscriminability by insisting that somewhere along the line the two samples in an indiscriminable pair must have different 'looks'. I concur, to the extent that I too hold there is a pair which are indiscriminable when viewed side-by-side but which will produce different categorial responses when viewed separately. The difference is that I do not see judgements of side-by-side indiscriminability as an *upshot* of the 'looks' produced when the samples are viewed separately. So I have an answer to the awkward question that so troubles the majority orthodox view, of explaining how the samples can possibly be indiscriminable, if they produce different 'looks'. My answer is that indiscriminability judgements depend on a different mechanism from the one that categorizes samples, and that this makes it perfectly possible for the former to detect no difference in some cases when the latter produces different classifications.

Here is an interesting question. How will it seem to you when you view the relevant pair of samples side-by-side? Will you *both* see the left-hand sample as orange and the right-hand sample as yellow, courtesy of the surface classifier, *and* see the two samples as indiscriminable in colour, courtesy of the difference detector? That would be strange, but we shouldn't rule it out a priori. There are other cases where distinct perceptual mechanisms produce judgements that contradict each other, for example the waterfall illusion (Crane 1988).

Still, I suspect that it won't work like this. I suspect that when the surface classifier is simultaneously presented with two side-by-side samples whose chromatic difference is below the just-noticeable threshold, it will always put them in the same colour category, even if these two samples mark the point where the surface classifier would switch categories if it were presented with a sequence of *single* samples successively. Think of it like this. Imagine now that you look at the whole sequence of side-by-side indistinguishable *pairs* of samples successively, starting with the first clearly orange pair, and ending with the last clearly yellow pair. Now again the surface classifier must switch from orange to yellow at some point. But if it is successively presented with the sequence of simultaneous pairs, then it seems likely that it will always switch *between* pairs, and never *within* them, not even within the pair of samples where it would have switched if the samples had been presented one by one.

If this is right, note that it follows that some particular sample$_n$ will be put in the category *orange* when it is juxtaposed to sample$_{n-1}$ and in the category yellow when it is juxtaposed to sample$_{n+1}$. So to this extent I am in a sort of agreement with the minority orthodox proposal; that the 'looks' of some samples changes with context. However, my view, unlike that earlier proposal, can explain why this happens. The earlier puzzle, recall, was to explain why sample$_n$ should be indistinguishable when juxtaposed with both sample$_{n-1}$ and sample$_{n+1}$, if the brain is capable of seeing it as a different colour from one of them when *not* juxtaposed. If judgements of colour sameness/difference derive from independent judgements about each sample's individual colour, as orthodoxy has it, then this seems mysterious.

But if independent mechanisms are responsible for judgements of sameness/difference and judgements of categorial colour, as I have suggested, then the puzzle disappears. The reason sample_n is indistinguishable from both sample_{n-1} and sample_{n+1} is simply that the differences within each pair are too small to trigger the difference-detector. And the reason sample_n is classified as in different colour categories when juxtaposed with sample_{n-1} and sample_{n+1} respectively is simply that the surface-classifier isn't going to reach different verdicts on unnoticeably different samples when they are presented side-by-side.

9.9 Conclusion

The existence of two distinguishable mechanisms of colour perception, giving rise to categorial and relational colour responses, respectively, is confirmed both by general functional considerations and by neurophysiological evidence. By distinguishing these two mechanisms, we can explain a number of puzzling features of colour perception, including the apparent ability of colour representation to outstrip conceptualization, and the intransitivity of colour indiscriminability.[24]

References

Abramov, I. (1997), 'Physiological Mechanisms of Color Vision', in C. Hardin and L. Maffi (eds), *Colour Categories in Thought and Language* (Cambridge: Cambridge University Press).

Armstrong, D. (1968), *A Materialist Theory of the Mind* (London: Routledge and Kegan Paul).

Brewer, A., Liu, J., Wade, A., and Wandell, B. (2005), 'Visual Field Maps and Stimulus Selectivity in Human Ventral Occipital Cortex', in *Nature Neuroscience* 8: 1102–9.

Brewer, B. (1999), *Perception and Reason* (Oxford: Oxford University Press).

Brewer, B. (2005), 'Perceptual Experience Has Conceptual Content', in E. Sosa and M. Steup (eds), *Contemporary Debates in Epistemology* (Oxford: Blackwell).

Chuard, P. (2006), 'Demonstrative Concepts without Re-Identification', in *Philosophical Studies* 130: 153–201.

Cohen, J. (2008), 'Colour Constancy as Counterfactual', in *Australasian Journal of Philosophy* 86: 61–92.

Crane, T. (1988), 'The Waterfall Illusion', in *Analysis* 48: 142–7.

[24] I have given versions of this chapter at King's College London, the Institute of Philosophy, Warwick, Stockholm, Cambridge, Rutgers, and the Phenomenal Qualities Project at Hertfordshire. I would like to thank all those who made comments on those occasions. I can particularly remember being helped by Peter Adamson, Charles Travis, Paul Coates, Philip Goff, Sam Coleman, Guy Longworth, Kranti Saran, Naomi Eilan, Åsa Wikforss, Kathrin Glüer-Pagin, Peter Pagin, Sören Häggqvist, Levi Spectre, Tim Crane, Will Davies, Hugh Mellor, Barry Loewer, Brain McLaughlin, Tim Maudlin, Barry Smith, David Chalmers, Michael Tye, Mike Martin, Ophelia Deroy, and Fiona Macpherson. I have also benefited from exchanges with Pete Mandik, Kevin O'Regan, Diana Raffman, Mohan Matthen, and Yasmina Jraissati.

Davidoff, J. (1997), 'The Neuropsychology of Color', in C. Hardin and L. Maffi (eds), *Colour Categories in Thought and Language* (Cambridge: Cambridge University Press).

Dummett, M. (1975), 'Wang's Paradox', in *Synthese* 30: 201–32.

Evans, G. (1982), *The Varieties of Reference* (Oxford: Oxford University Press).

Goodman, N. (1951), *The Stucture of Appearance* (Cambridge, MA: Harvard University Press).

Graff, D. (2001), 'Phenomenal Continua and the Sorites', in *Mind* 110: 905–35.

Hamwi, V., and Landis, C. (1955), 'Memory for Colour', in *Journal of Psychology* 39: 183–94.

Hardin, C. (1993), *Color for Philosophers*, 2nd edition (Indianapolis, IN/Cambridge: Hackett).

Heywood, C., and Kentridge, R. (2003), 'Achromatopsia, Color Vision and Cortex', in *Neurological Clinics of North America* 21: 483–500.

Heywood, C., Kentridge, R., and Cowey, A. (1998), 'Cortical Color Blindness Is Not "Blindsight for Color"', in *Consciousness and Cognition* 7: 410–42.

Hurvich, L., and Jameson, D. (1957), 'An Opponent-Process Theory of Color Vision', in *Psychological Review* 64: 384–404.

Keefe, R. (2011), 'Phenomenal Sorites Paradoxes and Looking the Same', in *Dialectica* 65: 327–44.

Kelly, S. (2001), 'Demonstrative Concepts and Experience', in *Philosophical Review* 110: 397–420.

Kentridge, R., Heywood, C., and Davidoff, J. (2003), 'Color Perception', in M. Arbib (ed.), *Handbook of Brain Theory and Neural-Networks*, 2nd edition (Cambridge, MA: MIT Press), 230–3.

McCamy, C. (1998), 'The Number of Discernible Colours', in *Colour Research and Application* 23: 337.

McDowell, J. (1994), *Mind and World* (Cambridge, MA: Harvard University Press).

Mandik, P. (2012), 'Color-Conscious Conceptualism', in *Consciousness and Cognition* 21: 617–31.

Peacocke, C. (1992), *A Study of Concepts* (Cambridge, MA: MIT Press).

Pointer, M., and Attridge, G. (1998), 'The Number of Discernible Colours', in *Colour Research and Application* 23: 52–4.

Raffman, D. (1995), 'On the Persistence of Phenomenology', in T. Metzinger (ed.), *Conscious Experience* (Exeter: Imprint Academic), 293–308.

Raffman, D. (2000), 'Is Perceptual Indistinguishability Nontransitive?', in *Philosophical Topics* 28: 153–74.

Regier, T., and Kay, P. (2009), 'Language, Thought, and Color: Whorf Was Half Right', in *Trends in Cognitive Sciences* 13: 439–46.

Roberson, D., Davidoff, J., and Braisby, N. (1999), 'Similarity and Categorisation: Neuropsychological Evidence for a Dissociation in Explicit Categorisation Tasks', in *Cognition* 71: 1–42.

Roberson, D., Davidoff, J., Davies, I., and Shapiro, L. (2004), 'The Development of Color Categories in Two Languages: A Longitudinal Study', in *Journal of Experimental Psychology: General* 133: 554–71.

Roberson, D., Davidoff, J. Davies, I., and Shapiro, L. (2005), 'Color Categories: Evidence for the Cultural Relativity Hypothesis', in *Cognitive Psychology* 50: 378–411.

Rosenthal, D. (2005), *Consciousness and Mind* (Oxford: Oxford University Press).

Shapley, R., and Hawken, M. (2011), 'Color in the Cortex: Single- and Double-Opponent Cells', in *Vision Research* 51: 701–17.

Sivic, L. (1997), 'Color Systems for Cognitive Research', in C. Hardin and L. Maffi (eds), *Colour Categories in Thought and Language* (Cambridge: Cambridge University Press), 163–93.

Werner, J. S., and Wooten, B. R. (1979), 'Opponent Chromatic Mechanisms: Relation to Photopigments and Hue Naming', in *Journal of the Optical Society of America* 69: 422–34.

Williamson, T. (2000), *Knowledge and Its Limits* (Oxford: Oxford University Press).

Winawer, J., Witthoft, N., Frank, M., Wu, L., Wade, A., and Boroditsky, L. (2007), 'The Russian Blues Reveal Effects of Language on Color Discrimination', in *Proceedings of the National Academy of Science* 104: 7780–5.

Wright, C. (1975), 'On the Coherence of Vague Predicates', in *Synthese* 30: 325–65.

Zeki. S. (1978), 'Functional Specialization in the Visual Cortex of the Rhesus Monkey', in *Nature* 274: 423–8.

Zeki, S. (1990), 'A Century of Cerebral Achromatopsia', in *Brain* 113: 1721–77.

10

The Nature of Pain and the Appearance/Reality Distinction

Michael Tye

You can feel hot without being hot. Perhaps an electrical probe is directly stimulating your brain, thereby triggering the experience while your body temperature is normal. You can also be hot without feeling hot. Perhaps your body temperature is greatly elevated but your nerve endings are damaged and you are insensitive to the heat with which you are in contact. Heat is one thing and the appearance of heat another.

It's not like this for pain. You can't feel pain without being in pain and you can't be in pain without feeling pain.[1] Why? Why is there no appearance/reality distinction for pain as there is for heat? The obvious answer is that pain, unlike heat, is a feeling. Being in pain and feeling pain are one and the same. For pain, *esse est percipi*.[2]

You can visually experience a dagger without there existing a dagger. Perhaps you have been reading *Macbeth* avidly and, after taking some LSD, you hallucinate a bloody dagger floating in space before you. You can also have a dagger before you without visually experiencing it. Perhaps your eyes are closed. A dagger is one thing and the appearance of a dagger another.

Not so in the case of a pain. If you have a pain then you feel a pain, and if you feel a pain then you have a pain. Why? The obvious answer is that having a pain and feeling a pain are one and the same.

We may now wonder what the relationship is between feeling *pain* and feeling *a pain*. The natural response, if pain is a feeling, is that feeling a pain is feeling a certain token feeling, namely a token of the pain feeling.

[1] Later on, I shall suggest that there are both sensory and affective dimensions to pain experiences (grounded in different neural regions) and that these can come apart. *Contra* Grahek (2007), this does not show that one can feel pain without being in pain (or vice versa). What it shows is that one can have an unpleasant experience that is not pain and that one can feel pain without its being unpleasant in the way that pains usually are. For more, see section 10.6.

[2] Arguably, it can seem to you that you are in pain when you aren't, as when you are expecting to feel a hot poker on your back and an ice cube is substituted without your seeing it. This is doxastic. You (briefly) believe that you are feeling pain, correcting yourself shortly thereafter.

But wait: if you feel a pain in a leg, you don't have a feeling in a leg! For one thing, feelings aren't in legs. If they are anywhere, they are in heads. For another, you can feel a pain in a leg even if you don't have a leg. You can have a phantom limb pain. And such a pain is not a feeling in a nonexistent leg. Something has gone wrong.

It has indeed. Some say that we need to distinguish pain qua feeling and pains qua intentional objects of pain (Harman 1998). The latter are nonexistent objects that enter into the contents of token pain feelings. They are like the dagger you hallucinate after reading too much *Macbeth*. This proposal has some virtues. For example, it explains why you can't feel my pains and why there can't exist a pain that no creature feels. These features flow from the nature of intentional objects. You can't hallucinate the dagger I hallucinate and there do not exist any such items as hallucinated daggers. But there are three problems. Firstly, there is no generally accepted theory of nonexistent intentional objects. Secondly, other things being equal, we should avoid bloating our metaphysics with nonexistent entities. Lastly, it must now be denied that pains are tokens of pain; for the latter are feeling tokens and the former are not. This seems very counter-intuitive.[3]

If pain is a feeling, then pains are naturally taken to be token feelings. A pain in a leg is then not a token feeling located inside the leg but rather a token of the leg pain (pain in a leg) feeling.

The view that pains are token feelings explains nicely two features of pains already noted: their necessary privacy and their necessary ownership. Pains cannot be shared for the reason that token feelings cannot be shared. You can't undergo my token feelings any more than you can laugh my token laughs or scream my token screams. Pains cannot exist un-owned for the reason that token feelings require subjects. There can no more be an un-felt feeling than an un-laughed laugh or an un-screamed scream.[4]

But just what is the nature of pain, conceived of as a feeling? That is the topic of this chapter.

10.1 Preliminary Remarks

Consider a pain in a leg. That's a leg pain feeling. There are two components to the feeling: there's the locational component and there's the painfulness of the feeling. The locational component can be shared with feelings that are not painful. A tickle in a leg, for example, is also a feeling. What makes a feeling an 'in a leg' feeling? Not that the feeling is in a leg, obviously. Nor that a disturbance is going on in a leg; for, as

[3] In an earlier essay, I tried to draw a distinction between pain *qua* feeling and pain *qua* intentional object. I now think that this was a mistake for the reasons given. It is also unnecessarily complicated.

[4] Token screams, laughs, and feelings belong to the general metaphysical category of event. A plausible requirement on all members of this category is that they cannot exist without some subject or other, and moreover that their actual subjects are essential to them.

noted above, one can feel a pain (tickle) in a leg even if one lacks a leg. A plausible answer is that a feeling is an 'in a leg' feeling just in case it is a feeling that *represents* that a disturbance or state or condition of some sort or other is to be found in a leg. Since misrepresentation is possible, there is now no difficulty in understanding how there can be a phantom leg feeling, be it a pain, a tickle, an itch, or whatever.

This proposal is naturally cashed out further by saying that it is the character of the disturbance that determines the character of the feeling. A pain in a leg represents a leg disturbance of one sort; a tickle in a leg represents a leg disturbance of another sort; and so on.

Suppose that you have a pain in a leg. You are told to pay attention to your pain. Where does your attention go? To the disturbance you feel to be occurring in your leg and its qualities. Those qualities, or at least some of those qualities, are ones that you dislike strongly. The disturbance itself is not a pain for reasons already given. Let me quickly add another. Suppose that you have a referred pain. You feel a pain in your left arm, but the disturbance you experience is actually in your heart. The case is one of misrepresentation. If the disturbance in your heart were a pain, then you would feel a pain in your heart. But you don't. You feel a pain in your arm.[5]

If the disturbance isn't a pain and the disturbance and its qualities are what you attend to when you are told to attend to your pain, it follows that your pain, and its qualities, are not the objects of your attention. Your pain and its intrinsic features are inaccessible to your introspective gaze. In this way, your pain, that is, your feeling or experience, is transparent to you. You 'see' right through it to what is represented.

But what exactly is represented by a feeling of pain? And what type of content is the content of a pain experience? Is it wholly indicative? Or is there an imperative content as well as an indicative one? Is the content singular or general? What is the relationship between the phenomenal character of a pain and its representational content? These are the topics of the next four sections.

10.2 On What Is Represented by a Pain Experience

Pain is Mother Nature's way of telling Her creatures that they have damaged, or are in the process of damaging, their bodies.[6] Pain is like the red warning light on the dashboard of your car that flashes when the oil level is too low (Byrne forthcoming).

[5] This answers Block who asks whether if the disturbance is in your heart, the pain is in your heart. See Block (2006). The *disturbance* of which you are conscious is in your heart but your experience 'places' it in your arm. The case is like that of experiencing someone as being straight ahead when in reality she is off to the right, a mirror having been placed in front of you at forty-five degrees. Of course, the disturbance of which you are conscious need not have the very non-locational properties you experience it as having any more than the person on the right need have all the non-locational properties you experience her as having. Perhaps, the mirror is slightly distorting, for example.

[6] Parts of this section and all of section 10.3 echo what is said in Cutter and Tye (2012).

The system has been designed so that the light (pain) is difficult to ignore. You may ignore it, of course, but the message is that you ignore it at your peril.

Pains represent tissue damage just as the flashing red warning light represents critically low oil.[7] Pains, of course, vary in how they feel; and this seems tied in part to variations in qualities of the represented tissue damage (notably, its shape, volume and intensity, and its location).[8] A stabbing pain represents tissue damage with a well-defined and bounded volume and a distinctive dagger-like shape occurring in a precise location; an ache represents tissue damage or irritation with a much vaguer shape and volume and (relatedly) a much less precise location.

Unfortunately, if the above is all that pains represent then it becomes very difficult to understand one salient aspect of their phenomenal character, namely their "negative affect".[9] Pains don't merely inform us of the presence of some disturbance at a location in our bodies; they *hurt*. A theory that says that pain experiences merely represent tissue damage at some location in one's body would seem to leave out the painfulness of pain.

Likewise, a theory that says that the feeling of orgasm only represents certain physical changes in the region of the genitals doesn't begin to explain the highly positive affect of orgasms.[10] What needs to be added?[11] Well, the obvious explanation of the popularity of orgasms is that they *feel* good and the obvious explanation for why people and other sentient creatures do their best to avoid pain is that pains *feel* bad. Feeling good and feeling bad are plausibly viewed as representational features of experiences. More specifically, my suggestion, in the case of pain, is that pains not only represent physical and locational properties of tissue damage, but (in first approximation) they also represent the valuational property of being bad.[12]

That valuational properties are represented in experience is supported by some recent work by Palmer and Schloss (2010) on color experience. Presented with a colored square on a monitor screen, when subjects are asked to rate how much they like the color, it was found that they tend to prefer blue, red, and green and they show least preference for dark yellow and brown. These preferences are based on how the

[7] One difference is that you, the driver of the car, are aware of the warning light. But if transparency holds, you, the subject of the pain experience, are not conscious of the pain. Rather you are conscious of what the pain represents.

[8] Pains may also represent whether the tissue damage is thermally, mechanically, or chemically produced. There is also a question as to whether the represented tissue damage has to be actual. It is certainly the case that pain is sometimes felt when the skin is under sharp pressure without having yet broken, as when one walks on a very sharply edged rock in bare feet. Here the tissue damage is impending.

[9] See, e.g., Aydede (2001).

[10] This, I take it, is what Burge (2003: 407) is getting at when he remarks: 'The representationalist treatment of orgasm would be apt for future joke books about analytic philosophy.' Unfortunately for Burge, no representationalist to my knowledge says that the represented physical changes exhaust the content of orgasm (not even Lycan who is rather explicit about the physical aspects of male orgasm, in Lycan (1995)). The joke is on Burge.

[11] Not, I take it, a sprinkling of mental paint. Orgasms are phenomenally rich but lacking in paint.

[12] More on this shortly.

colors look to the subjects. Some colors just look better than others. What does this involve? My proposal: some colors are represented as better or more pleasing to us than others. It is interesting to note, incidentally, that blue is the color of clear skies and clean water, red the color of ripe fruit, and green the color of fresh vegetation, whereas dark yellow is the color of vomit and rotten food, and brown the color of biological waste. Perhaps these facts play a role in accounting historically for why some colors look better to us than others.

Be that as it may, the valuational account of part of the content of pain experiences, with some further development, handles nicely the following imaginary case (due to Adam Pautz) which brings out very clearly the need for pains to represent more than physical and locational features of tissue damage, if the representational view is to pass muster. Imagine that there are two communities of creatures who feel pain. Mild is a member of one community and Severe is a member of the other.

> Both occasionally experience bodily disturbance *d* in the leg. In Mild's community, *d* is not very dangerous. So *d* normally puts his primary somatosensory cortex into state *m* involving a certain mild rate of firing of neurons [...] By contrast, in Severe's community, *d* is much more dangerous. For instance, maybe it is more susceptible to dangerous infections in this community because the community occupies an environment in which bacteria are more plentiful. In consequence, in Severe, *d* normally causes somatosensory state *s*, involving a rate of firing of somatosensory neurons which is twice as great as that which is involved in *m*.
>
> (Pautz 2010)

Let us agree that both of Mild's and Severe's experiences represent that there is tissue damage of a certain specific physiological sort ('*d*' above) at a certain bodily location. If that is all there is to pain experiences, then the pains of Mild and Severe should feel the same. But this prediction looks wrong; for we can imagine that when Severe undergoes *d*, he cries out in apparent agony, attending with great urgency to his wound, whereas when Mild undergoes *d*, he behaves as though he is only very slightly perturbed. Surely Severe is experiencing a very severe pain, while Mild is experiencing a very mild pain.

One reply that might be made to this case is that the difference between Mild and Severe lies in the strength of their desires to rid themselves of *d*, not in the way the pains themselves feel. This seems implausible. When people desire (and try) to rid themselves of pain, it is *because* the pain feels bad. Of course there will be a difference in the strength of their desires to rid themselves of *d*, but intuitively this difference should be explained by the difference in how bad their pains feel. Severe desires to rid himself of *d* much more strongly than Mild does because Severe's pain *feels much worse* than Mild's pain does. This is possible, I suggest, since pain experiences do not merely represent bodily disturbances as bad; they also represent them as bad to *some specific degree for their subjects*. Severe's experience represents *d* as bad to one degree for Severe and Mild's experience represents *d* as bad to another, lesser degree for Mild.

In taking this view, I am supposing that badness is a gradable determinable property. Its determinates are specific degrees of badness, and like other gradable determinable properties, our experiences can represent its various determinates. Consider, for example, brightness, loudness, or sweetness. Visual experience doesn't merely represent a stimulus as bright. It represents it as having some specific degree of brightness, such that while looking at two bright objects, one object can look brighter than the other. Similarly, auditory experience represents stimuli as being loud to some specific degree, so that some sounds can be experienced as louder than others; and taste experience can represent food as being sweet to some specific degree, so there can be two sweet things, one of which tastes sweeter than the other. Correspondingly, an adequate account of the content of pain experience must understand pain as capable of representing a range of specific degrees of badness.

Note that on the above proposal an individual's pain experience represents some bodily disturbance not as simply bad (to a certain degree), but rather as bad *for her* (to a certain degree). That is, the valuational property represented in pain experience is subject-indexed. This is needed since if Mild's experience just represents that the disturbance is bad to degree x and Severe's experience just represents that the disturbance is bad to different degree y, then, given that x is not identical with y, one of them must be inaccurate. The disturbance can't be both. But intuitively, there is nothing inaccurate in either of their experiences. We can allow that both of Mild's and Severe's experiences are veridical if we allow the relevant negative valuational property to be subject-indexed. There is no inconsistency about the co-instantiation of being bad for Mild to degree x and being bad for Severe to degree y, any more than it is inconsistent to have a single thing co-instantiate being five feet away from me and being ten feet away from you.

Furthermore, the supposition that the relevant valuational properties are subject-indexed is itself unproblematic.[13] Subject-indexed properties are ubiquitous in the contents of experience. Visual experiences represent one thing as to the left of another relative to their subjects; auditory experiences represent one noise as further away than another relative to their subjects; and so on.

But what is the property of being bad for a given individual? In your own case, patently some things are bad for you, e.g., undergoing tissue damage, eating poisonous mushrooms, and inhaling large quantities of smoke. Assuming a naturalistic worldview, this is not a matter of the things having a spooky or primitive non-natural property. Instead, the obvious proposal is that the property of being bad for you is

[13] What about the case of feeling pain in an alien limb, for example, an alien hand? Here, at least prima facie, the subject's experience does not represent a certain disturbance as being bad for *her* since she disavows ownership of the hand. We might respond that experience is nonconceptual and the difficulty lies with the subject's failure to conceptualize the represented individual as herself. An alternative is to say that her experience mistakenly represents the disturbance as being bad for a different individual, namely the possessor of the hand. Both alternatives are in keeping with the tendency of persons with alien limbs to personify the limbs, to take them to be possessed by an alien spirit or some other entity that can be named.

just the property of being apt to harm you. I shall not try to say here in any detail what it is for something to harm you. After all, there is no great mystery about what it is for something to harm something else, or about how it is consistent with a naturalistic worldview that something could be harmed. Still, *very* roughly, something harms a teleological system to the extent that it hinders that system (or one of its subsystems) from performing its function(s).

Some pain experiences feel bad even though they are not. The nurse punctures my arm with a needle in order to inject a vaccine. A man has his leg amputated (without anesthetic) to prevent a tumor from spreading to the rest of his body. In these cases, the resultant experience represents the bodily damage in question as bad for one, when in fact it is not bad for one in the circumstances. These cases are not a problem for the current proposal, since under optimal conditions (roughly, the conditions we were designed to operate in by natural selection), getting one's leg cut off or having one's skin punctured is bad for one.

What of cases in which the degree of felt badness of a bodily disturbance does not seem to correspond with the degree to which it is apt to harm one, even in design conditions? These are well illustrated by looking at pairs of bodily disturbances which vary considerably with respect to how harmful they are (in design conditions) but do not vary much with respect to their felt badness. Case 1: As a result of an accident, your leg is sliced open at the location of your great saphenous vein. Case 2: As a result of an accident, your leg is sliced open just next to the great saphenous vein. In the first case, the tissue damage is extremely harmful. In the second case, the damage is somewhat harmful, but much less so than in the first case. However, the felt badness of the pain is likely to be approximately the same in each case. Let d_1 and d_2 be the disturbance types represented, respectively, by your experiences in cases 1 and 2. Let's suppose also that the two experiences are identical with respect to felt badness, so each experience represents the relevant damage as being bad for you to the same (moderate) degree x. Let's also suppose that d_2 is in fact bad for you to degree x under design conditions. On the present proposal, your experience in case 1 represents d_1 as being bad for you to degree x, and does so (partly) in virtue of the fact that it is a token of a state S such that, under optimal conditions, S is tokened because d_1 is bad for you to degree x. But how can this be, since the disturbance you undergo in case 1 is bad for you (even under optimal conditions) to a degree much higher than x?

To understand what's going on here, we must take note of the fact that your current token bodily disturbance falls under multiple distinct types. For instance, it is a disturbance of the type *slice of the great saphenous vein*; this type of damage is bad for you (under optimal conditions) to a very high degree (a degree much higher than x). But it is also a disturbance of the types *slice of the leg*, and *slice of the skin*. These types of damage are bad for you to a much lesser degree. If your experience in case 1 represents your disturbance under the type *slice of the great saphenous vein*, then this would be a problem for the proposed view. But just because your (token) disturbance does belong to this type, it does not follow that your experience represents it under this type. It is quite plausible that the type under which your experience represents the disturbance in case 1 (namely d_1) is very similar to, or even identical to, the type under which your experience represents the disturbance in case 2 (d_2). (Perhaps they are both represented under a type like *slice of the skin*.) If so, then it's plausible to suppose that d_1 and d_2 in fact are equally bad for you under optimal conditions.

Consider next the case of the soldier in battle. He is shot in the torso and he experiences pain but in the heat of the battle the pain doesn't feel that bad to him. He fights on and it is only later after the battle ends that the pain overwhelms him. Here, it may said, it is optimal that the soldier does what he does; for if he does not continue to fight, he will not survive. But his pain experience is tracking bodily damage that is apt to harm him to a very great degree, and so, on the tracking account, since the soldier is in optimal conditions, it should feel very bad indeed.

One response to this case is to say that the problem is attentional. Given the intensity of the battle, all of the soldier's attentional resources are allocated to dealing with the enemy and so he fails to notice the intense pain that he is feeling. Were he to pause for a moment and attend to how he is feeling, he would be aware that the state he is in is very painful. As things actually are, that higher-level awareness is lacking.

Another response is to say that the pain sensory system is operating under abnormal conditions: the extreme endorphin rush the soldier is undergoing causes the system to generate a misrepresentation: the system simply misinforms the soldier as to how bad the damage is. Nonetheless, the inaccuracy has a pay-off. Lacking an accurate representation of the extent of the damage, the soldier continues to fight on, thereby behaving in a way that is conducive to his survival.

A third possible response is to maintain that the pain sensory system is still operating in design conditions but it is part of the design that when the level of endorphins is sky high, the soldier is not informed of how bad the damage is so that he can concentrate his resources on the more immediate threat. In this case, there is under-representation, not misrepresentation.

Here is another problem case (based on remarks made independently by Ned Block and Bill Brewer). Suppose that my left leg has been numbed and that I cannot feel bodily sensations in it. I see an evil-looking man take out a knife and make a nasty, jagged cut in my leg. The cut looks bad to me, and so, on a representational view of visual experience, I undergo an experience that represents the cut as bad (apt to harm) me. But I don't feel pain in the location of the cut. Apparently the painfulness of my experience has been left out of the account.

By way of reply, consider the following example: suppose that I have an ugly red rash on my left leg. The rash feels very itchy. Scratching the rash makes the itch worse. The bodily experience I undergo is very unpleasant but it isn't painful. Why not? The answer, I suggest, is that although the itch experience represents a certain bodily disturbance as bad to a certain degree for me, it does not represent that disturbance as involving a cluster of physiological properties of the sort represented in pain experiences. Being unpleasant is a necessary condition for being painful but it isn't sufficient. Correspondingly, my visual experience, as I view the cut in my leg, represents a disturbance in my leg as having various physiological features but these features do not make up a physiological cluster of the sort represented in pain experiences.

There is another way to make the point. Suppose that you see a coin and then you touch it. Your experiences are phenomenologically different. What grounds this difference? The representationalist says that there is overlap in the represented properties in the two cases but there is also difference. For example, the coin looks round and feels round but while it looks brown in color it doesn't feel brown in color and while it feels warm it doesn't look warm. Our visual systems are constructed to detect one range of properties; our tactual systems another. Some properties are represented by both systems but others are not.

Similarly, some properties represented by vision are not represented by the bodily sensation system and vice versa. This is a matter of system architecture. My visual experience, as I view the cut in my leg, represents its color, shape, length, width, etc.; were my leg to cease to be numb, my resultant pain experience would represent some of these properties (though not all) but others my pain experience would represent, for example, the chemical changes present in damaged tissue, indeed the property of being damaged tissue, are not represented in my visual experience at all. Of course, at a higher conceptual level, I might see the cut *as* having some of these distinguishing features (indeed I may see *that* the cut has the given features), but the experiences that are relevant to phenomenology are nonconceptual.[14, 15]

Here is a related problem case. Suppose that I have a cut on my face and also a cut of the same size and shape on my back. The former will feel much more painful than the latter. In what does the representational difference consist? My answer, in brief, is that, given the density of nociceptors on the face, the face-cut experience will represent the tissue damage in much more detail than the back-cut experience.[16] There is, then, no difficulty in finding a salient representational difference.

I have now provided an account of what it is that pain experiences represent. Further details remain to be filled in but the overall proposal should be clear. In the next section, I shall discuss an alternative approach to the painfulness of pain, one that tries to account for the negative affect of pains in terms of imperative content. After that I shall take up the question as to whether, on my account, the representational content of pain experiences is best viewed as singular or general and relatedly the question of which particulars, if any, enter into it. Before concluding this section, however, I want to address a worry that may linger.

[14] See Tye 2006.

[15] This brings out another way to respond to the above objection (suggested to me by Brian Cutter). Does the cut in my leg really look bad to me at a nonconceptual level? I certainly believe that it is bad for me, as I view it, and so in a doxastic sense of 'looks', it looks bad. But it is not so clear that in the phenomenal sense of 'looks', it looks bad.

[16] This, in turn, may result in the two experiences representing different degrees of badness.

The worry concerns the representation of valuational properties experienced. However the further story goes, it seems that a plausible constraint on any properties represented by experiences is that those properties be causally relevant to the internal state the person undergoing the experience is in. But how can a property like being bad be so relevant? The property of being bad for one does not supervene on the local physical properties of a bodily disturbance. Whether a disturbance is apt to harm an organism depends also on facts about the organism as a whole together with facts about the environment in which the organism is embedded. But according to some philosophers a property can only be causally relevant in producing an effect if the property supervenes on local physical properties.[17]

The problem with this argument is that it's just not true that a property can only be causally relevant in producing an effect if the property supervenes on local physical properties. When John tells Jane that she looks beautiful, Jane smiles at him. John's utterance causes Jane to smile at him, and does so in virtue of its semantic properties. But the semantic properties of an utterance do not supervene on its local physical properties; rather, they depend (perhaps inter alia) on facts about how words are used in one's community. Mental properties, like having the desire to drink water, are causally relevant in producing behavior. But if we accept the standard arguments for mental externalism, (many) mental properties, including the property of having a desire to drink water, do not supervene on local physical properties. But it would be silly to say that my having a desire for water has never caused me to drink water. Or consider properties, like the property of being a lion, which depend not just on an object's local physical properties but also on its historical origins. A herd of gazelles runs away upon encountering a lion. Surely the fact that the object they encountered was a lion causally explains (at least in part) their fleeing the scene. These are truisms about causation. There are theories of causation that entail that the only causally relevant properties are those which supervene on local physical properties, and therefore have the consequence that the cases listed above are not genuine cases of causation. It seems to me, however, a constraint on any adequate theory of causation is that it accommodate the truisms discussed above. That some theories of causation have the consequence that these cases are not genuine cases of causation should be taken as a reductio of those theories.

10.3 Imperative Content

Recently, a number of philosophers have invoked the notion of imperative content to account for the painfulness of pain.[18] Roughly, the idea is that we account for the

[17] Something akin to this line of thought is at play in the passage from Aydede (2001) quoted in this section.

[18] See, e.g., Martinez (2011) and Klein (2007). Hall (2008) proposes that other bodily sensations like the feeling of an itch or the feeling of hunger have imperative contents. The first criticism below of the

sensory dimension of pain experience in terms of the familiar indicative contents concerning the location and physiological type of some bodily disturbance, and we account for the negative affective dimension of pain in terms of imperative contents. So in addition to having the indicative content that a certain disturbance is in a certain location, pain experiences also have an imperative content like: stop that bodily disturbance! Such accounts are often motivated by the belief that there is serious difficulty in accounting for the negative affective dimension of pain by appeal to its indicative content. However, the imperative account faces two big difficulties.

First, the felt badness of pain comes in degrees. Any adequate account of the painfulness of pain must not only account for the fact that pain is painful, but also for the fact that pain can be painful to different degrees. The proposed account does so by holding that our pain experiences ascribe determinates of the gradable determinable property badness for oneself to bodily disturbances. But how can the proponent of imperative content account for this? Consider again Mild and Severe. Both have an experience as of a bodily disturbance of the same physiological type in the same location, and both undergo an experience with a negative affect. A proponent of imperative content should hold that the indicative contents of their experiences are the same, as both experiences should have as their indicative content that there is a disturbance *d* at such-and-such location (or something similar). They will then account for the negative affect of their pain experiences by saying that their experiences have, in addition, the imperative content: stop that bodily disturbance! But how, then, can they account for the felt difference in their experiences? To the extent that it is agreed that felt differences are or are at least accompanied by a difference in content, it doesn't look as if the proponent of imperative content has the resources to deliver a difference in content between Mild's experience and Severe's experience.

Perhaps the proponent of imperative content could say that states with the same imperative (and indicative) content can nonetheless differ along some other dimension—which we might call the urgency of the state—which is also relevant to determining phenomenal character. On such a proposal, the difference between Mild's experience and Severe's experience is analogous to the difference between the following two imperative sentences:

(1) (Please) stop that bodily disturbance.

(2) Stop that bodily disturbance!!!

But this approach is still objectionable.

First, the account I have given of the painfulness of pain has the advantage that its treatment of the various degrees of the felt badness of pain is structurally similar to

imperative content account of pain can be very naturally extended to an imperative content view of these other bodily sensations.

the most plausible treatments of, e.g., the various degrees of apparent brightness, loudness, and sweetness in experience. The most plausible account of the latter has it that experience represents determinates of the gradable determinable properties brightness, loudness, and sweetness. There seems to be no good reason to give a fundamentally different account of variation in pain intensity. To do so is to adopt a complex and inelegant theory when a simpler and more elegant theory is available.

A second reason to prefer my proposed account over the imperative content account is that it generalizes to other 'affectively valenced' experiences far more naturally than the imperative content account. I have focused on the painfulness or negative affective quality of pain experience. But pain is just one of a number of affectively valenced experiences. There are other experiences with a negative affect, such as the experience of smelling excrement or eating rotting meat. More importantly for the present discussion, there are also experiences, such as the experience of having an orgasm or eating a ripe strawberry, which have a positive affect. We say that strawberries taste good and orgasms feel good, and intuitively, when we say such things we are (at least obliquely) commenting on the phenomenal character of our experience of strawberries and orgasms. The proposed account of the content of pain experiences has a natural extension to affectively positive experiences: when an individual *A* has such an experience, the experience represents its object as good for *A* to a certain degree. The property of being good for *A* will be identified with the property of being apt to benefit *A*, and the explanation for how our experiences come to represent this property will proceed along the same lines as the explanation given above for how pain experience comes to represent the property of being bad for one. But how can the proponent of imperative content extend her proposal to account for the positive affect of some experiences?

Consider the experience one has when one chews on a delicious strawberry. On the imperative content view, presumably one's experience (in addition to whatever indicative content it might have) has an imperative content like: continue eating that strawberry! (Eat more of that kind of thing?) But what is it about this content that accounts for the positive affect of one's experience? It cannot be merely the fact that it is an imperative content, for the imperative content theorist holds that pain experiences, which are affectively negative, also have imperative content. So there must be some sort of relevant difference between the imperative content of pain experience (stop that damage!) and that of the experience of eating a strawberry (continue eating that strawberry!) that accounts for the fact that the former experience is affectively negative while the latter is affectively positive. Of course there are differences, but it is not at all transparent why any of these differences should be relevant to accounting for the difference in valence between the two experiences. By contrast, on the account being proposed, there is a very straightforward explanation for why our experience of pain has a negative affect and our experience of eating a strawberry has a positive affect. Pain feels bad to us and strawberries taste good to us because our experiences of pain represent their objects as bad for us and our experiences of strawberries represent their objects as good for us.

10.4 Content, Singular and General

If indeed the content of pain experience is wholly indicative, what sort of indicative content is it? Consider the case of your having a pain in a finger. Typically, in such a case there is tissue damage (or some closely related disturbance) in the finger causing your finger pain feeling. The particular disturbance in the finger—call it '*p*'—is naturally taken to be what your experience is about. Just as when you see a tomato, the tomato causes your 'tomato experience' and your experience represents the tomato as having various properties and a certain spatial position relative to you, so too intuitively in the pain case your experience represents *p* as having certain properties and a certain location within the relevant finger (call it '*f*').

One straightforward way to develop this view further is to hold that your pain experience has a singular content. Both *p* and *f* enter into the content together with various physiological and locational properties and a valuational property involving the subject of the experience. You are conscious of *p* just as you are conscious of the tomato. Likewise, you are conscious of your finger, *f*. Your pain experience locates *p* within *f* and attributes to it a range of properties.

Natural though this view is, it immediately creates difficulty; for suppose that there is nothing wrong with your finger and your experience of pain in your finger is brought about by direct stimulation of your brain via an electrical probe. In that case, there is no such thing as *p*. Alternatively, suppose that you no longer have a finger but you feel a pain in your finger. Now *f* does not exist. What is the representational content of your experience?

One line to take is to say that the content is gappy. It has holes in it where, in the normal case, a token disturbance and a bodily part go. This disjunctivist line on the content of pain experience has a counterpart in the case of visual experience. In veridical and illusory visual perception, the seen object enters into the content of the experience. In the hallucinatory case, the content is gappy. The key idea is that there is a common structure to the content in the veridical, illusory, and hallucinatory cases—I have called this elsewhere a 'content schema'—where this structure is to be conceived of as having a slot in it for an object. This slot is filled by an object in the veridical and illusory cases but it is left empty in the hallucinatory case.

Formally, there is no difficulty with the above disjunctivist line on content. To see this, suppose that the perceiver introduces the name '*a*' with the intention of using the name for the object he takes himself to be seeing. In the veridical and illusory cases, the name has a bearer. In the (standard) hallucinatory case, the name is empty. Suppose that the experience aims to attribute the property, *F*-ness, to the object putatively seen. Then the accuracy conditions for the experience in all three cases are just these:

(AC) Subject *S*'s experience is accurate if and only if *Fa*.

In the veridical case, '*Fa*' is true and *S*'s experience is accurate, so the biconditional (AC) is true. In the illusory case, '*Fa*' is false and *S*'s experience is inaccurate, so again (AC) is true. In the hallucinatory case, given a negative free logic (according to which all simple sentences with empty names are false), '*Fa*' is again false and *S*'s experience is inaccurate, so (AC) is true.

The difficulty with the disjunctivist view is metaphysical, not formal. Consider the visual singular content that object, *o*, is red. On the Russellian view of content, this content is complex, having object, *o*, and redness as its component parts.[19] A visual experience (or other mental state) having that content is accurate if and only if *o* is red. One way to think of the Russellian content here—the content that *o* is red—is as an ordered pair having *o* as its first member and redness as its second. Another way to think of the content is as a structured, possible state of affairs built out of *o* and redness.

Where a visual experience is hallucinatory, how should we think of its gappy content? Gappy content is supposed to be just like a singular content but with a gap or a hole in it where an object should go. But does this really make sense?[20] On the ordered pair conception of singular content, there must be two items to form the pair. Since a gap or a hole is not an item, or so it seems, there is no first member of the ordered pair and so no ordered pair at all. On the possible state of affairs conception, the relevant complex is structured out of *o* and redness in the singular case. But in the gappy case, there is no object *o*. So, how is there a *complex* entity structured out of its components?

A possible reply is to say that the missing item in both cases is the empty set. Where one hallucinates, the content is a complex entity built out of the empty set and various properties. But intuitively this is a bizarre proposal indeed. If the empty set is the gap filler, then the hallucinatory experience is about the empty set. So, in a hallucination, one experiences the empty set just as, in the veridical and illusory cases, one sees object *o*. Furthermore, if the hallucinatory experience is about the empty set then it is experienced as being some way or other, for example, red. So then the empty set looks red, just as the seen object, *o*, looks red when one sees *o* and experiences it as red! This is more than a little hard to swallow. Furthermore, the proposal effectively reconfigures hallucinations as illusions of a special sort. Instead of there being no object perceived, there is now an object of a special sort that is perceived, or if not perceived, at least experienced, and this object is not as it is experienced to be.

The empty set proposal is a desperate attempt to save the gappy content view. It confuses the truth that in hallucination one does experience something—for example, a ripe tomato—with the falsehood that there exists some thing one experiences, the empty set being proposed as the relevant thing since no ordinary object is available to do the job.

[19] Obviously, there are other views of singular content. For ease of exposition, I shall stick with the Russellian conception in what follows.

[20] This question is a pressing one for gappy proposition theorists (e.g., Braun 2005) generally.

Instead of the empty set, one might appeal to an absence or alternatively an empty space-time region. And there are other possibilities. But I have come to think that none of them works. And this problem, of course, generalizes to the pain case. There simply is no clear metaphysical account of the nature of the gappy content for your feeling pain in your finger, if there is no finger disturbance and/or no finger.

A possible reply to this problem is to say that there is no content at all unless the slot is filled so that in the hallucinatory case there is merely something that *would* be content, *if only* the slot were filled. But this fails to come to grips with the strong intuition many of us have that hallucinatory experiences are inaccurate. When one hallucinates, the world seems to one a certain way and it isn't that way. But this is not just an intuition. How, in the absence of an *F*, could one hallucinate an *F* unless one's experience were representational? And if one's experience is representational, then evidently it is a misrepresentation. To respond that in the hallucinatory case, there is not only no object but also no experience, and hence no experience that misrepresents, is obviously a non-starter. So, the challenge to those who deny that hallucinatory experiences are representations is to provide an alternative account of what is going on that not only explains away the above strong intuition but also explains why

Person *P* hallucinates an *F*

does not entail

There exists an *F* that *P* hallucinates.

Corresponding points can be made in the case of pain. Where one has a pain in a phantom limb, one feels a disturbance in a certain body part and there does not exist a body part in which that disturbance occurs. There may not even be a tissue disturbance if the experience results from direct stimulation of the brain.[21] How can one feel an *F* when there exists no *F* unless one's feeling is representational and it misrepresents the world? As in the visual case, the world seems to one a certain way and it isn't that way. The experience is inaccurate.

It is also worth thinking here about the red warning light model for pain. When the light on the dashboard for low oil flashes, it signifies something, namely that the oil level is too low and that this is a dangerous condition that needs attention. This is the case even if there has been an electrical malfunction and there is at that moment no oil level at all for the reason that the engine has been removed for work elsewhere on its cylinder heads, say. To suppose that in this scenario the oil light's flashing does not 'say' anything is surely a mistake. The red light's flashing 'says' what it always says. It's just that this time it is wrong.

[21] It might be replied that in such a case one is really feeling a disturbance in the stump. However, one need not be. We can imagine that there is direct neural stimulation causing the experience while messages from the nerves in the stump are blocked.

The conclusion to draw, I suggest, is that if there is singular content when there is a disturbance and a body part, then there must be gappy content when there is at most only one of the two. But gappy content is a chimera. What to do?

One possible solution is to embrace an existential view of content across the board for pain experience. There is a corresponding move in the case of visual experience. I reject this approach for reasons I have given elsewhere, but I shall return to it briefly below. The approach I now advocate is to take the content to be a set of possible worlds.[22] This gives straightforward accuracy conditions in the case mentioned earlier (given a negative free logic):

> (AC*) Subject *S*'s experience is accurate if and only if the actual world is a member of the set of possible worlds at which *a* is *F*.

It also removes the worry about structure. The content is now a set and sets are not structured entities. Of course, the seen object, *a*, is no longer a component of the content in the veridical and illusory cases, but this is compatible with holding that, in being seen, *a* is represented by the experience. For this is now cashed out further in terms of the experience having as its representational content the set of possible worlds at which *a* is a certain way (*F*).

To be sure, the set of possible worlds at which an experience that is about *a* is accurate has members, namely possible worlds, each of which has *a* as a component part (whether one supposes that worlds are maximal states of affairs or (implausibly) concrete configurations of objects). But *a* is not a component part of that set, any more than my heart is a component part of the set whose members are myself and my mother.[23] So, *a* is not a part of the content of the experience.[24]

Even though, on my current view, *a* is not a part of the content of the experience, the experience remains crucially dependent on *a*. This is because the content of the experience is specified by reference to *a* as the set of worlds at which *a* is red. Thus, given that in actuality there is such an object as *a*, had things been different and *a* not existed, neither would the experience occasioned in actuality by the subject's seeing *a*.[25]

The same points can be made in the case of pain on an austere view of pain content. My having a pain in my finger is an experience about a certain disturbance,

[22] For a detailed elaboration of this view, see Tye (2014).

[23] Set membership should not be confused with the part-whole relation. The former is irreflexive, asymmetric, and intransitive; the latter reflexive, asymmetric, and transitive.

[24] In the foregoing, I assumed that the members of an ordered pair are parts of the ordered pair. This assumption might be challenged on the grounds that ordered pairs can be defined set-theoretically (e.g., on Wiener's definition, <a,b>:= (((a), the empty set), ((b))), in which case they have sets as their parts. The trouble here is that there are too many equally good definitions and thus too many equally good candidates. We should accept all or none of them. We can't accept all of them because they are in conflict. So, we should accept none.

[25] Assuming that the content is essential to the experience.

p, and my finger, *f*. The experience attributes certain properties to *p*, some in relation to *f*. The content of the pain is the set of possible worlds at which *p* and *f* have the relevant properties and the experience is accurate (let us suppose) since the actual world is a member of that set. The content does not contain *p* or *f* as a component part even though the experience is about both *p* and *f*. And an experience with that very content would not have existed had either *p* or *f* not existed.[26]

This brings out an important advantage the proposed view has over the existential account. Even though in the above visual case the object, *a*, is not part of the representational content of the experience in the case that one sees *a*, the accuracy conditions for the experience essentially involve *a*. In this way, *a* is crucial to the matching of the experience with the world in the case that the experience is accurate. Not so on the existential account. According to the existentialist, the experience is accurate if and only if there is some object or other that has the relevant feature or features to which the subject is appropriately related. So, the experience can be fully accurate even if *a* does not exist. This (by my lights) is unsatisfactory. It is not an *accident* that the experience one has in seeing *a* is accurate if and only if *a* is the way it looks. *a* is essential to the world's being as the experience 'says' it is.

Likewise in the pain case. The disturbance *p* and the finger *f* are essential to the world's being as the pain experience 'says' it is. If *p* does not exist or *f* does not exist, the experience is not accurate.

There is one complication I have ignored in the above proposal. For reasons given earlier (in section 10.2), it seems to me a mistake to hold that the pain experience represents the token disturbance as apt to harm one to degree so-and-so. Instead, I suggest that the experience represents the token disturbance as having certain physiological properties and as being located in a particular bodily location and it further represents that the tokening of those physiological properties is apt to harm one to such-and-such a degree. The full content, then, has two components to it, one sensory and one evaluative. This is reflected in the neurophysiological basis of pain experience, as we shall see in section 10.6.

The case of veridical hallucinations, I might add, is also handled in a straightforward way. Take the visual case first. Suppose that it seems to me that President Obama is before me, and in fact he is though I am not seeing him. No light from Obama reaches my eyes. Instead a neuroscientist is causing my visual cortex to go into just the state it would, were I genuinely seeing Obama. My experience is accurate then just in case the actual world belongs to the set of worlds at which Obama is before me. Since Obama is before me, my experience is accurate or veridical. But I am hallucinating, for the conditions necessary for seeing Obama are not met.

[26] The view that the content of a thought is a set of worlds is part and parcel of a view defended with Mark Sainsbury in our book, Sainsbury and Tye (2012). It is crucial to the plausibility of this proposal that thoughts not be individuated by their contents but rather by the concepts they exercise and the ways they are combined.

There can also be veridical hallucinations in the case of pain experiences. Suppose that I feel a pain in my left big toe. I have a left big toe and tissue in it has just been damaged, but the messages from my toes to my brain have been blocked. My pain experience is caused by a neuroscientist who is stimulating my brain with a probe. My pain experience is accurate; even so I am not conscious *of* my toe or the disturbance there, for there is no causal connection of a sort necessary for consciousness of these things.

That, then, is the approach I favor to the content of pain experiences. But as with most things in life, it does not come for free.

10.5 The Price You Pay

Suppose that you feel a throbbing pain in your left foot and a little later you feel a stinging pain in your right arm. You have no left foot or right arm, both having been amputated after a car accident. Your pains are triggered by the operation currently being performed on your brain. Here there is no tissue damage in your legs or your arms. Accordingly, the representational content of each pain is the same: the empty set. But your pains certainly feel different. It follows that experiences that have the same representational content can differ phenomenally.

Strong representationalism in its classic formulation identifies the phenomenal character of an experience with a certain sort of representational content the experience has. Weak representationalism, unlike strong representationalism, is not an identity thesis. It does not purport to identify phenomenal character with representational content. It is rather a supervenience thesis. In its classic formulation, it asserts that necessarily experiences with the same representational content have the same phenomenal character. This more modest thesis offers no real illumination about the nature of phenomenal character.

The proposed view of pain entails that both strong representationalism and weak representationalism, in their classic formulations, are false. This is the price you pay.

One reaction is to say: so much the worse for representationalism! An even stronger reaction is to say that the proposed view has eaten its own tail: if content does not ground phenomenology, then it is left with no real role to play in pain experience. Pain content might just as well be eliminated. Let me take the latter reaction first.

I accept that the view that pain experiences have accuracy conditions is not one and the same as the view that pain experiences have representational content, at least if the second view is taken to entail that there exist representational contents that pain experiences have. The reflections of the previous sections seem to me to provide strong support for the first view but not the second. I have simply taken it for granted that where a representation has accuracy conditions, this is grounded in the fact that there is a content the representation has, a content that itself has the relevant accuracy conditions. Given this assumption, I have discussed how best to understand the nature of pain contents. However, I remain non-committal here on whether it is ultimately possible to do away with pain contents in our ontology.

Turning to the initial reaction above, and assuming as above that pains have representational contents, let me first note that representationalists generally accept that persons, in undergoing experiences, are conscious of a range of properties or features that may or may not be instantiated in the surrounding environment or their bodies.[27] These properties or features are predicatively represented by the experiences. One way to cash out further the claim that experiences predicatively represent properties even though the properties so represented are not components of the representational contents of the experiences is via the accuracy conditions for the experiences. To see this, consider the earlier statement of accuracy conditions:

(AC*) Subject *S*'s experience is accurate if and only if the actual world is a member of the set of possible worlds at which *a* is *F*.

(AC*) provides a canonical statement of the accuracy conditions for *S*'s experience. According to (AC*), the property, *F*-ness, enters into the accuracy conditions for *S*'s experience without entering into the content of *S*'s experience (the relevant set of possible worlds). We may say, then, that what it is for *S*'s experience to predicatively represent *F*-ness is for *F*-ness to be a property expressed by some predicate that is used in a canonical statement of the accuracy conditions for the experience and that also distinguishes that experience's accuracy conditions from those of others.

Now we can formulate weak representationalism in an alternative way that eschews the notion of representational content (without thereby doing away with contents) as follows:

(R) Necessarily, experiences that predicatively represent the same property complex have the same phenomenal character.[28, 29]

[27] Along with (most) other representationalists, I am happy to say that, in the hallucinatory case, the perceiver is conscious of an un-instantiated property. This seems to me to be part of naïve common sense. Suppose that you had never seen any red things and then, one day, you hallucinated a red car. Did you not then encounter redness in your experience? Did you not then 'get a good look' at redness (Hawthorne and Kovakovitch 2006), one that enabled you then and there to know what it is like to experience red? Of course, some further account needs to be given of what it is for an experience to represent or be about a property that does not require that the property be instantiated. But there are several such accounts in the literature. Take, for example, the Normal tracking account of basic sensory representation (in first approximation, a sensory state is about a property, *P*, just in case the state is of a type that is Normally tokened if and only if *P* is tokened and because *P is* tokened). This relationship between the state and the property can obtain even if in some Abnormal situations the property is not instantiated. The same is true if we think of property representation by experiences in terms of indicator function (see Dretske 1995). For more on the tracking account, see Cutter and Tye (2012).

[28] The thesis that visual experiences involve awareness of property complexes is endorsed by Mark Johnston (2004) and Colin McGinn (1996), though neither would cash out this awareness representationally. Johnston writes of 'sensible profiles' and McGinn of 'clusters of properties'.

[29] In my view, visual experiences are *nonconceptual* representations. (This is another way in which visual experiences differ from thoughts.) So, where properties are conceptually represented in perceptual acts, they are not represented by perceptual experiences proper but rather by associated judgments or beliefs (within, for example, hybrid mental acts of seeing-that).

(R) is the thesis of weak *property representationalism*. Unlike the earlier *content representationalism* theses, (R) is not threatened by the case of phenomenally different hallucinatory experiences. Such experiences predicatively represent different property complexes.[30] Strong property representationalism is the thesis that what it is for an experience to have a certain phenomenal character is just for it to represent a certain property complex.[31]

There remains the task of spelling out how the relevant property complexes are to be understood. Consider the visual case. The scene before one's eyes is usually made up of a number of different objects arranged in various spatial relationships. Suppose that the scene one is viewing consists of a red, triangular thing to the left of a green, round thing. Evidently, what it is like for one to view this scene is different from what it is like to view a second scene containing the same things but with the green, round item on the left. What is the property complex represented by the first experience? It cannot just be the complex:

Being red and being triangular and being green and being round.

For this complex does not distinguish one's experience phenomenally from one's experience of the second scene. Nor is the following complex any better:

Being red and being triangular and being to the left of and being green and being round.

For the constituents of this complex, like those of the first one, can be commuted and so again no distinction has been drawn between the phenomenal characters of the two experiences.[32]

Suppose we complicate things by saying that the relevant property complex is as follows:

Being red and being triangular and being to the left of a green round thing and being green and being round and being to the right of a red triangular thing.

[30] Likewise the visual experiences undergone in perceptually different waterfall illusion scenarios do not present a problem for (R). Although the content of these experiences is the same—the empty set—the property complex predicatively represented is different.

[31] This thesis does not say what makes an experience an experience. My own view is that a state gets to be an experience by being a *nonconceptual*, suitably *poised* representation predicatively representing a property complex. For more on what it is for a representation to be nonconceptual and poised, see, for example, Tye (1995) and Tye (2009).

[32] Of course, these property complexes are much too coarse-grained to capture phenomenal character anyway, since the experiences predicatively represent determinate shades of color, determinate shapes, location, and many other details. But this makes no difference to the point I am currently making and so I ignore it.

In the case of the second experience, the property complex is different with respect to the left/right relations, so this proposal at least has the virtue of keeping the phenomenal characters of the two experiences distinct. But it seems ad hoc. Why pick the above property for the first experience? Why not pick this one instead, say?

Being red and being triangular and being to the left of a green round thing that is to the right of a red thing and being green and being round and being to the right of a red triangular thing that is to the left of a green thing.

And there are indefinitely many other equally good candidates.

So, what is the right account of the relevant property complex? Let us call the two objects in the scene 'O_1' and 'O_2'. One's first experience is not about an ordered pair composed of O_1 and O_2. Intuitively, it is simply about O_1 and O_2. What one's experience does is to attribute a complex property to O_1 and O_2. Since one's first experience is accurate if and only if the actual world belongs to the set of worlds at which O_1 is red and triangular and O_2 is green and round and O_1 is to the left of O_2, the property so attributed is as follows (using '%*xFx*' as a singular term abbreviating an expression of the form 'the property of being an *x* such that *x* is *F*'):

(P1) %*x*%*y*(*x* is red and *x* is triangular and *y* is green and *y* is round and *x* is to the left of *y*).

That complex property is not a property of O_1 in the veridical case nor is it a property of O_2. It is a property of objects, O_1 and O_2.[33] It is also not the property one's experience of the second scene attributes to objects, O_1 and O_2. The property in that case is this:

(P2) %*x*%*y*(*x* is green and *x* is round and *y* is red and *y* is triangular and *x* is to the left of *y*).

So, the two phenomenal characters are in no danger of being conflated. And evidently the above points generalize to other more complicated visual experiences and also to bodily experiences such as pain.[34] This, then, is how the notion of a property complex is to be understood in thesis (R).

The question of whether the advocate of (R) should embrace the view that what it is for an experience to have a certain phenomenal character just is for it to represent a certain property complex or whether she should hold instead that the relationship is

[33] O_1 and O_2 jointly instantiate (P1). It is an interesting further question in metaphysics as to how to understand what is involved in O_1 and O_2 having a property that is not possessed either by O_1 alone or by O_2 alone or by the ordered pair $<O_1, O_2>$. Here are some further examples of joint instantiations: John and Jane together lifted the piano; the children stood in a circle.

[34] In the case of pain, the valuational component complicates things still further, but it can be incorporated without much difficulty.

one of supervenience is left open in the above account. I myself prefer the former option.[35] The latter incurs the burden of explaining how and why the phenomenal character of an experience is fixed by the experience's representing a given property complex. Failure to provide such an explanation naturally leads to the thought that there is no explanation to provide. That, then, demands primitivism about phenomenal character—and primitivism leaves the world shrouded in mystery.

10.6 The Neurophysiological Basis of Pain

Modern neuroscience has focused for the most part on the sensory aspect of pain. Historically, this was not the case. The ancient Greeks, for example, took pain to be the opposite of pleasure. They classified it with the emotions and appetites rather than the sensations. The problem with the modern sensory view is that it leaves out the unpleasant aspect of pain. Many bodily sensations are affectively neutral; what is it about pain that makes it unpleasant? On the other hand, there are unpleasant somatic sensations that are not pain.[36] What is it about pain that makes it distinctively painful? In the earlier sections, I have tried to provide answers to these questions. In this section, I want to discuss the neurophysiological bases for the aspects of pain I have distinguished.

The sensory aspect of pain is generated by activity in the primary and sensory somato-sensory cortices of the parietal lobe (SI and SII). The contributions to pain of activity in these areas have been extensively studied in animals. The unpleasantness of pain—what I have called its 'felt badness'—seems closely tied to activity in the anterior cingulate cortex (ACC). Human functional imaging studies show that there is a significant correlation of the felt badness of pain with ACC activation (Devinsky et al. 1995; Rainville et al. 1992). Further, when subjects feel pain from a stimulus that is held constant and a hypnotic suggestion is used to increase or decrease subjective unpleasantness, a correlation is found in regional cerebral blood flow in ACC but not in primary somato-sensory cortex (SSC) (Fields 1999). Also patients with ACC lesions say that their pain is 'less bothersome'.

If regions of SSC are damaged but not ACC, what results is an unpleasant sensation that is not pain. For example, a laser was used to deliver a thermal stimulus to a fifty-seven-year-old man with most of SI damaged as a result of a stroke (Ploner et al. 1999). When the stimulus significantly above normal threshold on the right hand was delivered to his left hand, the man reported an unpleasant sensation but he denied that it was a case of pain.[37]

[35] It is important to appreciate that, on this option, what it is for an experience to have a phenomenal character is on a par with what it is for a linguistic expression to have a semantic value. It is not to be understood on the model of what it is for an entity to have a property.

[36] H. L. Fields reports that a patient with nerve injury described the sensation of gently stroking her skin as 'like someone scratching a chalkboard with their fingernail'. The sensation she underwent was certainly very unpleasant but not a case of pain.

[37] Asked to classify his sensation from a list of terms that included 'hot', 'burning', and 'pain', the patient picked none.

It appears, then, that the painfulness of pain is based on activity in two different neural regions: somato-sensory cortex (SI and SII) and ACC. Activity in the former area issues in a representation to the effect that a certain disturbance has such-and-such physiological properties in so-and-so bodily region. Activity in the latter area issues in a representation of unpleasantness to so-and-so degree. It is a consequence of the views taken in this essay that these representations are somehow combined via mechanisms as yet unknown to produce a further representation that a certain disturbance is taking place with such-and-such physiological properties in so-and-so bodily region and that the tokening of those properties is unpleasant to such-and-such degree. Once that representation is generated, so long as it arises at the right stage in the overall information processing and it is in the right format, the experience of pain occurs.[38]

References

Aydede, M. (2001), 'Naturalism, Introspection and Direct Realism about Pain', in *Consciousness and Emotion* 2 (1): 29–73.

Block, N. (2006), 'Bodily Sensations as an Obstacle for Representationism', in M. Aydede (ed.), *Pain: New Essays on Its Nature and the Methodology of Its Study* (Cambridge, MA: MIT Press).

Braun, D. (2005), 'Empty Names, Fictional Names, Mythical Names', in *Nous* 39: 596–631.

Burge, T. (2003), *Reflections and Replies: Essays on the Philosophy of Tyler Burge*, edited by M. Hahn and B. Ramberg (Cambridge, MA: MIT Press).

Byrne, A. (forthcoming), 'Hmm... Hill on the Paradox of Pain'.

Cutter, B., and Tye, M. (2012), 'Tracking Representationalism and the Painfulness of Pain', in *Philosophical Issues* 21 (1): 90–109.

Devinsky, O., Morrell, M., and Vogt, B. (1995), 'Contributions of Anterior Cingulate Cortex to Behavior', in *Brain* 118: 279–306.

Dretske, F. (1995), *Naturalizing the Mind* (Cambridge, MA: Bradford Books, MIT Press).

Fields, H. (1999), 'Pain: An Unpleasant Topic', in *Pain Supplement* 6, S61–9.

Grahek, N. (2007), *Feeling Pain and Being in Pain* (Cambridge, MA: MIT Press).

Hall, R. (2008), 'If It Itches, Scratch!', in *Australasian Journal of Philosophy* 86 (4): 525–35.

Harman, G. (1998), 'The Intrinsic Qualities of Experience', in N. Block, O. Flanagan, and G. Guzeldere (eds), *The Nature of Consciousness* (Cambridge, MA: MIT Press).

Hawthorne, J., and Kovakovitch, K. (2006), 'Disjunctivism', in *Proceedings of the Aristotelian Society*, Supplementary Volume, 80: 145–83.

Johnston, M. (2004), 'The Obscure Object of Hallucination', in *Philosophical Studies* 103: 113–83.

Klein, C. (2007), 'An Imperative Theory of Pain', in *Journal of Philosophy* 104 (10): 517–32.

[38] Earlier versions of this chapter formed the basis for a talk at MINDGRAD at the University of Warwick, a symposium on pain at Stanford and a colloquium talk at the University of Oklahoma. I am grateful to Bill Brewer, Todd Ganson, Mike Martin, Lucy O'Brien, Howard Fields, John Perry, and Matthew Soteriou for comments and/or discussion.

Lycan, W. (1995), *Consciousness* (Cambridge, MA: MIT Press).

McGinn, C. (1996), 'Another Look at Color', in *Journal of Philosophy* 93 (11): 537–53.

Martinez, M. (2011), 'Imperative Content and the Painfulness of Pain', in *Phenomenology and the Cognitive Sciences* 10 (1): 67–90.

Palmer, S. and Schloss, K. (2010), 'An Ecological Valence Theory of Human Color Preference', in *Proceedings of the National Academy of Sciences of the United States of America*, 107: 8877–88.

Pautz, A. (2010), 'A Simple View of Consciousness', in R. Koons and G. Bealer (eds), *The Waning of Materialism* (Oxford: Oxford University Press).

Ploner, M., Freund, H-J., and Schnitzler, A. (1999), 'Pain Affect without Pain Sensation in a Patient with a Postcentral Lesion', in *Pain* 81: 211–14.

Rainville, P., Feine, J., Bushnell, M., and Duncan, G. (1992), 'A Psychological Comparison of Sensory and Affective Responses to Four Modalities of Experimental Pain', in *Somatosensensory Motor Research* 9: 265–77.

Sainsbury, M., and Tye, M. (2012), *Seven Puzzles of Thought* (Oxford: Oxford University Press).

Tye, M. (1995), *Ten Problems of Consciousness* (Cambridge, MA: Bradford Books, MIT Press).

Tye, M. (2006), 'Nonconceptual Content, Richness and Fineness of Grain', in T. Gendler and J. Hawthorne (eds), *Perceptual Experience* (Oxford: Oxford University Press).

Tye, M. (2009), *Consciousness Revisited: Materialism without Phenomenal Concepts* (Cambridge, MA: MIT Press).

Tye, M. (2014), 'What is the Content of a Hallucinatory Experience?', in B. Brogaard (ed.), *Does Perception Have Content?* (Oxford: Oxford University Press).

11

The Life of the Mind

Michelle Montague

11.1 Introduction

A subject who consciously sees a red rose in front of her in normal conditions has a visual experience as of a red rose. This conscious visual experience involves certain kinds of distinctively visual phenomenology, e.g. color phenomenology and (visible) shape phenomenology. Each sensory modality has certain phenomenological features typically—indeed essentially—associated with it, and color and shape are the phenomenological features centrally associated with vision.[1]

Conscious seeing is an occurrent mental process, an occurrent mental phenomenon. As such it needs to be clearly distinguished from non-conscious occurrent mental processes that take place during vision, and are indeed an essential part of it.[2] When a subject sees a red rose, a great deal of non-conscious processing takes place, processing of the kind postulated by computational theories of vision.[3] This non-conscious processing is essential to her having the conscious visual experience she does, and I am going to assume that at least some of it is rightly called 'mental'.

Consider now a subject who is consciously judging that grass is green, or consciously comprehending the English sentence 'Hillary Clinton may be the next US president'. Consciously comprehending the English sentence about Hillary Clinton involves a lot of non-conscious mental processing, and, just as in the case of conscious seeing, conscious occurrent thought (of the sort involved in consciously understanding the proposition that Hillary Clinton may be the next US president) needs to be distinguished from any non-conscious occurrent mental processing that takes place during conscious thought and is essential to its occurrence.

[1] For the purposes of this chapter, I will put aside the possibility of cross-modal phenomenological effects.

[2] Those who doubt this can simply call them neural. I use 'non-conscious' and 'unconscious' interchangeably, unlike Searle (1992), for example, who uses 'non-conscious' to designate neural processes that are not mental.

[3] None of the processing in V1, for example, is conscious in any way at all (Koch 2012). Milner and Goodale (1995) have argued forcefully that the visual information processed in the dorsal stream responsible for the visual control of action is non-conscious.

Given that not every non-conscious occurrent process in the brain that is involved in the production of mental phenomena is itself a mental phenomenon (the processing of blood sugar, for example), there is a very general question about what makes a process *mental* when it is non-conscious.[4] I won't, however, attempt to answer this general question here. In this chapter, I am assuming that there is a class of non-conscious occurrent mental phenomena, however exactly the class is delineated.

Suppose we allow, as I think we can and should, that at least some non-conscious occurrent processing can count as thought (and *a fortiori* as mental). Then the question I am interested in is, what is distinctive of *conscious* thought? Given that there are occurrent non-conscious thoughts, what is it about a thought that makes it a *conscious* thought? I can't hope to give a complete answer to this question, and will only focus on certain features that I take to be essential.

Let me stress again that the question I am concerned with is different from the general question of what makes a conscious mental phenomenon (event, state, or process) conscious. The latter question is concerned with a general theory of consciousness; my question is less ambitious and is concerned only with conscious thought. The answers to these two questions may, however, overlap in various ways, and I will address the overlap when it is relevant to my purposes.

I am going to argue that a successful account of what makes an occurrent thought a conscious thought must appeal to phenomenological features. If this is right, a further question arises: which kind of phenomenological features? I will argue that sensory phenomenology cannot do the job, and that we cannot give an adequate account of what conscious thought is without appealing to what is now called 'cognitive phenomenology'.[5] I am therefore arguing that the notion of 'phenomenal' or 'phenomenological' must be extended beyond the sensory, i.e. sensory phenomenological properties are not the only kinds of phenomenological properties there are.

In arguing for cognitive phenomenology's essential role in accounting for what makes an occurrent thought a conscious thought, I will criticize two opposing views. The first view grants that an occurrent thought's being conscious must consist partly in its possessing phenomenological features, but insists that that phenomenology is sensory. Understanding the exact nature of the relationship between the conscious thought in question and the associated sensory phenomenology is crucial for understanding what this kind of view amounts to, and why it is ultimately implausible.

The second view attempts to give an account of what makes an occurrent thought a conscious thought in non-phenomenological terms. The central claim of this view is that there is a non-phenomenological kind of consciousness, and that this non-phenomenological kind of consciousness is what accounts for conscious thoughts

[4] On this topic, see e.g. Searle (1992: ch. 7), Strawson (1994: 158–74), Kriegel (2011).

[5] I am assuming that there is no such thing as unconscious or non-concious phenomenality, i.e. if a state has phenomenological features, then it is conscious.

being conscious. Block (1995, 2002) and Dennett (1991, 2009) have given the most influential non-phenomenological accounts of consciousness. For ease of exposition I will focus on Block's notion of 'access-consciousness', although I will briefly discuss a central aspect of Dennett's view.[6, 7]

Whether one is giving a phenomenological account or a non-phenomenological account of what makes occurrent thought conscious thought, I will argue that it is essential for a thought's being conscious that the content of the thought be consciously entertained. This seems intuitively obvious.[8] The content of the thought is essential to the thought's being the thought it is, and I will argue in section 11.4 that to assert that a thought can be conscious without the content of the thought being consciously entertained is really to deny that the thought is conscious. (In what follows I will say that the content of the thought itself is consciously occurrent when it is being consciously entertained.)[9]

The overall plan of the chapter is as follows. In section 11.2, I briefly introduce the notion of cognitive phenomenology and mention a few standard motivations for it. In section 11.3, I argue that Block's notion of access-consciousness fails to give an adequate account of what it is for a thought to be a conscious thought. Indeed, if I am right, the argument shows that the label 'access-consciousness' is a misnomer. The strategy is two-fold. First, I argue that there are examples of mental states that fulfil Block's conditions for a state's being access-conscious but are clearly non-conscious. Second, I argue that Block has not provided us with good reason to think that 'access-consciousness' is really consciousness in any sense.

In section 11.4, I argue against the proposal that what makes an occurrent thought a conscious thought can consist in sensory phenomenology that is somehow 'tied up' with the thought. I suggest that this proposal faces a dilemma. On the first horn, the danger is that the sensory phenomenology appealed to in accounting for the thought's property of being conscious has only an arbitrary relation to the thought. That is, the sensory phenomenology supposedly responsible for making a particular occurrent thought conscious seems unconnected to the (content of the) thought itself. In an attempt to avoid this arbitrariness, the proposal faces the second horn, on which the thoughts themselves are not really conscious at all; all that is really conscious is the associated sensory phenomenology.

[6] I will briefly consider a higher-order thought theory of consciousness in section 11.4.

[7] Although Dennett claims that all consciousness can be accounted for in non-phenomenological terms, Block holds that in addition to 'access consciousness' there is 'phenomenal consciousness', predominately associated with sensory states. I'll come back to this distinction in section 11.3.

[8] One might argue that a thought's syntactical structure is part of what a thought is. Since its syntactical properties need not be conscious when the thought is conscious, why should its content be conscious? A brief response to this objection is that access to a thought's content is essential for entertaining the thought in question, whereas a thought's syntactical properties need not be available to the subject for entertaining the thought.

[9] Both Block and Dennett speak freely of a content's being conscious in addition to a thought's being conscious.

In section 11.5, I introduce the strategy of appealing to cognitive phenomenology. Appealing to cognitive phenomenology accounts for what makes an occurrent thought a conscious thought without any worries about arbitrariness and without being forced into a position that ultimately denies the existence of conscious thought.

11.2 Cognitive Phenomenology: The Basics

Since the term 'cognitive phenomenology' is relatively new to contemporary analytic philosophy, it will be helpful to say briefly what I take it to mean.[10] It is useful to begin by defining it in contrast to sensory phenomenology. Sensory phenomenology is the kind of phenomenology we typically associate with our sensory modalities, e.g. color-shape phenomenology, sound phenomenology, and so on. In what follows, I will construe sensory phenomenology broadly to include imagery, e.g. visual and auditory imagery, including 'inner speech'. It is important to emphasize that visual imagery and auditory imagery are instances of sensory phenomenology in the following sense. Inner speech, construed in a purely sensory manner, is just particular kinds of sounds with no meaning attached to those sounds. Sensory imagery, visual or otherwise, construed in a purely sensory manner, is just e.g. color, shape, and sound phenomenology with no 'meaningful object' attribution. I take cognitive phenomenology to be a kind of phenomenology that is essentially something over and above sensory phenomenology and that is paradigmatically associated with conscious thought, but also occurs in perception and emotion. On this view, there is something it is like to consciously think that 2+2=4 or to consciously think that temperance is a virtue that is irreducible to any sensory phenomenology that may be associated with these thoughts.

One way of arguing for cognitive phenomenology is by appealing to 'phenomenological contrasts'. Contrast arguments involve the presentation of two scenarios that allegedly differ in phenomenological character but not in sensory features. Since there is by hypothesis no difference in sensory phenomenology, the phenomenological contrast between them can be accounted for only by appealing to some form of non-sensory phenomenology. One kind of case concerns two subjects who hear the same sounds and have the same auditory experience but have different experience overall, because one of them experiences the sounds as words that they understand (see e.g. Moore 1910–11/1953: 58–9, Strawson 1994: 6–7, Siewert 1998: 274–83). Another kind of case involves 'perceiving as', as in the famous duck/rabbit case. The idea is that although the sensory phenomenology remains essentially the same, when one perceives the picture now as a duck, now as a rabbit, there is an experiential

[10] Cognitive phenomenology was completely accepted by many phenomenologists and early twentieth-century philosophers, see e.g. Brentano (1874), Husserl (1900–1/2001), and James (1890). The denial of its existence seems to be a symptom of the dominance of behavioral/functionalist conceptions in contemporary philosophy of mind.

difference and this difference is a cognitive-phenomenological difference. I'm not going to go into an analysis of these arguments. I mention them only to give a better initial sense of what cognitive phenomenology is supposed to be.[11]

This standard use of the term 'cognitive phenomenology' needs to be carefully distinguished from certain deflationary uses. Joe Levine (2011) offers one such deflationary use in allowing that there may be such a thing as what he calls 'impure cognitive phenomenology'. Levine's impure cognitive phenomenology is the phenomenon of sensory experience being 'cognitively inflected'. The idea is that although all phenomenology is sensory phenomenology, cognitive states can influence the way the 'sensory manifold' is experienced in such a way that two distinct thoughts or conceptual sets result in the same set of sensible features being experienced differently. For example, a fake barn façade 'looks' different to a subject once she knows it is a fake barn façade, not a real one. That is, somehow, the colors or shapes or arrangements of the colors and shapes 'look' different to one when one knows one is looking at a fake barn façade. I think, however, that this kind of phenomenon is better labeled 'cognitive penetration'. The idea behind cognitive penetration is that beliefs, for example, can affect the way the sensory manifold (e.g. shapes and colors) is experienced. But one need only be committed to the existence of sensory phenomenology in order to accept the reality of cognitive penetration.[12]

A closely related but distinct issue from cognitive penetration is the idea that in addition to representing 'low-level' properties such as colors and shapes in visual experiences, for example, we also typically represent so called 'high-level' properties such as natural kinds, e.g. being a pine tree, or a tiger. In so far as the representation of high-level properties is part of visual experience itself, some have wished to categorize these as instances of sensory phenomenology. This is a terminological mistake. High-level perceptual phenomenology is best understood as an instance of cognitive phenomenology given the close connection between high-level content and concepts.

Another suggestion is that we use the term 'cognitive phenomenology' to denote any phenomenology whatever that is experienced as somehow intimately or constitutively 'tied up' with particular conscious thoughts, even if in the end all phenomenology is sensory. I'll come back to the question of what exactly this might amount to. For the moment, I'll say only that this use of the term 'cognitive phenomenology' obscures the central issue in the cognitive phenomenology debate, which is precisely whether there is a kind of phenomenology distinct from and irreducible to sensory phenomenology.

[11] See Carruthers and Veillet (2011), Levine (2011), Prinz (2011), and Strawson (2011), and Wittgenstein (1953) for a discussion of these kinds of cases.

[12] For more on this notion see e.g. Macpherson (2012) and Siegel (2012).

Two key questions here, which I will discuss in more detail in sections 11.4 and 11.5, are, first: is there a sense in which the conceptual content of conscious thought is experienced directly, or is it only ever experienced indirectly? Second, and connectedly: is the conceptual content of conscious thought ever itself consciously occurrent? As for the contrast between direct and indirect, I take it that in the case of impure cognitive phenomenology in Levine's sense, the conceptual content of thought is only experienced indirectly, because it is only experienced in as much as it is something that can affect the sensory manifold. Correspondingly, I take it that the conceptual content of conscious thought is not itself consciously occurrent in this case. Against this, I will argue that cognitive phenomenology, in the sense I have defined it, allows a subject to experience aspects of conceptual content of conscious thought directly, and, correspondingly, that the content of a conscious thought can in such a case itself be consciously occurrent.

11.3 Access-Consciousness and Cognitive Accessibility

As I said, I am concerned with conscious occurrent thought, understood generally to cover conscious judging, contemplating, wondering, and so on. This cluster of mental states brings to mind Block's notion of access-consciousness, or 'A-consciousness' for short.[13] Many philosophers believe that the notion of A-consciousness gives an adequate account of what one of these mental states' being conscious consists in. Carruthers, for example, seems to endorse such a view:

> Most theorists believe that there are mental states—such as occurrent thoughts or judgments—that are access-conscious (in whatever is the correct functionally-definable sense), but that are not phenomenally conscious. (2001/2007: 1)

The idea is that there is a class of conscious mental states that are conscious in a non-phenomenological sense, which is accounted for in terms of the notion of 'access'. (For my purposes here, I am taking a state's being 'phenomenally conscious', 'P-conscious' for short, to mean that there is 'something it is like' to be in that state, experientially speaking: the state has a phenomenology.) According to this approach, there are two ways for a state to be conscious; it can be access-conscious or it can be phenomenally conscious. For the most part, philosophers have taken it that sensory experiences are P-conscious, and that conscious thoughts are A-conscious but not P-conscious.[14]

[13] 'The paradigm A-conscious states are "propositional attitude" states like thoughts, beliefs, and desires' (Block: 2002: 281).

[14] Block doesn't rule out the possibility that conscious thoughts, in addition to being A-conscious, may also be P-conscious and vice versa.

The reason I am focusing on Block's notion of A-consciousness in particular, rather than the account offered by Dennett, is because most philosophers do think there is such a thing as phenomenology, but only want to acknowledge the existence of sensory phenomenology. So there is an immediate issue with conscious thought: either conscious thought is conscious because it involves some sort of sensory phenomenology, or it must be possible to give a wholly non-phenomenological account of conscious thought. (The only other alternative is that there is really no such thing as conscious thought.) With Block's notion of A-consciousness, it is easy to think that we already have a credible account of conscious thought, which does not appeal to phenomenology. I want to block this lazy inference.

What is it for a state to be access-conscious? In his original 1995 definition, Block defined A-consciousness as '(roughly) being "poised for control of speech, reasoning and action"', but in 2002 he added the following:

> A representation is A-conscious if it is broadcast for free use in reasoning and for direct "rational" control of action (including reporting)...[A]-conscious representations are ones that are broadcast in a global workspace. What makes a typical A-conscious representation A-conscious is what getting to the Executive module sets it up to do, namely affect reasoning and action. (Block 1995/2002: 206–9)

Block added the notion of being 'broadcast in the global workspace' to capture the idea that A-consciousness is an occurrent phenomenon. He says:

> My guide in making precise the notion of A-consciousness is to formulate an information processing correlate of P-consciousness that is not ad hoc and mirrors P-consciousness as well as a non-ad hoc information processing notion can...A flaw in both my definition and Chalmers' definition is that they make A-consciousness dispositional whereas P-consciousness is occurrent...that makes the relation between P-consciousness and A-consciousness the relation between the ground of a disposition and the disposition itself...I have dealt with the issue here by using the term 'broadcast' as in Baars' (1988) theory that conscious representations are ones that are broadcast in a global workspace. (Block 2002: 208)

There seem, then, to be the following central elements to a state's being A-conscious:

(i) *that it be poised to play a certain causal role in the overall cognitive system*;

and

(ii) *that it be broadcast.*

I take it that (ii) implies

(iii) *that it is occurrent (non-dispositional).*

In subsequent writings, Block has (temporarily) replaced the phrase 'access-consciousness' by the phrase 'cognitive accessibility'. Recently he wrote that 'access-consciousness was my term for approximately what I am calling "cognitive accessibility" here' (Block 2007: 486), and argued that phenomenal consciousness can occur in the absence of cognitive accessibility, understood as that which underlies reporting.[15] I mention this change in terminology because I believe it is more apt, and because the term 'cognitive accessibility' does not imply that there are fundamentally different 'kinds' of consciousness, as the term 'access-consciousness' seems to. 'Cognitive accessibility' simply picks out a functional property that certain mental states have, and I believe, and am going to argue, that this is all that the term 'access-consciousness' really does.

The notion of 'action' in Block's phrase 'direct "rational" control of action' denotes 'intentional action', and includes bodily action, mental action involving relations between mental states, responses to requests to perform certain mental actions, and so on. For example, I can form the intention to begin thinking about my lecture on functionalism or I can imagine a green river upon a request to do so. The reference to 'rational' is meant to rule out the kind of behavior that occurs in typical blindsight cases. In these cases subjects' actions or behavior are either reactions to verbal prompts asking the blindsighter to guess what's in the 'blind' portion of his visual field, or to physical objects the blindsighter can successfully navigate around. In the case of verbal prompts, the fact that the blindsighter guesses means that, from his own perspective, he does not have a reason for answering as he does. In the case of physical prompts, the blindsighter does not, from his own perspective, have a reason to move as he does. The blindsighter may be completely surprised that he is able to successfully navigate around physical objects.[16]

We have, then, the notion of access-consciousness or cognitive accessibility, and we can now ask about the relationship between a thought's being access-conscious or cognitively accessible and its being conscious. (For the moment I will use the term 'cognitive accessibility', for reasons that will become clear below.)

It's plausible that

(a) *if a thought T is conscious at time t_1, then T is cognitively accessible at time t_1.*

There are certain kinds of cases that may call (a) into question. For example, there may be cases where conscious thought is not appropriately connected to action due to some sort of impairment. In this situation we would have a conscious thought

[15] In this paper he also gives up the term 'phenomenal consciousness' in favor of 'phenomenology' (Block 2007: 484).

[16] There is a remarkable video of a blindsight patient who is surprised at his ability to navigate around objects: <http://www.youtube.com/watch?v=xekRNLNzrr8&feature=related>.

without it being poised for global control. However, adding certain qualifications may easily put such worries to rest.

It should also be noted that cognitive accessibility only underlies one's ability to report one's conscious thoughts; it should not be identified with one's ability to do so. A 'locked-in' patient may become incapable of reporting on their conscious thoughts, but it would be implausible to deny that they were having conscious, and thus cognitively accessible, thoughts simply because they couldn't report them. This can also be true in the case of children. They may see something without being able to put what they saw into words. Sometimes one has a thought and finds it hard to put it adequately into words. Experience is often richer than anything that can be put into words.

The notion of cognitive accessibility Block has in mind also allows him to capture the following case. Owen et al. (2006) plausibly show that a woman in a vegetative state was able to respond to requests to imagine certain activities. (The same areas of her brain lit up that light up in normal patients.) 'The evidence is that the patient is capable of an intentional act, namely, the act of imagining something described. That should be considered no less an indication—though of course a fallible indication—of consciousness than an external behavioural act.'[17] So, the patient is having conscious thoughts, and thus cognitively accessible thoughts, but she cannot report on them verbally nor indicate them non-verbally.

So (a) seems plausible given certain qualifications and clarifications. But what really concerns us here is the conditional going in the other direction:

(b) *if T is cognitively accessible at time t_1, then T is consciously thought (is a conscious thought) at time t_1.*

(b) seems false. I will argue that a thought T can fulfil the condition of being

(i) *poised for global control*

without being conscious, and can fulfil the condition of being

(ii) *broadcast for free use in reasoning*

without being conscious, and can also fulfil both (i) and (ii) together without being conscious.

Consider (i), a state's being poised for global control, first. As stated, (i) is a very weak claim. Suppose that at t_1 I believe that Barack Obama has two lungs, although I have never explicitly entertained this thought. (It is what used to be called an

[17] Block (2007: 484).

'implicit' belief as opposed to an 'explicit' belief, where an explicit belief is one that has at some point been consciously entertained.) This thought is poised for control of speech and action in the clear sense that if someone asks me how many lungs Obama has, I can *immediately* respond with the correct answer. (The same qualifications concerning reportability discussed above apply here.)

In one sense, having an 'implicit' dispositional belief is similar to the blindsight case, because prompting is required in both cases. However, it is unlike the blindsight case in that the subject, after prompting, is aware of having the belief in question at t_1, whereas the blindsighter lacks awareness of the informational state that allows him to answer questions about objects in the blind field correctly, or avoid objects placed in his path. That is, the blindsighter is aware of his report that the object in the 'blind' part of his visual field is circular, for example, but he is unaware of the state that undergirds his report.

Presumably, Block had something other than these kinds of dispositional thoughts in mind. Perhaps we should strengthen (i) to

(i*) *optimally poised for global control*

where 'optimally' obviates the need for direct prompting. In light of this slight change, however, consider Strawson's 1986 notion of 'explicit^{+}'.

> If you are reviewing two courses of action, X and Y, which you believe to be the best (or only) ones open to you, and if, having assessed the pros and cons of X in conscious, occurrent thought, you then pass to the assessment of Y in the same way, your belief that you can perform an action of kind X may... be explicit^{+} in the present sense... [it may be]—here the ineliminable vagueness—'near at hand' in the mind, present to the mind in some way in which a belief or thought can be present to mind without actually being [consciously] occurrent.
>
> (Strawson 1986: 117–18)

Clearly there is a difference between my belief about Obama's lungs and my belief or thought that I can do action X (one of the differences is that my belief that I can do action X does not require any prompting), and Strawson's case seems to cast doubt on the idea that replacing (i) by (i*) can rescue (b) (the view that access-consciousness (or cognitive accessibility) is sufficient for conscious thought).

How should we interpret the case? One view is that my belief or thought that I can do action X can't be occurrent at all, in the case described, simply because human beings can only really think one thing at a time. On this interpretation, Strawson's case involves the claim that a state can be optimally poised for global control without being occurrent. It follows that being optimally poised for global control is not sufficient on its own to account for what makes a thought a conscious thought, since a state must also be occurrent, in order to be conscious. Block agrees. The occurrentness requirement is built into the broadcasting requirement, on his view.

This brings me to the second interpretation of Strawson's case. On this interpretation, when a thought is explicit⁺, 'near at hand in the mind', it is occurrent, perhaps as a state of activation of working memory, and it is broadcasting in Block's sense, but it is below the threshold of consciousness: after all, you are now thinking about action Y and you can't think two conscious thoughts at the same time. This suggests that the addition of broadcasting to being optimally poised for global control is compatible with non-conscious occurrent dissemination. If so, broadcasting doesn't suffice for what makes a thought a conscious thought.

In fact, Block's own 'superblindsight' case seems to tell against taking access-consciousness as an account of conscious thought, and in particular as an account of the cases that are my main concern, e.g. consciously thinking 2+2=4, or judging that temperance is a virtue. An ordinary blindsight patient can only guess what's in the blind portion of his visual field upon prompting, but a superblindsighter can be trained to prompt himself to guess what's in the blind portion of his visual field, without being instructed to guess. He spontaneously offers that he thinks that there is an 'X' in his visual field although he can't see it. Visual information about the blind portion of his visual field just pops into his thoughts. Block characterizes the case as follows:

> Of course, the superblindsighter has a thought that there is an 'X' in his blind field that is both A-conscious and P-conscious. But I am not talking about the thought. Rather, I am talking about the state of his perceptual system that gives rise to the thought. It is this state that is A-conscious without being P-conscious. (Block 1995/2002: 21)

In order for this non-P-conscious state of his perceptual system to give rise to a thought as it does, it seems it must be occurrent, and it's broadcast by the definition of 'A-consciousness'. But the question remains: is there any good sense in which it is conscious, now that Block has argued that it isn't P-conscious?

The key difference between the superblindsighter and the typical blindsight patient is that the relevant state of the superblindsighter does not require external prompting. But this lack of need for *external* prompting doesn't seem to result in that state's being conscious. The fact that prompting is needed at all seems to show that the state is not conscious in any sense; it is not part of the conscious field.

This, perhaps, is the kind of consideration that motivates Block's switch back to the term 'cognitively accessible'. Using this term, we can simply and clearly say that the state of the superblindsighter that gives rise to the thought that there is an X is his visual field is cognitively accessible and occurrent and even 'broadcasting', but not conscious. What these cases show is that we can make sense of a state, e.g. a thought, being broadcast and optimally poised for global control independently of the idea that it is conscious.

Although Dennett may not agree with my particular diagnosis of the superblind-sight case, he does in general agree that, 'arrival in the global workspace is necessary but not sufficient for consciousness of some content, since not all contents vying in the global workspace achieve fame' (Dennett 2009: 454).

So, my question is, what then does it take to make a content (or a thought) part of the conscious field? In answering this question, Dennett and I part ways. He considers this an ill-posed question. He says of the contents that arrive in the global workspace: 'Precisely when do these winning contents become conscious? That is an ill-posed question' (Dennett 2009: 453). According to Dennett, there are multiple streams of content taking place simultaneously and

> these are the multiple drafts out of which the appearance of a final draft…is created by the occurrence of 'probes' that retrospectively elevate some drafts at the expense of others. In the absence of such probes, the question of whether or not a content was conscious is ill-posed…achieving fame (or 'clout') in the brain is not a precisely datable transition in the brain…consciousness is only retrospectively determinable. Since it is constituted by its sequelae…a content cannot be conscious for 15ms and utterly forgotten afterwards; that would not be consciousness.
>
> (Dennett 2009: 452–4)

The idea seems to be that a conscious thought, a conscious content, is not after all a dateable, clockable occurrence. Dennett compares a conscious thought to fame: one cannot be famous for only fifteen minutes. But this seems a bad analogy. Fame is a vague concept—how many people does it take to recognize you for you to be famous? The vagueness involved in answering this question at least partly accounts for the vagueness in answering the question about how long you are famous. But conscious thoughts aren't like this at all. There is nothing inherently vague in my right now thinking about the snow in my back garden. I am now clearly thinking about the snow in my back garden and as my train of thought continues on, that thought will no longer be part of my conscious field. In short, there seems to be nothing at all wrong with asking the question, what pushes a non-conscious thought or content into the conscious field, and that's the question I'm trying to answer.

11.4 Sensory Phenomenology and Conscious Thought

It's a necessary condition on a thought's being conscious that it is occurrent, and it also seems plain that there is a difference between conscious occurrent thought and non-conscious occurrent thought. The conclusion from the previous section is that being optimally poised for global control and being broadcast in the workspace, although perhaps necessary conditions for conscious thought, are neither individually sufficient nor jointly sufficient. Since this account seems to be as good a functional account as any, it is difficult to see how any additional functional property can push a non-conscious occurrent thought into the conscious field.[18] The obvious suggestion is that phenomenological properties are needed to push a thought into the conscious field. The question now becomes, which kind of phenomenological properties?

Most philosophers accept that there are sensory-phenomenological properties, but of those who do, many reject that there are cognitive-phenomenological properties. So, if one accepts that phenomenological properties are necessary for conscious thought, and rejects the existence of cognitive-phenomenological properties, one must hold that what makes occurrent thought conscious thought must be its being somehow intimately associated with, or indeed partly constituted by, sensory-phenomenological properties.

But what exactly is the nature of this intimate association between thoughts and sensory phenomenology? I'll begin with what I will call the 'simple sensory' proposal, according to which what makes an occurrent thought conscious is the thought's having sensory-phenomenological properties of some sort. (I suppose no one actually holds this simple sensory approach, but it is nonetheless instructive.)

Consider the following example. At t_1 John thinks that grass is green and has a green patch image; let's suppose that it's acceptable to say that the green patch image is a sensory phenomenological *property of the thought*, the conscious thought-episode. (For simplifying purposes, we may suppose that he has no other images or sensory experiences at this time. This kind of restriction will be assumed for all of the cases considered below.) The current proposal is that what makes John's occurrent thought a conscious thought is that it essentially involves, or is partly constituted by, his having a green patch image, whatever else it also necessarily involves.

It seems clear, however, that an image of a green patch is not the only kind of sensory phenomenology that could be associated with John's thought that grass is green. Suppose at t_2 John thinks that grass is green, but this time he imagines a patch of *green grass*. In this case, therefore, the claim is that what makes John's occurrent thought a conscious thought is the fact that it essentially involves, or is partly constituted by, his imagining a patch of *green grass*, whatever else it also involves or necessarily involves.

[18] One might wonder if a higher-order thought theory of consciousness might not fare better than a Block-inspired account. I don't think so. Firstly, the higher-order thought theory seems implausible on other grounds. It was intended to give a general theory of consciousness, and given problems such as the 'mismatch' problem (see e.g. Block 2011 and Van Gulick 2006), I think it fails to do so. Secondly, it is quite mysterious how an unconscious higher-order thought directed at an unconscious lower-order thought results in the lower-order thought's being conscious. Thirdly, the same sort of case that shows access-consciousness fails to give an account of conscious thought applies to a higher-order theory as well. Consider cases where one is not actively trying to solve a problem, but has put it aside to let one's unconscious mind work on it for a while. After some period of time, suppose the solution to the problem just comes to one. During the unconscious period of working on the problem, it is plausible that one has higher-order thoughts directed at lower-order thoughts, e.g. thoughts of the form 'How does thought A fit with thought B?', without thereby making thoughts A and B conscious.

Now, that John could have these different images while thinking that grass is green is undeniable. But even if sensory images are part of what makes occurrent thoughts conscious thoughts, it's hugely implausible that you *have* to have an image of green grass, or a patch of green, in order to consciously think that grass is green. At the very least, there is presumably some possible variation in what these images can be. John could have various associations with grass. For example, his summer months spent mowing lawns, the story he wrote about a red dragon that was afraid of grass, and the taste of grass open up a whole range of possible sensory-phenomenological goings-on that could accompany the thought that grass is green and thus be the sensory phenomenology that makes John's occurrent thought a conscious thought.

On the face of it, it seems we can imagine the same sort of cases for verbal imagery. While having the thought that grass is green, John could have the verbal image of the word 'green'. So, John's conscious occurrent thought that grass is green essentially involves his having a verbal image of 'green'. But if John understood German, the verbal image that makes his occurrent thought conscious could be 'grün'. Moreover, the same sort of variety of associations mentioned above (e.g. lawnmowers, red dragons, a tangy taste) could also result in a plethora of possible word tokens, e.g. 'lawnmower', 'red dragon', and 'tangy'.[19] At this point it is important to emphasize that inner speech, understood solely as a sensory-phenomenological phenomenon, is not intrinsically contentful, and so meaningful content cannot be appealed to to restrict the variation of word tokens. I'll come back to this point below.

Given the cases so far considered, the following seems true

(1) *There seems to be an unlimited kind of variation of verbal and non-verbal sensory imagery that could accompany any given conscious occurrent thought, and could indeed be part of what constitutes a conscious thought.*

The 'simple sensory' proposal under discussion is that if a particular conscious thought requires phenomenology to be conscious, and the kind of phenomenology in question must be a particular instance of sensory phenomenology, then that sensory phenomenology is an essential part of that particular conscious thought. What (1) asserts is that on different occasions the particular sensory phenomenology that is essential for making the particular occurrent thought in question conscious could vary.

(1) taken on its own without any further qualifications seems to lead to (2):

(2) *that some instance of sensory phenomenology makes some particular occurrent thought conscious seems arbitrary.*

[19] By the phrase 'verbal image' I mean something like inner speech. Exactly what inner speech is and what it involves is very hard to say, but in using the phrase 'verbal image' I do not mean that one has to have anything like a visual image of the word in question.

That is, since it doesn't seem to matter whether it's a green patch image, or an image of green grass, or an image of a lawnmower, not to mention the variety of word tokens, that makes John's thought that grass is green a conscious thought, the *relationship* between the phenomenology and the thought seems not to matter. If one instance of sensory phenomenology is as good as any other, if an instance of sensory phenomenology is replaceable with any other, what kind of connection can there be between the sensory phenomenology instanced and the thought itself?

This lack of connection between the thought and phenomenology seems problematic. It can't just be a lucky accident that some piece of sensory phenomenology makes a thought conscious. One is bound to wonder exactly how an image of a green patch accounts for John's conscious occurrent thought at t_1 being the conscious thought that grass is green. How exactly does it account for John's conscious occurrent thought at t_1 being the conscious thought that grass is green in a way in which John's image of a red dragon at t_2 does not? What's the connection between the image and the thought? Presumably, some sort of connection between the thought and the particular sensory phenomenology in question must be made.

The mere fact of variability on its own does not always lead to arbitrariness. For example, the realizers of some functional role can be variable, but there is no arbitrariness involved. Consider the concept of employment. There are many ways of being employed: banker, lawyer, philosopher, etc. The charge of arbitrariness is avoided in this example, because realizing the same functional role unifies the realizers. But this is precisely what seems to be missing from the simply sensory approach. To see this more clearly, consider Loar's (2003: 3–4) proposal:

> Thinking is something lively—there is something that it is like to engage in it. So phenomenological reflection on thinking hardly conceives its properties in purely dispositional terms... We might then think of perceptual states and other phenomenal states as among the realizers of conceptual roles, or somehow intimately connected with such realizers. The liveliness of thinking in general would stem from perceptual states, linguistic states, various forms of imagery, with conceptualizing supplied by their connections within an interlocking network of conceptual roles.

In order for sensory phenomenology instances to be the realizers of conceptual roles, they would have to have all of the interconnected relations that conceptual roles do, but this seems most implausible. And to simply assert that sensory phenomenology is somehow intimately connected with such realizers amounts to an empty promise. Much of the preceding discussion has been dedicated to pointing out the lack of 'intimate connection' between sensory phenomenology and 'conceptualizing'.

So we can conclude that

(3) *the sensory phenomenology that is supposed to be what makes a particular occurrent thought a conscious thought cannot be arbitrary.*

It may be a very personal matter, but something needs to show how the phenomenology in question is explanatorily or intelligibly connected to the thought in question being conscious. With (3), therefore, we can conclude that the 'simple sensory' proposal fails: the assertion that what makes an occurrent thought conscious is the thought's having sensory-phenomenological properties of some sort is not adequate.

One obvious problem with the simple sensory approach is that the *representational content* of John's thought *can be* completely divorced from the kinds of *sensory phenomenology* whose occurrence is being supposed to be what makes it true that the thought is conscious. If, for example, in the case of John having an image of a red dragon, the connection between it and the thought that grass is green is a personal symbolic connection, then we need to see how the connection works. And this is long before we consider conscious thoughts with more abstract content, like 'ought implies can' or 'democracy is the least worst political institution'.

The natural proposal is that an explanation of how phenomenology can be involved in giving an adequate account of what makes an occurrent thought that *p* a conscious thought that *p* must somehow link the phenomenology component of the thought to the representational content component of the thought. So,

> (4) *The phenomenology that makes a particular occurrent thought a conscious thought must be explanatorily or intelligibly linked to the representational content of that thought. That is, the phenomenology that makes some essential contribution to a particular occurrent thought's being the conscious thought that p must be explanatorily linked to the content*: that p.

So what could this connection between the phenomenology of a thought and the content of the thought be? It seems clear that appealing to a (the) causal connection between the content of the thought and the associated sensory phenomenology is just not enough to establish the right type of connection. One possibility is this: that the content of the thought should simply cause one to have some sensory phenomenology without making the thought conscious at all. In this case the content (*green grass*) is simply causing a (possibly co-occurring) green patch image or perhaps causing a thought about green patches.

One proposal for satisfying (4) is to link the content of thought to verbal imagery—to occurrent images of sentences, which could be acoustic. For example, Prinz (2011: 187) suggests that

> sentences do not merely stand in for thought, but actually constitute thoughts. When we produce sentences in silent speech, they issue forth from *unconscious representations* that correspond to what those sentences mean (these are perceptual representations if empiricism is true). Sentences inherit their truth conditions from the unconscious ideas that generate them. So produced, these sentences aren't arbitrary marks, but rather meaningful symbols. If we define a thought as a mental state that represents a proposition, then mental sentences qualify as thoughts. (italics my emphasis)

There are two initial problems with this proposal. First, it may be the case that in having conscious thoughts we often have verbal imagery of the words we would use to express them. But is this always and necessarily the case? I take it that it is not. Sometimes thought is simply too quick. But then this proposal will need to appeal to non-verbal sensory imagery as well, given that it has conceded that conscious thought must involve phenomenology, and is now allowing that this phenomenology may not always be verbal. And so it will be faced with the challenge of variation of such sensory imagery already presented.[20]

The second, and more serious, worry is based on the following simple claim.

(5) *If an occurrent thought is to be a conscious thought, the content of that thought must in some manner be consciously occurrent.*

A conscious thought must somehow involve conscious entertaining of the content. (5) seems true, although 'in some manner' needs careful spelling out. (In what follows I shall sometimes say that the content of the thought itself is consciously occurrent when it is being consciously entertained.) For what can it mean (now that 'A-consciousness' has been ruled out) for a thought to be conscious if the content of that thought weren't itself conscious? It is generally accepted that a particular thought is the thought it is because of the particular content it has. And if what a thought is depends on its content, then a thought's being a conscious thought must somehow involve the conscious occurrence (entertaining) of its content.

This raises a doubt about the precise role played by non-conscious or unconscious content in Prinz's account of how it is that phenomenology makes an occurrent thought a conscious thought. If Prinz's proposal is committed to a thought's content being non-conscious, it looks as if his claim is that the thought is really non-conscious and that there is some associated sensory phenomenology that is conscious. On this proposal, conscious thoughts come out as non-conscious. In fact, according to this proposal, it looks as if there is no such thing as conscious thought at all.

One may challenge the claim that the content of a conscious thought is itself conscious on the following grounds. Suppose that one is an externalist about content, so that the thought that the Eiffel Tower is tall has the Eiffel Tower as part of its content. In what sense is the Eiffel Tower conscious? The point, already stated in effect, is simply that the content *that p* for any given conscious thought itself has got to be *entertained* ('live') in some way analogous to the way in we experience greenness in a sensory state.

[20] I assume that Prinz would deny that one could have the conscious thought that grass is green while tokening the verbal image 'red dragon'. Prinz can intelligibly make this denial because he has tied verbal images to content, and in English 'red dragon' is not tied contentfully to the thought that grass is green.

We must allow, then, that the content itself is indeed conscious in the case of conscious thought, in the sense just given: we must allow that the content is consciously entertained. And this takes us back to our original question. With a slight variation, our original question becomes, what accounts for the content of a conscious thought being conscious?

One might again propose that the non-conscious content causes some co-occurrent sensory phenomenology, and that it is in virtue of this causal relation that the sensory phenomenology makes the content conscious. But, first, rather than explaining the sense in which content is conscious, this proposal seems again like the claim that the content is in fact non-conscious although it does cause some conscious sensory phenomenology.

Second, it is hard to see how a particular instance of sensory phenomenology being an effect of some cause can make that cause, e.g. a certain content, conscious. At the bare minimum, the effect, i.e. the sensory phenomenology, would need to be lawfully linked to the cause, i.e. the content. However, this kind of lawful correlation between particular instances of sensory phenomenology and particular kinds of content seems utterly implausible, given the possible variation already pointed out. (The phenomenon of variation tells against general lawful correlation between content and sensory phenomenology and personal lawful correlation.)

One might maintain that an image of a green patch *is* the content of the thought *that grass is green*, but this proposal runs into all of the well-known problems faced by the British Empiricists' 'picture theory of thinking'.[21]

Despite the apparent implausibility of sensory phenomenology actually being the content of thought, Prinz offers a version of this view. (According to Prinz's view, consciousness takes place at the 'intermediate level'.)[22]

> If concepts are acquired by storing percepts, then concepts may be encoded in a high-level perceptual format that is not consciously accessible, if the intermediate-level theory is right. But I think concepts can be conscious, because, in occurrent acts of conceptualization, we use the high-level representations that are stored in long-term memory to construct temporary mental images of what our concepts represent... These temporary images can be conscious because imagery can be generated using intermediate-level representations... I think we should regard images generated from long-term conceptual memory as occurrent tokens of the stored concepts used to generate them. Thus, I think that concepts can be conscious... I think that the images generated from stored concepts inherit semantic properties from those concepts... So an image of a walrus represents that natural kind, and an image of an electron

[21] See e.g. Mackie (1976).

[22] Prinz accepts Jackendoff's 1987 thesis that perceptual systems are hierarchicially organized. At the low level there is response to stimulus features, but no integration of these features into wholes. At the intermediate level there is feature integration such that in vision, for example, 'we experience stimuli as bounded wholes from a specific vantage point, occuping a specific size and position within the visual field' (Prinz 2011: 177). At the high level the system abstracts away from many details and produces representations that remain stable across many vantage points.

circling a proton represents these particles. But I think these images also retain their sensory content. I endorse a Lockean notion of double reference according to which images represent both "real" natural kinds with unobservable essences and their "nominal" appearances ... Put simply, images refer to their conceptual contents by means of representing sensory contents. A mental image represents walruses by representing how they look, and an image represents subatomic particles by representing swirling circles. (Prinz 2011: 189–90)

Roughly, according to Prinz's view, there are two levels of content, non-conscious conceptual contents and sensory phenomenology which can refer to what conceptual contents refer to. The first question is, how exactly does the sensory phenomenology manage to refer to what conceptual contents refer to? In the case of thinking of a walrus, Prinz gives us a clue: a mental image represents a walrus by representing how a walrus looks. So, is Prinz proposing a version of the resemblance theory of representation? If so, this view seems totally implausible. Surely it isn't going to be the case that every conscious thought is conscious in virtue of an image resembling what the thought is about. What if I have a Picassolike image in mind whenever I have a thought about my best friend Lisa? Prinz's example of an image of an electron circling a proton representing subatomic particles is another case of non-resemblance. Moreover, Prinz's proposal will somehow have to restrict the kinds of sensory phenomenology that can accompany different thoughts. But how is he going to do that, given the possible variation of sensory phenomenology given any particular thought pointed out at the beginning of this section?

The situation so far seems to be the following. Either sensory phenomenology is in some sense representing content and thus (somehow) making content conscious, or the relationship between content and sensory phenomenology is a causal relationship. If the former, the question simply arises again about what a content's being conscious consists in. Prinz offers a version of sensory phenomenology actually representing what our non-conscious concepts represent. But this proposal is at worst very implausible or at best requires a great deal more elaboration. And the latter is just a version of a content's being non-conscious, which violates (5).

What about once again appealing to inner speech, conceived of as a phenomenological occurrence? Isn't there something like a lawful correlation between words and their meanings, at least within the system constituted by a given individual language speaker's psychology? Perhaps. But even if there is, lawful correlation on its own still doesn't make content conscious. Perhaps the point can be put as follows. Is the tokening of some inner speech in conscious experience making *the content* of the thought in question conscious? If yes, this is a variation of my proposal, and so we need to hear more about what content being conscious consists in. By appealing to inner tokens of sentences 'inheriting' truth conditions, Prinz may be sneaking in content as conscious. That is, something more is conscious than just inner speech, given that inner speech is not itself intrinsically contentful. If the answer is 'no' and the content remains unconscious, then it seems that all we really have is some associated sensory phenomenology that is conscious and the thought itself, with the content that it has, remains unconscious.

Finally, one may claim that one is simply aware of some content in having conscious thought. That is, the content of some given thought is conscious because one is aware of that content. But now the question arises, what does this 'awareness' amount to? On one very natural understanding, awareness is simply a synonym for experiential awareness (putting aside blindsight cases for the moment). And since experiential awareness involves phenomenology, so does awareness. Take the case of perceptual experience. In having a visual experience of a red round ball, one is aware of the content, the red round ball, at least partly in terms of experiencing certain kinds of sensory phenomenology, e.g. what it's like to see red, what it's like to see a color-shape, etc. Similarly, then, in genuinely consciously thinking that temperance is a virtue, one must be aware of the content in question, being temperate and being virtuous, at least partly in virtue of experiencing certain kinds of phenomenology.

I have been arguing that the phenomenology that must be present if a thought is to be conscious cannot be sensory phenomenology. If some other notion of awareness is appealed to in order to explain the sense in which awareness accounts for a thought's content being conscious, we need an account of it (keeping in mind I have rejected A-consciousness or 'cerebral celebrity' accounts as adequate).

11.5 Cognitive Phenomenology and Conscious Thought

I have argued that any adequate account of what makes occurrent thought conscious thought must satisfy two requirements: (a) *the phenomenology that is proposed as part of what the thought's being conscious consists in must be explanatorily or intelligibly linked to the content of that thought*; and (b) *the content of the thought in question must itself be conscious or consciously entertained.*

I propose now that the only plausible way to explain how a thought can be conscious, and hence how the content of a thought can be conscious, is to claim that there is cognitive phenomenology associated with, and indeed essentially constitutive of, all conscious thoughts. That is, for any content that is consciously occurrent, consciously entertained, there must (trivially) be some distinctively *cognitive phenomenological* apprehension of that content. What does that entail?

(6) *associated with each (conscious) content are some non-sensory cognitive-phenomenological properties that are possessed by conscious thoughts with those contents.*

As stated, (6) asserts a fairly weak connection between content and cognitive-phenomenological properties. (7) provides a stronger statement of the link

(7) *associated with each (conscious) content are non-sensory cognitive-phenomenological properties that are essentially possessed by any conscious thought that is a thought with that content.*[23]

Moreover,

(8) *if and in so far as we gain direct experiential access to the contents of our conscious thoughts, we do so via the cognitive-phenomenological properties of the thoughts.*

In the bulk of this chapter, I have argued that cognitive phenomenology is necessary for giving an adequate account of conscious thought. A full treatment of this issue, which is beyond the scope of this chapter, must address whether (6) or (7) is more plausible. In the end, I believe that we must accept (7), although it needs considerable refinement before it is acceptable.

For now my conclusion is that conscious thought must indeed involve phenomenology (contrary to functional/informational notions of consciousness), and sensory phenomenology is not enough. If I am right, one must either grant that there is such a thing as cognitive phenomenology, or deny that there is such a thing as conscious thought. A number of philosophers who have heard this argument have chosen the second option, denying that there is really any such thing as conscious thought. I think that there is certainly such a thing as conscious thought, and that one must therefore admit the existence of cognitive phenomenology.[24]

References

Block, N. (1995), 'On a Confusion about a Function of Consciousness', in *Behavioral and Brain Sciences* 18: 227–87.

Block, N. (2002), 'Concepts of Consciousness', in D. Chalmers (ed.), *Philosophy of Mind: Classical and Contemporary Readings* (Oxford: Oxford University Press).

Block, N. (2007), 'Consciousness, Accessibility, and the Mesh between Psychology and Neuroscience', in *Behavioral and Brain Sciences* 30: 481–548.

Block, N. (2011), 'The Higher Order Approach to Consciousness Is Defunct', in *Analysis* 71 (3): 419–31.

Brentano, F. (1874/1973), *Psychology from an Empirical Standpoint*, translated by L. McAlister (London: Routledge and Kegan Paul).

Carruthers, P. (2001/2007), 'Higher-Order Theories of Consciousness', in Edward N. Zalta (ed.), *Stanford Encyclopedia of Philosophy*, at <http://plato.stanford.edu/archives/fall2009/entries/consciousness-higher/>.

[23] See David Pitt (2004) for a discussion of this claim.

[24] I would especially like to thank Paul Coates and Sam Coleman for helpful comments on earlier drafts of this paper and for all of their hard work on this volume. I'd also like to thank Ned Block, Dave Chalmers, Daniel Stoljar, Susanna Siegel, and Galen Strawson.

Carruthers, P., and Veillet, B. (2011), 'The Case against Cognitive Phenomenology', in T. Bayne and M. Montague, (eds), *Cognitive Phenomenology* (Oxford: Oxford University Press).

Dennett, D. (1991), *Consciousness Explained* (Boston, MA: Little Brown).

Dennett, D. (2009), 'Multiple Drafts Model', in T. Bayne, A. Cleeremans, and P. Wilken, (eds), *The Oxford Companion to Consciousness* (Oxford: Oxford University Press).

Husserl, E. (1900–1901/2001), *Logical Investigations*, Vols 1 and 2. Translated by J. N. Findlay with revised translations by Dermot Moran (London and New York: Routledge).

Jackendoff, D. (1987), *Consciousness and the Computational Mind* (Cambridge, MA: MIT Press).

James, W. (1890), *The Principles of Psychology* (Cambridge, MA: Harvard University Press).

Koch, C. (2012), *Consciousness: Confessions of a Romantic Reductionist* (Cambridge, MA: MIT Press).

Kriegel, U. (2011), 'Cognitive Phenomenology as the Basis of Unconscious Content', in T. Bayne and M. Montague (eds), *Cognitive Phenomenology* (Oxford: Oxford University Press).

Levine, J. (2011), 'On the Phenomenology of Thought', in T. Bayne and M. Montague (eds), *Cognitive Phenomenology* (Oxford: Oxford University Press).

Loar, B. (2003), 'Phenomenal Intentionality as the Basis of Mental Content', in M. Hahn and B. Ramberg (eds), *Reflections and Replies: Essays on the Philosophy of Tyler Burge* (Cambridge, MA: MIT Press).

Mackie, J. L. (1976), *Problems from Locke* (Oxford: Clarendon Press).

Macpherson, F. (2012), 'Cognitive Penetration of Color Experience: Rethinking the Issue in Light of an Indirect Mechanism', *Philosophy and Phenomenological Research* 84 (1): 24–62.

Milner, A. D., and Goodale, M. A. (1995), *The Visual Brain in Action* (Oxford: Oxford University Press).

Moore, G. E. (1910–11/1953), 'Propositions', in his *Some Main Problems in Philosophy* (London: Allen and Unwin).

Owen, A. M., Coleman, M. R., Boly, M., Davis, M. H., Laureys, S., and Pickard, J. D. (2006), 'Detecting Awareness in the Vegetative State', in *Science* 313 (5792): 1402.

Pitt, D. (2004), 'The Phenomenology of Cognition or What Is It like to think that P?', in *Philosophy and Phenomenological Research* 69: 1–36.

Prinz. J. (2011), 'The Sensory Basis of Cognitive Phenomenology', in T. Bayne and M. Montague (eds), *Cognitive Phenomenology* (Oxford: Oxford University Press).

Searle, J. (1992), *The Rediscovery of the Mind* (Cambridge, MA: MIT Press).

Siegel, S. (2012), 'Cognitive Penetrability and Perceptual Justification', *Noûs* 46 (2): 201–22.

Siewert, C. (1998), *The Significance of Consciousness* (Princeton, NJ: Princeton University Press).

Strawson, G. (1986), *Freedom and Belief* (Oxford: Oxford University Press).

Strawson, G. (1994), *Mental Reality* (Cambridge, MA: MIT Press).

Strawson, G. (2011), 'Cognitive Phenomenology: Real Life', in T. Bayne and M. Montague (eds), *Cognitive Phenomenology* (Oxford: Oxford University Press).

Van Gulick, R. (2006), 'Mirror Mirror—Is that All?', in U. Kriegel and K. Williford (eds), *Self-Representational Approaches to Consciousness* (Cambridge, MA: MIT Press).

Wittgenstein, L. (1953), *Philosophical Investigations* (Oxford: Blackwell).

SECTION IV

Phenomenal Qualities and Empirical Findings

12

A Function-Centered Taxonomy of Visual Attention

Ronald A. Rensink

It is often said that appearances can be deceiving. This is certainly true in regards to what they convey about the world. But appearances can also deceive in regards to what they convey about the processes that create them. For example, our visual experience of the world is so immediate and effortless that it tends to engender a belief that scene perception results from a single unitary system that lets us immediately experience everything in our field of view. But a host of experiments in vision science have shown this not to be the case. Instead, scene perception appears to rely on the co-ordinated operation of several systems: an *early* system that rapidly creates a dense and volatile representation across much of the visual field,[1] an *attentional* system that selects a small part of this and forms it into a coherent visual object, and a *setting* system that guides this selection so that the right item is attended at the right time (e.g. Rensink 2000a and 2010).

The possibility considered here is that this is not the end of the line—that we may likewise have an incorrect belief about visual attention itself. Although 'attention' is easy enough to understand at a subjective level, it has been notoriously difficult to characterize in an objective way (e.g. Allport 1993; Chun et al. 2011; Jennings 2012). Difficulties have also been encountered in reconciling various proposals about how attention relates to conscious perceptual experience (cf. e.g. Cohen et al. 2012; De Brigard and Prinz 2010; Kentridge 2011; Koch and Tsuchiya 2007; Lamme 2003). It has been suggested that many of these difficulties exist because—contrary to common belief—'attention' does not refer to a single process, but is an umbrella term referring to *several* processes (Allport 1993; Treisman 1969). This chapter explores

[1] 'Dense' means that when a quantity is present in some area, it exists at most points in that area. 'Volatile' means that the representation is not robust, being overwritten by subsequent input, or in the absence of that, quickly dissipating. Dissipation is typically complete within a few hundred milliseconds. The trace—while it remains—corresponds with iconic memory (Rensink 2002).

one way of developing this idea, and discusses how it might help us better understand conscious visual experience.

In particular, it is suggested here that visual attention may best be viewed in terms of the co-ordinated operation of a set of processes, each with a distinct function and underlying mechanism. A key concern is then to develop a taxonomy that can describe each process and relate it to others. Towards this end, a set of constraints is first proposed on the nature of any such taxonomy, centered around the function of each process—viz. the kind of structure it outputs. A particular set of processes is then presented that is consistent with these constraints and that provides a coherent grouping of many (if not most) experimental results to date. Finally, it is suggested that a similar fractionation may apply to conscious visual experience. Among other things, this creates the possibility of reducing the problematic relationship between visual attention and visual experience to a set of simpler issues, each concerned with the relationship between a particular kind of attentional process and a particular kind of visual experience.

12.1 The Nature of Visual Attention

Performance in many visual tasks is governed by a factor within the observer that enables certain operations to be carried out, but is limited in some way. For example, when keeping track of several automobiles in traffic, only a small number can be handled simultaneously; if more are attempted, performance begins to fail. This limited factor is generally referred to as *attention*. But what exactly is it?

Considerable work has been carried out on this question over the years (see e.g. Itti et al. 2005; Jennings 2012; Pashler 1999; Wright 1998). At various times, visual attention has been associated with things such as clarity of perception, consciousness, or a limited 'resource' that enables particular kinds of operations to be carried out (see Hatfield 1998). But perhaps the greatest amount of progress has been achieved by focusing on the idea of *selection* (Broadbent 1982).

In what follows, an attentional process is taken to be one that is *contingently selective, controlled on the basis of global considerations* (Rensink 2013)—e.g. tracking a particular item based on its importance.[2] Global considerations include not only cognitive factors such as the importance for the task at hand, but also perceptual factors such as *salience*—the visual distinctiveness of an item with respect to all others in the visual field. These are largely handled via two kinds of attentional control: *endogenous* (via top-down cognitive mechanisms subject to conscious volition), and *exogenous* (via bottom-up perceptual mechanisms that operate automatically, although still in terms of global considerations).

[2] This is somewhat similar to the proposal of Jennings (2012), except that no explicit mention is made here of a 'subject' that controls the process. The emphasis here is instead on objective factors that are non-local, such as responding to the brightest dot in an image.

In this view, 'attention' is more an adjective than a noun—an attentional process is one that is selective and subject to a particular kind of control; 'paying attention' is exerting that control, resulting in a particular kind of selection. One advantage of this characterization is that it allows 'attention' to be implemented in different ways—there need not be a single process that can be identified with it, nor a single site where it operates (cf. Allport 1993; Tsotsos 2011: ch. 1). This characterization excludes processes such as the transduction of light by photoreceptors: although this process is selective (in that it has a differential sensitivity to wavelength), its selectivity is not contingent. On the other hand, this characterization includes any globally-controlled process of limited capacity (such as storing information into visual short-term memory), since limited capacity necessarily results in selectivity of some kind. And although this definition can apply to the controlled allocation of a single resource or process, it is not limited to this—it can also apply to the control of several processes, provided this is done in a co-ordinated way.

This characterization departs somewhat from the traditional notion of attention as a simple 'stuff' or 'resource'. This notion, however, does not always help make sense of experimental results, nor does it always lead to interesting experimental questions (Allport 1989; Franconeri 2013; Navon 1984). Even more importantly, the traditional view has been unable to engender a comprehensive framework capable of providing a good understanding of attention (see e.g. Allport 1993) or its connection to conscious experience. It may therefore be time to give serious consideration to the alternative.

12.2 Constraints on Potential Taxonomies

If different kinds of attentional process exist, a taxonomy of some kind could help delineate what these are and how they relate to each other. But, creating such a system involves addressing several taxonomic issues, such as the nature of the main categories and the appropriate granularity for each. How might this be done?

12.2.1 General principles

A reasonable constraint for any potential taxonomy is that it be based on principles that are relatively general, and so unlikely to significantly change as new facts are discovered. Several such principles appear relevant:

1. Function-centeredness: The specification of each process must center around its *function*—e.g. selecting information from a particular part of the visual field, or explicitly linking estimates of orientation and color at a given location. Such a focus provides greater generality than if the taxonomy were organized around type of perceptual effect or experimental task used. As mentioned earlier, the function must be more than just selective: it must also be controllable on the basis of global considerations, such as those conveyed by task instructions.

2. *Maximal functionality*: The processes contained in the taxonomy must include—in one form or other—as many useful distinctions as possible in terms of function. This might include, for example, selection of items in a given area of space, or of a particular color. (Assuming that these can be controlled via global considerations.) No important ability should be neglected. Following the principle of function-centeredness, the articulation of these should be done in terms of function alone, without regard to implementation.

3. *Minimal mechanism*: The taxonomy must posit as few underlying mechanisms as possible. (In essence, this is a form of Occam's razor.) Here, *mechanism* refers to the set of operations, implemented in a neural substrate, that carry out the function under consideration. When description is in terms of observable properties alone (e.g. time taken, number of operands), this can be viewed as a *specification*; a more complete characterization would include the *algorithm* used, along with a description of the representation(s) involved. Some mechanisms can support several functions, although not necessarily concurrently (e.g. a computer operating system). The complete set of functions associated with a mechanism—along with the mechanism itself—corresponds to a single attentional *process*.

4. *Computational analysis*: Each process should be described in terms of (i) function, (ii) perceptual effects, (iii) mechanism (algorithm and representation), and (iv) neural implementation. The need for a functional description is clear from the above. The requirement for perceptual effects operationalizes these functions so as to guarantee they can be measured. The other two requirements are part of the computational analysis of any visual process (Marr 1982); the result could be viewed as an *augmented computational theory* of attention. A complete analysis from all four perspectives is more of an ideal than a reality—in practice, only some of these may be possible. But following the principle of function-centeredness, analysis at the functional level should always be included.

12.2.2 Distinctions concerning function

The maximal-functionality principle requires that a taxonomy make as many functional distinctions as possible. But what should these be? And how should they be grouped? One possibility (Chun et al. 2011) is to begin by distinguishing between functions involving information *external* to the observer (e.g. collecting it from a selected location in the environment) and information that is *internal* (e.g. transmitting it along particular pathways). In what follows, consideration will be limited to external functions, which are better understood and arguably more closely related to perceptual experience.

External functions can be subdivided (Rensink 2009 and 2013) into *orientation* (selective access to a particular set of data from the environment) and *integration*

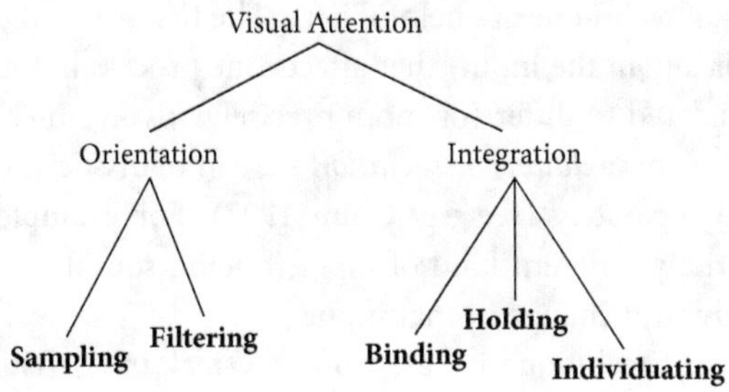

Figure 12.1 Potential subdivisions of external functions associated with visual attention. This reflects functional aspects only; these divisions correspond to different processes only if the mechanisms that underlie them are different. Many of these distinctions could be further subdivided.

(selection of a particular set of spatiotemporal associations for this data). Orientation can in turn be subdivided into two sub-functions:

- *sampling* (collection of sufficient information from the world);
- *filtering* (discarding of unnecessary information).

Ideally, these result in the collection of exactly the information necessary for the task at hand. For integration, various sub-functions can likewise be defined:

- *holding* (association across both time and space);
- *binding* (association across space alone; minimal temporal extent);
- *individuating* (association across time alone; minimal spatial extent).

Figure 12.1 shows the result.[3] Nothing prevents these functions from being subdivided further; indeed, the principle of maximal functionality would require making any distinction that is useful. For example, binding could be separated into more specialized forms such as linking items with a given color, or associating an item to a particular location in space. The ultimate granularity of such distinctions will likely be determined by practical considerations. In any event, the relationships established between these functions on the basis of such refinement form a 'shadow taxonomy', which can specify the relationships of any processes subsequently posited as being distinct.

12.2.3 Distinctions concerning mechanism

The minimal-mechanism principle requires assuming as few underlying mechanisms as possible. This may be done by initially assuming a single underlying mechanism and positing separate mechanisms only when there is sufficient evidence for doing so.

[3] In the nomenclature used here, individual processes end in '-ing', the participle indicating their status as active entities; higher-level, more abstract groupings end in '-tion'.

Two general kinds of technique are helpful here. The first is based on *dissociation*—a manipulation (typically in the input) that affects one process but not the other. Two processes are considered to differ (or more precisely, involve mechanisms not used by the other) if they show a *double dissociation*—a pair of dissociations such that each process is affected separately (see e.g. Chun 1997). For example, if each process operates on an entirely different kind of input (one on sound, one on light, say), it will be affected only by a change in that input.

The second kind of technique is based on *dual-task interference* (see e.g. Braun 1994; VanRullen et al. 2004). Here, performance on two tasks carried out concurrently is compared to when they are carried out separately one at a time. If no detriment exists, the processes involved do not use a common resource, and thus do not draw upon common mechanisms. A popular form of this is the *attentional operating characteristic* (Sperling and Dosher 1986), which describes the extent to which two attentional tasks interfere with each other.

12.3 A Provisional Taxonomy

Although the considerations above constrain any potential taxonomy, they are not enough to specify it uniquely. A provisional candidate is therefore suggested here, consistent with all the above constraints and capable of organizing most known perceptual effects (including deficits) related to visual attention (Rensink 2013). Although unlikely to completely capture all aspects of attention, it will serve to keep discussion focused, and provide a basis of comparison for any proposed improvement.

Note that some of the processes described have a nonattentional component to their control—for instance, they could be controlled *reflexively*, via a precompiled routine that operates automatically on the basis of local visual properties such as edges of sufficient contrast.[4] This does not prevent them from being attentional, however, in that they can still be controlled on the basis of global considerations whenever necessary.

12.3.1 Attentional sampling

A: FUNCTION

Visual perception begins with the pick-up of information via the selective *sampling* of incoming light by the eye. Because the eye has high resolution only in the few degrees around the point of *fixation*, it must be continually repositioned via brief jumps, or

[4] Reflexive control is similar to exogenous control (section 12.1) in that both are automatic and can be driven by the contents of the image. However, exogenous control involves *global* considerations (e.g. processing the highest-contrast item in an image as part of a given task) whereas reflexive control only involves *local* ones (e.g. processing any item with sufficient contrast, no matter what). Reflexive control would likely be overridden by global control in most situations. But it would generally be difficult to empirically determine whether the control used in any particular situation is exogenous or reflexive.

saccades; when controlled appropriately, these allow the right information to be obtained from the environment at the right time (Ballard et al. 1997; Carpenter 1988). Although the control of this process can be reflexive, it often involves global considerations—e.g. fixating or pursuing the object needed for the task at hand. In such situations, this process is attentional in the sense used here.[5] It is also attentional in the traditional sense, which refers to it as *overt attention*. To make more explicit its functional role, it is referred to here as *attentional sampling*.

Other selective processes exist that are entirely internal to the observer; their operation is often referred to collectively *as covert attention*. Overt and covert systems are only partly correlated: they need not—and often do not—act on the same information (e.g. Juan et al. 2004). Put another way: if an observer is fixating (and thus sampling) a given item on the basis of some global consideration, it does not necessarily follow that they are 'attending' to it in all other possible ways.

B: PERCEPTUAL EFFECTS

Attentional sampling has been the subject of considerable work by vision scientists, in large part because its external (overt) character allows direct observation and manipulation of its operation. Selectivity can be measured when eye movements are prevented, such as having the observer view an image during a brief flash. Acuity and color perception are best in the central few degrees (or *foveal* area), falling off rapidly with eccentricity in the outer parts (or *periphery*). Information is thus of maximal resolution. Conversely, motion perception is poor in the fovea and better in the periphery (see e.g. Barlow and Mollon 1982).

C: MECHANISM

The systems underlying sampling are reasonably well understood. Incoming light is picked up by two interleaved arrays of photoreceptors: *rods* and *cones*. Rods are located mostly in the periphery, cones—which alone can distinguish color—in the fovea. The eye itself is moved via three pairs of muscles, controlled via areas in the brain such as the superior colliculus and the frontal eye fields (see e.g. Crowne 1983); these are in turn controlled via several different neural pathways. (For more information, see e.g. Henderson and Hollingworth 1998; Krauzlis 2005).

12.3.2 Attentional filtering (gating)

A: FUNCTION

Although a vast amount of information is picked up via sampling, most is irrelevant for any given task. This irrelevant information can significantly degrade performance, essentially acting as a form of noise (see e.g. Rensink 2013). As such, it must

[5] It may be worth emphasizing that according to the definition used here, a selective process is attentional only when global control is in effect.

be filtered out as much as possible, improving the *quality* of the information used. (This is sometimes referred to as applying 'selective attention'.) A simple way of doing so is *gating*—transmitting only the information at a particular location or containing a particular property, such as color or size. Various subdivisions are possible, depending on the parameter(s) controlled. These include:

- *spatial filtering* (selection of information from a particular region of space; sometimes referred to as 'spatial attention');
- *feature filtering* (selection of information containing a simple property, or *feature*; sometimes referred to as 'feature-based attention');
- *ocular filtering* (selection of information from a particular eye).

An important issue for most of these is the extent of selection. At one extreme, selection can be *diffuse*, with a relatively broad range of inputs. In the case of space, for example, information can be accessed from a large area of the visual field, allowing some processes to speed up by operating in parallel; the downside, however, is that more noise is introduced. Selection can also be *focused*, with input taken from a relatively restricted range—e.g. from a small region of space. This reduces noise, but may cause processing to slow down. (These extremes are sometimes referred to respectively as *diffuse* and *focused attention*.) The extent of selection essentially involves a trade-off between speed and accuracy, with the optimal choice depending upon details of the task and the environment.

B: PERCEPTUAL EFFECTS

Attentional filtering lies at the heart of various effects associated with the *quality* of the information transmitted. These include *interocular suppression* (items not seen if originating in the unattended eye), *enhancement* (attended items have greater apparent contrast), and *inattentional blindness* (items not seen if not attended). All can be characterized in an objective way. (For details on these and related effects, see e.g. Itti et al. 2005 and Rensink 2013.)

Several deficits can be traced to difficulties with filtering. Damage to the right posterior parietal cortex can result in *neglect*—the absence of visual experience in some part of space (Bartolomeo and Chokron 2002; Bisiach 1993). A related condition is *extinction*, where an item vanishes when a competing item is placed on the opposite side of the visual field. Both deficits appear to result from a failure to gate information from the appropriate area (or representation of the item), causing either an outright failure to access the information it contains, or at least a slowdown of processing (Posner et al. 1984).

C: MECHANISM

Although the phenomena above superficially have little in common, several commonalities exist in their mode of operation:

- can be controlled on the basis of global considerations;
- inputs can be switched very quickly (typically, within 30–50 milliseconds);
- selection is of simple properties (e.g. spatial locations or simple features);
- for space, a contiguous area is involved, akin to a spotlight (1° in size at fixation; increases with retinal eccentricity);
- transmitted information is poorly localized (can't precisely establish position on retina).

Although the parameters that *control* filtering are simple, the structures *acted upon* are not,[6] generally having at least some degree of organization (see e.g. Driver et al. 2001; Rensink 2013). For example, filtering can be affected by background structures (*segments*) formed on the basis of luminance or texture boundaries at early 'pre-attentive' stages of vision, before attentional filtering has had time to act (Driver et al. 2001). Transmitted information can be measurements of relatively complex structures of limited extent (*proto-objects*) formed at early levels (Rensink and Enns 1995). Consistent with this, these effects tend to operate over perceived rather than 'raw' retinal space (Robertson and Kim 1999).

12.3.3 Attentional binding

A: FUNCTION

Ideally, the representations of all properties in an image that are relevant for a task should be explicitly associated or linked so as to adequately capture the structure of the world at each moment—i.e. they should be *bound*. Some degree of reflexive binding is already apparent in the creation of preattentive background segments and proto-objects (section 12.3.2). But to better capture structure, more sophisticated control is often needed. For example, if a line segment can be assigned equally well to either of two groups on the basis of purely local factors, determination of its placement will need to be based on non-local considerations. In other words, it will need to involve *attentional binding*.

As in the case of filtering, several kinds of binding can be distinguished, many of which can be subdivided in turn. For example:

- *feature binding*
  - across-feature binding (e.g. color and orientation);
  - within-feature binding (e.g. horizontal and vertical lines in a 'T');
- *part binding* (or *connecting*)
  - binding across space (i.e. grouping);
  - binding across levels of hierarchical structure;

[6] As used here, 'structure' can refer either to structure in the external world or the corresponding structure that is part of representational content. It will hopefully be clear from context which meaning is intended.

- *position binding* (or *positioning*)
  - binding to a precise location in space.

Attentional binding is often associated with filtering. For example, the feature integration theory of Treisman and Gelade (1980) posits that the linking of different kinds of features in an item (e.g. blue and horizontal) occurs via the focused gating of information over a small area at their location, which enables their representations to be activated simultaneously. But from a functional point of view, binding differs substantially from filtering: it is concerned not with *access*, but with *construction*.

B: PERCEPTUAL EFFECTS

As in the case of filtering, effects involving attentional binding show up in various ways, all of which can be characterized objectively. But rather than involving the *quality* of information, they involve—via success or failure—its *integration*. These include *conjunction detection* (detection of items with a unique combination of features), *illusory conjunctions* (inappropriate linking of features in briefly-presented items), and *repetition blindness* (failure to distinguish similar stimuli within a brief time). (For more information on these and related effects, see e.g. Kanwisher et al. 1999, Rensink 2013, and Wright 1998.)

Several perceptual deficits can be ascribed to failures of binding. For example, damage to the inferior temporal lobe can result in *integrative agnosia*, an inability to perceive overall shape or configuration; perception is only of simple features, such as color or texture (Farah 2004; Riddoch and Humphreys 1987).

C: MECHANISM

Attentional binding creates representations that support processes such as the recognition of complex shapes and characters. These appear to depend on a mechanism—or set of mechanisms—having the following characteristics:

- can be controlled on the basis of global considerations;
- medium-speed operation (complete in about 100–150 milliseconds);
- operates on organized structures (e.g. segments, proto-objects);
- involves only a small number of such structures at any time.

In some cases attentional binding may be carried out via filtering (e.g. Treisman and Gelade 1980). In other cases, however—such as those involving non-local structure—different mechanisms are used (e.g. Maddox et al. 2002; VanRullen et al. 2004).

12.3.4 Attentional holding (stabilizing)

A: FUNCTION

When a physical object changes over time (e.g. a bird taking flight), it is often useful to represent it not as a set of unrelated structures, but as a single persisting object.

Continuity of this sort can be captured via a representation that is *coherent* (or *stabilized*). Here, properties are linked not only across space but also across time, so as to refer to an object with a substrate that endures, even across eye movements (Kahneman et al. 1992; Rensink 2000a).[7] Owing to the complexity of the processes involved in constructing the underlying representation, such *holding* may require a considerable amount of computational resources. It is therefore unlikely that much of it is done reflexively.

Two kinds of continuity can be distinguished: *perceptual* continuity, where the perceptual representation of an object is continually maintained, and *conceptual* continuity, where this representation is recreated and matched with a trace in long-term (semantic) memory. The first corresponds to the perception of *dynamic change*, where an object is seen to dynamically transform; the second to *completed change*, where the object is simply perceived as having changed at some point in the past (Rensink 2002).

B: PERCEPTUAL EFFECTS

Attentional holding links properties across both space and time. Effects involving its failure or success include *object-specific preview benefit* (faster detection of stimuli located inside objects in which they appeared previously), *attentional blink* (failure to create a second visual object if presented less than 250–300 milliseconds after the first), and *change blindness* (failure to detect clearly-visible change in an object over time). All can be characterized in an objective way. (See e.g. Jensen et al. 2011 and Rensink 2013 for more complete descriptions of these and related effects.)

Several deficits caused by damage to the occipital region of the brain may be linked to mechanisms that enable holding. Among the more striking of these is *dorsal simultanagnosia*. Here, observers cannot recognize more than one object (or part of one object) at a time, with the rest of the input simply not being experienced (Coslett and Saffran 1991; Farah 2004). A variant is *ventral simultanagnosia*, in which observers cannot recognize more than one object, but can still experience several simple (bound) shapes simultaneously (Farah 2004).

C: MECHANISM

Each of the effects associated with attentional holding appears to involve a mechanism with most (if not all) of the following properties:

- can be controlled on the basis of global considerations;
- relatively slow operation (250–300 milliseconds);

[7] Eye fixations require an exposure of no more than about 150 milliseconds if eye movements are to be optimally guided (Rayner et al. 2009). This suggests that the bound structure generated at each fixation suffices for most aspects of perception. Persistence across eye movements would then involve the representation of a different kind of structure.

- operates on organized structures (e.g. segments, proto-objects);
- accesses up to 3–4 such structures (only a small amount of information from each);
- only one structure in play at a time (accessed structures act as 'parts');
- stability across interruptions for several seconds (access to visual short-term memory).

Such a mechanism can represent at most only a few aspects of a physical object at any time. Although the situation here is not as well understood as it is for the others, indications are that attentional holding is also a distinct process (Rensink 2013).

One model of this is the *object file*, a temporary representation of (bound) properties that captures the continuity of an object as it transforms or changes position (Kahneman et al. 1992). Another is the *coherence field*, in which information is 'held' in a reverberating circuit created by feedforward and feedback connections between selected proto-objects and a higher-level collection point, or *nexus* (Rensink 2000a and 2001).

12.3.5 Attentional individuating (indexing)

A: FUNCTION

It is sometimes useful to *individuate* a physical object—to see it not just as *an* object, but as a *particular* object. This can be important when more than one object must be dealt with, such as determining a 'between' relation, or ensuring that the items in an image are processed in an efficient sequence (Pylyshyn 2003; Ullman 1984). In contrast to other attentional functions, individuating—or 'indexing' (Pylyshyn 2003)—is not concerned with visual structure per se, but with *process*, e.g. applying a particular operation to a particular item at a particular time.

Although individuating could in principle be done via coherent representation, it is difficult to create more than one such representation at a time (section 12.3.4). Fortunately, complete coherence is rarely needed: it is often sufficient to consider an item considered distinct at some point, and then *track* it on the basis of its position.[8] If this can be done successfully, the item can be immediately accessed or operated upon whenever needed.

B: PERCEPTUAL EFFECTS

Several effects involve items which persist over time, but for which physical properties are unimportant, or even irrelevant. These include *multiple-object tracking* (immediate report about selected items that move about), *prioritization of search* (faster search for items in locations shown ahead of time), and *subitizing* (rapid

[8] Tracking may be a distinct process concerned with temporal continuity only (cf. the separation of binding into several possible processes). However, invoking the principle of minimal mechanism, tracking will be assumed to be an aspect of individuating until evidence is found for a distinct underlying mechanism.

counting of a small number of items). (For further details on these and other related effects, see e.g. Rensink 2013 and Scholl 2009).

C: MECHANISM

The mechanism that underlies the various effects involving individuating appears to have many—if not all—of the following characteristics:

- can be controlled on the basis of global considerations;
- operates quickly (approximately 30–50 milliseconds per item);
- operates on organized structures (e.g. segments, proto-objects);
- accesses up to 7–8 such structures (via location of their centers of mass);
- only one overall structure at a time (locations organized into a 'virtual polygon');
- based on an environment-centered frame (not 'raw' retinal space).

Coherent representations are not necessarily individuated, suggesting that individuating and holding involve different mechanisms (see e.g. Bahrami 2003; Scholl 2009). However, individuating does appear to facilitate the control of filtering, suggesting at least some interaction of these (see Rensink 2013).

12.3.6 Nonattentional processing

As the above survey indicates, all attentional processes appear to be influenced by organized structure determined rapidly at early levels, before any process has had much time to act. Although such effects have sometimes been ascribed to 'object-based attention', it may be that they originate at a stage used by *all* attentional processes (or at least, all those beyond sampling). In this view, considerable processing takes place reflexively and rapidly across the visual field, resulting in a substrate upon which attentional processes can draw. An interesting issue is the extent to which an attentional process could affect this substrate itself. In the extreme, it might be able to do so substantially, with the resultant structure possibly reverting to its original form after attentional processing ends (see Rensink 2009, 2010, 2013).

12.3.7 Dependencies

How might the various attentional processes depend on each other? The simplest set of possible relations—those among the processes themselves, whether or not global control is in effect—is shown in Figure 12.2. Here, sampling and filtering are posited as acting prior to the others, since no process can proceed without adequate input. Reflexive gating of information is possible: for example, everything around the edges in an image could simply be transmitted. But global control would help ensure that the transmitted information is exactly what is needed.

The outputs of sampling and filtering are similar in that both involve a dense array of simple quantities. However, the information transmitted by filtering is not tightly

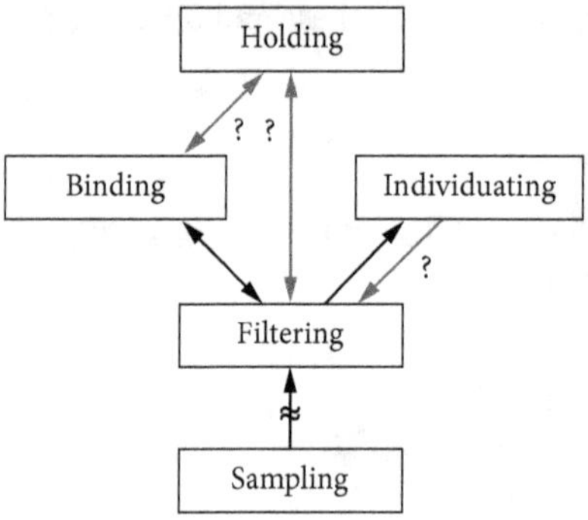

Figure 12.2 Possible set of dependencies between attentional processes. (Arrows with question marks denote connections for which insufficient evidence exists.) All processes depend on transmission of information at the filtering stage, which in turn depends on sampling. Between sampling and filtering exist processes that enable positional invariance. (Wavy lines indicate that correspondence to retinal position is via a transform to more object-centered co-ordinates.) It is unclear whether the dependence of holding on filtering is direct, via binding, or both.

bound to retinal position (section 12.3.2). Note that the poor localization of filtered output is a natural consequence of positional invariance, which allows processes such as recognition to give much the same result regardless of the exact position of the target in the image (Tsotsos 2011).

The relationships between the other three processes are largely unknown; functional specifications do not completely constrain the situation. For example, although binding involves spatial structure, and holding involves both spatial and temporal structure, the type and extent of spatial structure in each need not be the same. If binding involves more extensive spatial structure than holding, say, its outputs are unlikely to be directly drawn upon by holding. However, many of these dependencies are likely reciprocal—for example, in several models (e.g. Tsotsos 2011), binding depends upon filtering, and vice versa.

A key issue is whether these dependencies also hold when global control is involved. For example, although attentional binding may require filtering, does it require *attentional* filtering? Experimental results currently provide only limited guidance, in large part because of the practical difficulties involved. However, a case might be made for an *alignment thesis*: each attentional process requires attentional control of the contingently selective processes upon which it depends, so as to ensure that all the relevant processes operate on the appropriate inputs.

12.4 Relation to Visual Experience

Having defined a set of attentional processes, the next step is to examine how they might relate to conscious visual experience—or more precisely, to its representational content.[9] Consciousness is often believed to participate in the consolidation of information over a global scale (Baars 1988; Cohen and Dennett 2011; Dehaene

[9] Or more precisely yet—to the representational content of experience that is *sensory*, i.e. that results when our eyes are open and is used for getting around in the world. The phenomenal experience encountered in dreams or mental imagery, for example, is not considered here.

and Changeux 2011). As such, it could be involved in a given process in several ways. It could, for example, participate in the global *transmission* of information associated with that process, such as the information input or output—e.g. results that are broadcast to other areas. Or it could participate in the control of the *process itself*—e.g. override particular bindings made reflexively at early levels (cf. Libet 1985). The extent to which conscious visual experience is involved in such functions appears to be a contingent matter, as is the extent to which these functions involve visual attention. Such issues have proven difficult to resolve (see e.g. De Brigard and Prinz 2010; Kentridge 2011).

A potential way to simplify this problem is to reduce it to parts that are each concerned with a particular aspect of conscious experience. Two types of consciousness are often distinguished: *P-consciousness* (phenomenal consciousness), involving the phenomenal aspects of experience, and *A-consciousness* (access consciousness), involving the representational aspects that can be reported verbally (Block 1995). But given that different kinds of structure are created by different attentional mechanisms, another—possibly complimentary—set of distinctions might be drawn, based on the kinds of structures involved. Just as the experience of color and motion are distinct kinds (or at least aspects) of experience concerned with distinct *physical* properties of the world, so might there be kinds of experience concerned with distinct *structural* properties. Such distinctions might in turn be associated with differences in the properties of the experience itself (e.g. different time constants, due to different underlying processes). If so, there may well result a clustering of properties that could allow various kinds of experience to be defined, and related to each other.

12.4.1 Attentional sampling/visual uniformity

Information pick-up—and thus, sampling—is necessary for any kind of visual perception. But although our visual experience can be vivid and compelling, it does not usually correspond directly to what is picked up at the retina. For example, although the eyes generally saccade several times a second (often over several degrees of visual angle), our subjective impression is of a single, stable 'picture'. In addition, variations across the eye in the range of colors and motions sampled (section 12.3.1) are never part of this picture—a uniform resolution and range is experienced throughout. The mechanisms that create such stability and uniformity are largely unknown (Bridgeman et al. 1994; O'Regan and Noë 2001), although they may depend in part upon the positional invariance established during attentional filtering (e.g. Tsotsos 2011). If so, their involvement suggests that although attentional sampling (via the alignment thesis) may be necessary for visual experience, it cannot be sufficient.

It has been argued that the need for attentional sampling does not apply at a local level. For example, although the retina contains a *blind spot* where no photoreceptors exist (and thus no sampling occurs), what is experienced at that location appears to be 'filled in' on the basis of adjacent information, so that the gap is not noticed (Ramachandran 1992). However, the nature of such filling-in is problematic; it has been argued that there may actually be no experience of the missing information (see e.g. Dennett 1992; Pessoa et al. 1998).

12.4.2 Attentional filtering/fragmentary experience

Filtering—or at least, gating—appears necessary for conscious visual experience of any kind. In binocular rivalry, for example, observers fail to experience anything from the unmonitored eye, in which the output has likely been suppressed (see Rensink 2009). A similar failure occurs in inattentional blindness when an unattended item smaller than a few degrees in size disappears completely (Mack and Rock 1998), and in the neurophysiological condition of *neglect*, in which items in one hemifield are not seen at all (Bisiach 1993). In all these conditions, gating has presumably shut down entirely.

Although it has been claimed that visual experience can occur without 'attention' (Braun and Sagi 1990; Koch and Tsuchiya 2007), it may be that attentional gating is still required. In the dual-task design typically used in such experiments (Figure 12.3), observers given the task of identifying a pattern at the center of a display cannot also report the shape of an item located outside this zone. But they *can* report—and presumably experience—its color and orientation (Braun and Sagi 1990; Fei-Fei et al. 2002). Likewise, when observers track one event and do not recognize another in the background (suggesting a limit in holding or individuating), they occasionally report seeing 'something' of the background, even though they cannot say what it is (Neisser and Becklen 1975). Such reports suggest that what is limited in these dual-task conditions is not attentional processing in its entirety, but only attentional *binding*.

A similar experience of localized properties without sophisticated structure is encountered during the perception of briefly-presented images. Observers can reliably determine the meaning (or *gist*) of an image presented for 30–60 milliseconds

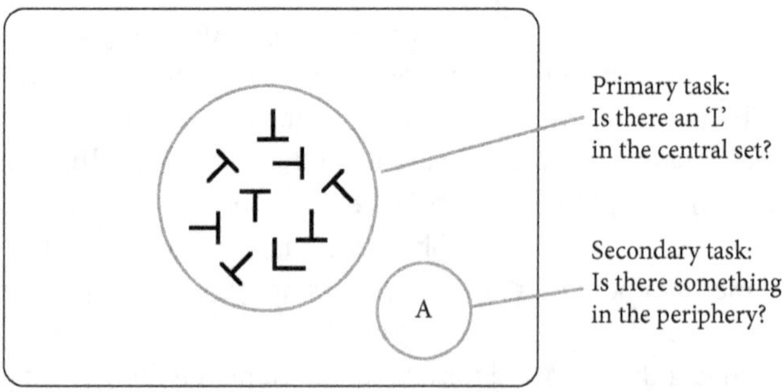

Figure 12.3 Example of dual-task design often used in investigations into how perception relates to attentional processing, e.g. Braun and Sagi (1990), Fei-Fei et al. (2002).

(Loschky and Larson 2009; Thorpe et al. 1996); they can even detect the presence of animals under such conditions (Fei-Fei et al. 2002), as well as relatively abstract quantities such as the average size of a set of items (Chong and Treisman 2003). The experience reported for such brief exposures in all these situations is one of a fleeting array of simple colors and shapes, with relatively little sophisticated structure (e.g. Fei-Fei et al. 2007).

Such results therefore suggest the possibility of a distinct kind of visual experience—*fragmentary experience*—in which the observer has access primarily to a dense array of simple localized features with little intrinsic structure (Rensink 2010 and 2013);[10] in some ways, it is similar to what is experienced when viewing an Impressionist painting. The content of such experience contains only those properties (such as color, motion, and orientation) that can be measured on the basis of local information, assigned to each point in the image, represented as scalars or low-dimensional vectors, and for which well-defined distance measures exist. The simplicity of these properties is consistent with the fact that they can be experienced in stimuli presented for as little as 30 milliseconds. Their simplicity is also consistent with the fact that in terms of phenomenal character, they are unproblematically visible, constituting the 'raw stuff' of visual experience.

Fragmentary experience may be similar to the 'background consciousness' thought to occur in iconic-memory displays, where contents are fleeting and appear to contain more than can be reported (Iwasaki 1993). It may also include the 'partial awareness' of word fragments experienced in brief displays (Kouider et al. 2010), provided these are limited to simple components such as oriented line segments or localized structures (e.g. corners) formed by reflexive binding. Its focus on 'raw' sensory qualities suggests that fragmentary experience may also be related to P-consciousness (Block 1995), although it does not include non-local structures and shapes: if a set of blue patches, say, is arranged into a triangle, that triangle will not be explicitly represented—and thus not experienced—at this level. Note that fragmentary experience can be accompanied by abstract categorization (e.g. identification of scenes and animals) even if there is little or no conscious experience of the non-local structure of the underlying stimuli.

Fragmentary experience often involves gating that extends over a relatively wide expanse, possibly allocated in a sequential way (VanRullen et al. 2004). As the primary task becomes more demanding, fragmentary experience of the scene—along with the perception of its gist—begins to fail (Cohen et al. 2011). If this is

[10] This is referred to as *ambient experience* in Rensink (2013). An interesting issue is whether this is best viewed as a distinct kind of *experience* or an experience of a distinct kind of *structure*. In a similar vein: does someone suffering from integrative agnosia (who can experience only simple features) have an experience different in kind from that of most observers, or the same experience that is more restricted in its structure? Owing to the clustering of traits sketched here, it appears more appropriate to describe fragmentary experience as differing in kind. Similar considerations apply to the other kinds of experience described in the following sections.

because the extent of gating has been reduced to remove noise in order to facilitate the primary task (cf. Lavie 1995), it would suggest that filtering—or more precisely, the information that filtering transmits—is needed for *any* process involving the fragmentary properties of an image, including the generation of fragmentary experience.[11] This is compatible with the suggestion that such filtering must be attentional in order to yield at least a fragmentary experience of a stimulus (Mack and Rock 1998).

12.4.3 Attentional binding/assembled experience

When given the task of identifying a pattern at the center of a briefly-presented display (Figure 12.3), observers can still detect simple fragmentary properties outside this zone, such as localized colors or orientations (Braun and Sagi 1990; Braun 1994). This has sometimes been considered evidence for visual experience without attention (Braun and Sagi 1990). But given the distinctions made here, a more nuanced possibility arises: without attentional binding, fragmentary experience is still possible, but nothing more.

The kind of experience that *is* encountered when binding succeeds is that of simple sensory properties such as color and motion (fragmentary experience) along with a 'layer' of static structure. Given its involvement with structure, this might be termed *assembled experience*. In some ways, it is similar to what is experienced under stroboscopic conditions, where brief flashes of light remove the information needed to perceive motion, yet still allow other basic properties—including form—to be seen. It can be encountered in displays presented for 100–150 milliseconds (Fei-Fei et al. 2007), the time needed for binding. Although structures bound pre-attentively (and thus, reflexively) can pre-empt immediate access to their components, their components can be accessed—and thus, experienced—by further (attentional) control of the binding process (Rensink and Enns 1995).

In this view, any aspect of static organization is manifest only in assembled experience, which requires binding.[12] Note that for many aspects of binding (section 12.3.3), local information does not suffice. In the case of shape, for example, although some properties can be defined locally (e.g. orientation or curvature at a point), others cannot (e.g. symmetry or size). Moreover, the explicit representation of bound structure involves associations, which cannot always be well represented by scalars or low-dimensional vectors.[13] Nor is there always a well-defined distance measure

[11] Given that filtering operates on representations that contain a degree of organization, it follows that what is experienced in a fragmentary way is not the raw information that enters the eye, but a quantity that has already been abstracted to some extent.

[12] There may be sub-types of assembled experience, corresponding to sub-types of attentional binding (section 12.3.3). In the interests of simplicity, this possibility is not discussed here.

[13] A shape could be represented as a scalar or vector under some conditions—e.g. a closed curve could be described in terms of its compactness. But unless there are tight constraints on the set of possible shapes, such a measure will capture only one aspect of its structure.

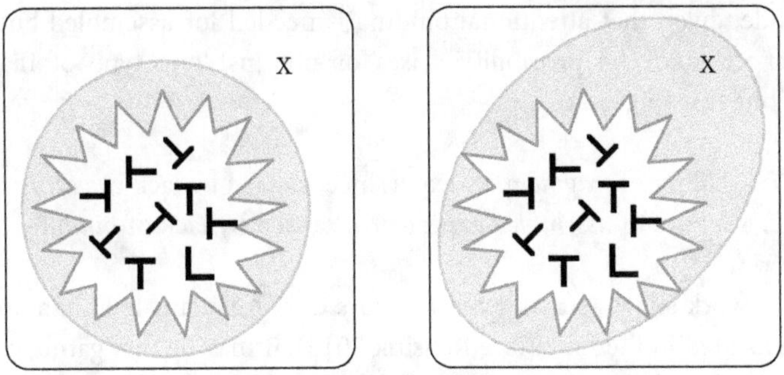

(a) Inattentional blindness Type 1 (b) Inattentional blindness Type 2

Figure 12.4 Types of inattentional blindness. (a) Type 1: Allocation of both attentional binding (jagged border) and filtering (smooth border) is limited to the central group, resulting in a failure to transmit any information about the 'X'. This causes a failure to experience the 'X' even in a fragmentary way. (b) Type 2: Attentional filtering extends to the 'X', but binding is still absent. This causes a failure to experience the 'X' in an assembled way, although a fragmentary experience of it is still possible.

between structures. The structures experienced—such as shapes that extend over space—also differ from fragmentary properties in that they need not be dense (i.e. not present at each point in the image), but can be distinct elements that cover the visual field in a much sparser way. Finally, more sophisticated processing is likely involved; indeed, if the perception of shape is taken to be the beginning of concept formation (Arnheim 1969), assembled experience may be the first stage (or level) where the perception of concepts occurs (cf. Prinz 2006). It is likely that binding must be attentional if a viewer is to have an assembled experience of the stimulus (Treisman and Gelade 1980).

The view of assembled experience as a combination of unstructured sensory properties and superimposed form is vaguely reminiscent of the hylomorphism of Aristotle, where substance is considered to be a compound of unstructured matter and superimposed form. But although assembled experience may contain form, it is not limited to this; other types of bound structure can also be experienced (e.g., a particular juxtaposition of two colors). Moreover, structure can largely be experienced on its own—e.g. the perception of a group that transcends the visible fragments it links. Assembled experience may be related to P-consciousness in that it includes the experience of both fragmentary properties and non-local shapes; the difference between the experience of sparse assembled structure and dense fragmentary properties may be related to the proposal that perceptual consciousness overflows cognitive access (Block 2011). Like fragmentary experience, assembled experience can be accompanied by semantic categorization—e.g. identification of animal species (Fei-Fei et al. 2007). In such cases, the combination of raw sensory experience, structure, and semantic attribution might be considered a more 'complete' form of static perception (cf. Prinz 2006).

Meanwhile, given that attentional binding is needed for assembled but not fragmentary experience, the possibility arises of not just one type of inattentional blindness, but *two* (Figure 12.4):

- *Type 1*: a failure of *fragmentary* experience, caused by lack of *gating*.
- *Type 2*: a failure of *assembled* experience, caused by lack of *binding*.

Empirical work suggests that Type 1 occurs only for items less than about 1°, at least when located in the fovea (see Rensink 2013); it may be that gating can be shut down completely only if an item is in a single 'gating zone'. If so, Type 2 would be the only type of inattentional blindness encountered for larger stimuli (e.g. Neisser and Becklen 1975; Simons and Chabris 1999). This may explain the common belief that 'inattentional blindness seems at odds with introspection' (Wolfe 1999): since many tests involve relatively large stimuli, the observer might have inattentional blindness Type 2 while still having a fragmentary experience of the stimulus, since conditions would not be suitable for inattentional blindness Type 1.

12.4.4 *Attentional holding/coherent experience*

In the same way that assembled experience involves static structure, another kind of experience could involve dynamic structure. This would include not only what is contained in fragmentary (and perhaps assembled) experience, but also an impression of *continuity*—of an object or event persisting over time. Such *coherent experience* is similar in some ways to the *object consciousness* proposed on the basis of verbal reports of structure, which likely involve visual short-term memory (Iwasaki 1993). It may also connect to the idea of A-consciousness (Block 1995), provided the latter concept applies to reporting the structure of objects or events that extend over time. Indeed, the apparent difference in capacities between this and fragmentary experience might account for the impression that an observer can report much less than what is experienced in a momentary glance (Block 2011; see Kouider et al. 2010 for a somewhat similar proposal).

Attentional holding appears necessary for the coherent experience of an object (Rensink 2002).[14] Whether it is also *sufficient* depends on what is meant by 'object'. If this refers to the physical object, holding will generally be insufficient: relatively little information can be maintained in coherent form, preventing most properties of a physical object from being represented at any given time. But if 'object' refers to the *representation* of the object (i.e. the corresponding visual object) that is always available for conscious report, then holding would be sufficient (Rensink 2002; see also De Brigard and Prinz 2010). Either way, given the necessity for attentional

[14] In the view proposed here, change blindness—the failure to see change caused by a lack of attentional holding—could be described as 'inattentional blindness Type 3'.

holding (and the complexity of the associated processes), this kind of experience is relatively time-consuming, taking up to 250–300 milliseconds to emerge.

As mentioned in section 12.3.4, two kinds of continuity can be distinguished, based on whether the representation of an object is maintained throughout time, or whether it is recreated and matched with a trace in long-term memory, with differences then noted. These likely form the basis for different kinds of experience: *dynamic change*, where an object is experienced as dynamically transforming, and *completed change*, where the object is simply perceived as having changed at some point (Rensink 2002). The former is encountered in coherent experience; the latter might involve a higher-level feeling of recognition.

Another kind of experience possibly related to these may underlie reports from some observers that they sometimes 'sense' or 'feel' a change in an image without having any clear idea of exactly what or where it is (Rensink 2004). This *sensing* may be a distinct form of awareness involving some of the mechanisms that underlie coherent experience, although it likely also draws upon mechanisms that are different (Busch et al. 2010).

12.4.5 *Attentional individuating/perceptual continuity*

At a subjective level, individuating requires effort, consistent with it involving a form of attention (Scholl 2009). It can also be accompanied by—at least during tracking—an experience of perceptual continuity somewhat similar to that experienced during holding. However, there is no experience here of the structure of the items individuated (e.g. their shape); for example, when an item is tracked, the only relevant property appears to be the position of its center of mass (Scholl et al. 2001).

It is unclear whether attentional individuating is associated with a distinct kind of experience—e.g. a continuity different in some way from that encountered in holding. Because individuating enables more effective control, its effects are likely to be exhibited mostly—if not entirely—via the facilitation of other kinds of attentional process. And if no new kinds of basic control are involved, it may be that no new kinds of conscious visual experience are needed. In any event, further progress on this issue will likely require additional empirical work to separate out the effects of individuating from those of the processes that it facilitates.

12.4.6 *Nonattentional processing/dark structure*

Many visual processes appear to operate in the complete absence of visual experience (see e.g. Dehaene and Changeux 2011). For example, in inattentional blindness Type 1, an unseen item can affect the treatment of a subsequently-presented item that is semantically related to it (Mack and Rock 1998). Likewise, although observers generally fail to visually experience a target presented for an extremely brief duration (15–20 milliseconds), such an unseen item can speed up the identification of a subsequent item related to it (e.g. Naccache et al. 2002).

An important issue concerns the status of such unseen stimuli. One possibility is that their contents are not consciously experienced until some kind of attentional process operates on them; in analogy with 'preattentive', these could be said to be *preconscious* (see, e.g. Dehaene and Changeux 2011). However, there is also the possibility of *dark structure*: representational content (formed reflexively) that can *never* be part of conscious visual experience (Rensink 2013). Dark structure might exist in various parts of the nervous system—e.g. the dorsal stream, which is believed to be exclusively concerned with action (see Goodale and Milner 1992).

An interesting possibility is that conscious experience might participate in the control of dark structure to some extent—e.g. adjusting filter parameters or undoing binding that was created reflexively—with only the controlled aspects of the end results being consciously experienced. In the extreme version of this, conscious visual experience would essentially be a 'control panel' that enables important aspects of fine-grained (and likely sophisticated) control, but does not participate in the bulk of visual processing, which would operate in the dark, as it were (cf. Norretranders 1999). From this point of view, the conscious experience of a property would be inextricably linked with the control of its associated attentional processes. (If control of those processes were not sufficient for that kind of experience, it would imply that other, nonconscious, forms of attentional control also exist.) Various forms of nonattentional processing, meanwhile, could still take place in the background.

12.4.7 Visual attention/visual experience

Bringing together the points above, a pattern begins to emerge in the way that visual attention relates to visual experience (Figure 12.5). First, attentional filtering appears to be necessary for all three kinds of experience, and is the only attentional process needed for fragmentary experience. Next, attentional filtering and binding are necessary for assembled experience, while filtering, holding, and possibly binding are needed for coherent experience. (Because sampling is necessary for

	Filtering	Binding	Holding	Individuating
Coherent	Yes	?	Yes	No
Assembled	Yes	Yes	No	No
Framentary	Yes	No	No	No

Figure 12.5 Dependence of kinds of visual experience on kinds of attentional process. Each rectangle indicates whether the given kind of attentional process necessarily accompanies the given kind of experience. Status is based on data drawn from the sources discussed in section 12.3 and Rensink 2013.

visual perception in general, its status is not discussed in detail here.) As such, the results of experimental work to date seem consistent with a simple principle: *for any kind of conscious experience, a distinct kind of attentional process is necessary* (see also Cohen et al. 2012). Consistent with the alignment thesis, the various kinds of attentional processes appear to form a cascade, with the more complex drawing upon the less complex. If so, this suggests that the different kinds of visual experience might correspond to *grades* that involve increasingly complex levels of structure.

The extent to which each kind of attentional process suffices for visual experience is less clear. Holding may be sufficient for coherent experience, given that its outputs are visual objects (section 12.4.4). And since visual short-term memory is needed to form verbal reports, which are often used as an indicator of conscious processing (see e.g. Dehaene and Changeux 2011), this could account for the proposal that attention—or more precisely, attentional holding—is both necessary and sufficient for conscious experience (De Brigard and Prinz 2010). Meanwhile, filtering can be controlled in the absence of consciously experienced stimuli (Kentridge, et al. 2008), suggesting that while attentional filtering may be necessary for conscious (fragmentary) experience, it is not sufficient. There is also some evidence that binding can occur for unseen stimuli (see Kentridge 2011), although it is unclear whether such binding is attentional or reflexive. More work is needed on these issues.

12.4.8 Co-ordination

Given the various kinds of visual experience posited here, how might these enter into our everyday experience of the world? It may be best to begin by considering how scene perception is believed to work. One proposal involves three systems co-ordinated so that attention—or more precisely, attentional holding—creates the right visual object at the right time; if this process is managed sufficiently well, the result is a *virtual representation* of the scene, which can be treated as if it were coherent everywhere (Rensink 2000a). Such co-ordination can also be applied *within* an object: even though only a small amount of information can be held in coherent form at any time, if this is done for the right part at the right time, the result would effectively be a coherent, detailed representation of the entire object (Rensink 2001). An important consequence of this proposal is the constraint that while any visual representation can be dense (and volatile) or nonvolatile (and sparse), no visual representation can be both dense *and* nonvolatile.[15]

[15] The triadic architecture posited that the representation of dynamic structure in a scene was sparse. It also posited that the representation of static structure—experienced or not—could not be both dense and nonvolatile. But although the existence of change blindness can provide empirical support for assertions about dynamic structure, it was acknowledged that it cannot do so for static structure (e.g. Rensink 2000b: 1475; Rensink 2002: 266). This amounted to a claim that the attentional processes for dynamic structure

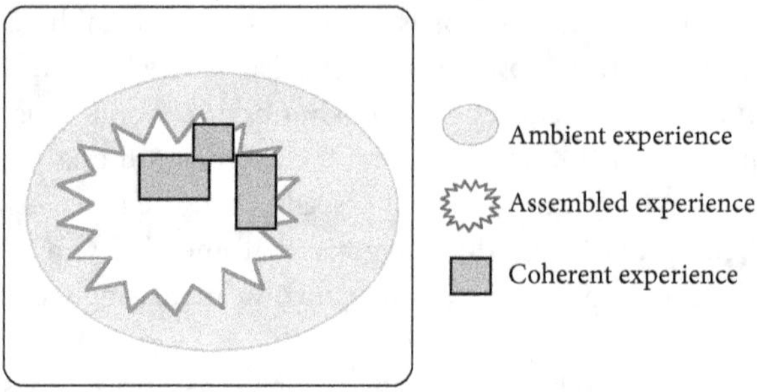

Figure 12.6 Zones of different kinds (grades) of visual experience. This assumes that each kind aligns reasonably closely with the extent of its corresponding attentional processes. The zone of fragmentary experience extends over the area gated by attentional filtering; assembled and coherent experience are located within it. If coherent experience involves bound structure, the zone of coherent experience would likewise exist within the zone of assembled experience.

If several kinds of attentional processes exist, a similar kind of co-ordination might be possible among these, and thus, among the corresponding kinds (or grades) of visual experience. Assuming that each kind of experience aligns reasonably closely with its corresponding attentional processes,[16] their distribution across space would be subject to particular constraints (Figure 12.6). To begin with, a zone of fragmentary experience would correspond to the area of spatial filtering. Given that filtering is necessary for binding and holding, zones of assembled and coherent experience would necessarily be located within the zone of fragmentary experience. Likewise, if attentional binding is needed for holding, the zone of coherent experience would need to be within the zone of assembled experience. Ideally, the intersection of all three zones would align with the center of fixation, so that the information contained within would have maximal resolution. Such an arrangement would allow coherent experience to remain relatively sparse in content and limited to the items held, while concurrently supporting other kinds of (static) experience with greater informational density or extent.[17]

If the appropriate attentional process could be applied to the appropriate part of the input at the appropriate time, it would create a *virtual experience* of all aspects of structure existing everywhere. It is only when such co-ordination breaks down—such as under the demanding conditions encountered in a controlled experiment on

differed in some ways from those for static. As such, it could be seen as the first step in the development of the framework presented here.

[16] Even if an attentional process is necessary for its corresponding kind of experience, it may not be sufficient. As such, there may not be a 1:1 mapping between the spatial distributions of the two.

[17] The extent of fragmentary and assembled experience is an open issue. But given that a large image can be experienced in a fragmentary way when presented briefly, fragmentary experience likely extends over a considerable area, at least when attentional filtering is diffuse.

attentional allocation, or when a brain lesion interferes with control processes—that the separate components of visual experience would become evident.

12.5 Prospects

The relationship between visual experience and visual attention is a complex one. Determining its nature has proven to be a challenge, in terms of both the conceptual issues addressed and the empirical issues faced. This chapter has explored one possible way of handling this challenge: fractionating both attention and visual experience into components, each concerned with a different kind of structure in the world. In this approach, the original issue of how attention relates to visual experience is replaced by a set of simpler issues, each concerned with how a particular kind of attentional process relates to a particular kind of visual experience. As the discussion here has shown, such an approach is not only feasible and helps cast light on the relationship between attention and visual experience, but also raises new issues such as the existence of different kinds of inattentional blindness. As such, it appears to be worth developing further.

Of course, such an attempt is at heart a gamble: nature may simply not be this way. But even if this approach does not succeed entirely, parts may still be helpful. For example, regardless of any connection with visual experience, it may still be useful to characterize 'paying attention' as the co-ordinated control of several processes, each concerned with a particular aspect of structure. And if the particular groupings proposed here do not turn out to capture reality sufficiently well, the principles suggested here as the basis of a taxonomy might still help create an improved classification.

Similar prospects exist for the proposal that conscious visual experience might be fractionated into distinct components (or possibly, grades). If nothing else, this view raises several interesting questions: To what extent is the experience of color the same 'kind' of experience as that of motion? Is the experience of continuity over time 'perceptual' in the same way as the experience of the color blue? Similar considerations apply regarding the extent to which conscious visual experience is a virtual phenomenon: What kinds of co-ordination exist? How might these break down? And even if visual experience does turn out to match our impressions and actually be a unitary phenomenon, there would still be great value in knowing this, and knowing why this should be so.

Acknowledgements

This work was supported by the Natural Sciences and Engineering Research Council of Canada. Many thanks to Paul Coates, Carolyn Dicey Jennings, Minjung Kim, and John Tsotsos for their helpful comments on earlier versions of this chapter. Thanks also to Paul Coates for providing this vision scientist with an opportunity to interact with an interesting group of philosophers; I hope that in return they find something of interest here.

References

Allport, A. (1989), 'Visual Attention', in M. I. Posner (ed.), *Foundations of Cognitive Science* (Cambridge, MA: MIT Press), 631–82.

Allport, A. (1993), 'Attention and Control: Have We Been Asking the Wrong Questions? A Critical Review of Twenty-Five Years', in D. E. Meyer and S. Kornblum (eds), *Attention and Performance XIV: Synergies in Experimental Psychology, Artificial Intelligence, and Cognitive Neuroscience* (Cambridge, MA: MIT Press), 183–218.

Arnheim, R. (1969), *Visual Thinking* (Berkeley, CA: University of California Press), ch. 2.

Baars, B. J. (1988), *A Cognitive Theory of Consciousness* (Cambridge: Cambridge University Press).

Bahrami, B. (2003), 'Object Property Encoding and Change Blindness in Multiple Object Tracking', in *Visual Cognition* 10: 949–63.

Ballard, D. H., Hayhoe, M. M., Pook, P. K., and Rao, R. P. N. (1997), 'Deictic Codes for the Embodiment of Cognition', in *Behavioral and Brain Sciences* 20: 723–67.

Barlow, H. B., and Mollon, J. D. (eds) (1982), *The Senses* (Cambridge: Cambridge University Press).

Bartolomeo, P., and Chokron, S. (2002), 'Orienting of Attention in Left Unilateral Neglect', in *Neuroscience and Biobehavioral Reviews* 26: 217–34.

Bisiach, E. (1993), 'Mental Representation in Unilateral Neglect and Related Disorders: The Twentieth Bartlett Memorial Lecture', in *Quarterly Journal of Experimental Psychology* 46: 435–561.

Block, N. (1995), 'On a Confusion about a Function of Consciousness', in *Behavioral and Brain Sciences* 18: 227–47.

Block, N. (2011), 'Perceptual Consciousness Overflows Cognitive Access', in *Trends in Cognitive Sciences* 15: 567–75.

Bridgeman, B., van der Heijden, A. H. C., and Velichkovsky, B. M. (1994), 'A Theory of Visual Stability across Saccadic Eye Movements', in *Behavioral and Brain Sciences* 17: 247–92.

Braun, J. (1994), 'Visual Search among Items of Different Salience: Removal of Visual Attention Mimics a Lesion in Extrastriate Area V4', in *Journal of Neuroscience* 14: 554–67.

Braun, J., and Sagi, D. (1990), 'Vision outside the Focus of Attention', in *Perception and Psychophysics* 48: 45–58.

Broadbent, D. E. (1982), 'Task Combination and Selective Intake of Information', in *Acta Psychologica* 50: 253–90.

Busch, N. A., Fründ, I., and Hermann, C. S. (2010), 'Electrophysiological Evidence for Different Types of Change Detection and Change Blindness', in *Journal of Cognitive Neuroscience* 22: 1852–69.

Carpenter, R. H. S. (1988), *Movements of the Eyes* (2nd ed.) (London: Pion).

Chong, S. C., and Treisman, A. (2003), 'Representation of Statistical Properties', in *Vision Research* 43: 393–404.

Chun, M. M. (1997), 'Types and Tokens in Visual Processing: A Double Dissociation between the Attentional Blink and Repetition Blindness', in *Journal of Experimental Psychology: Human Perception and Performance* 23: 738–55.

Chun, M. M., Golomb, J. D., and Turk-Browne, N. B. (2011), 'A Taxonomy of External and Internal Attention', in *Annual Review of Psychology* 62: 73–101.

Cohen, M. A., and Dennett, D. C. (2011), 'Consciousness Cannot Be Separated from Function', in *Trends in Cognitive Sciences* 15: 358–64.

Cohen, M. A., Cavanagh, P., Chun, M. M., and Nakayama, K. (2012), 'The Attentional Requirements of Consciousness', in *Trends in Cognitive Sciences* 16: 411–17.

Coslett, H. B., and Saffran, E. M. (1991), 'Simultanagnosia: To See but Not Two See', in *Brain* 114: 1523–45.

Crowne, D. P. (1983), 'The Frontal Eye Field and Attention', in *Psychological Bulletin* 93: 232–60.

De Brigard, F., and Prinz, J. (2010), 'Attention and Consciousness', in *Wiley Interdisciplinary Reviews: Cognitive Science* 1: 51–9.

Dehaene, S. and Changeux, J.-P. (2011), 'Experimental and Theoretical Approaches to Conscious Processing', in *Neuron* 70: 200–27.

Dennett, D. C. (1992), '"Filling in" versus Finding out: A Ubiquitous Confusion in Cognitive Science', in H. L. Pick Jr., P. van den Broek, and D. C. Knill (eds), *Cognition: Conceptual and Methodological Issues* (Washington, DC: American Psychological Association), 33–49.

Driver, J., Davis, G., Russell, C., Turatto, M., and Freeman, E. (2001), 'Segmentation, Attention and Phenomenal Visual Objects', in *Cognition* 80: 61–95.

Farah, M. J. (2004), *Visual Agnosia* (2nd ed.) (Cambridge, MA: MIT Press).

Fei-Fei, L., VanRullen, R., Koch, C., and Perona, P. (2002), 'Rapid Natural Scene Categorization in the Near Absence of Attention', in *Proceedings of the National Academy of Sciences USA* 99: 9596–601.

Fei-Fei, L., Iyer, A., Koch, C., and Perona, P. (2007), 'What Do We Perceive in a Glance of a Real-World Scene?', in *Journal of Vision* 7 10: 1–29.

Franconeri, S. L. (2013), 'The Nature and Status of Visual Resources', in D. Reisberg (ed.), *Oxford Handbook of Cognitive Psychology* (New York: Oxford University Press), 147–62.

Goodale, M. A., and Milner, A. D. (1992), 'Separate Visual Pathways for Perception and Action', in *Trends in Neurosciences* 15: 20–2.

Hatfield, G. (1998), 'Attention in Early Scientific Psychology', in R. D. Wright (ed.), *Visual Attention* (Oxford: Oxford University Press), 3–25.

Henderson, J. M., and Hollingworth, A. (1998), 'Eye Movements during Scene Viewing: An Overview', in G. Underwood (ed.), *Eye Guidance in Reading and Scene Perception* (Oxford: Elsevier), 269–93.

Itti, L., Rees, G., and Tsotsos, J. K. (2005), *The Neurobiology of Attention* (Burlington, MA: Academic).

Iwasaki, S. (1993), 'Spatial Attention and Two Modes of Consciousness', *Cognition* 49: 211–33.

Jennings, C. D. (2012), 'The Subject of Attention', in *Synthese* 189: 535–54.

Jensen, M. S., Yao, R., Street, W. N., Simons, D. J. (2011), 'Change blindness and inattentional blindness', in *Wiley Interdisciplinary Reviews: Cognitive Science* 2: 529–46.

Juan, C.-H., Shorter-Jacobi, S. M., and Schall, J. (2004), 'Dissociation of Spatial Attention and Saccade Preparation', in *Proceedings of the National Academy of Sciences USA* 101: 15541–4.

Kahneman, D., Treisman, A., and Gibbs, B. J. (1992), 'The Reviewing of Object Files: Object-Specific Integration of Information', in *Cognitive Psychology* 24: 175–219.

Kanwisher, N., Yin, C., and Wojciulik, E. (1999), 'Repetition Blindness for Pictures: Evidence for the Rapid Computation of Abstract Visual Descriptions', in V. Coltheart (ed.), *Fleeting Memories: Cognition of Brief Visual Stimuli* (Cambridge, MA: MIT Press), 119–50.

Kentridge, R. W. (2011), 'Attention without Awareness: A Brief Review', in C. Mole, D. Smithies, and W. Wu (eds), *Attention: Philosophical and Psychological Essays* (Oxford: University Press), 228–46.

Kentridge, R. W., Nijboer, T. C. W., and Heywood, C. A. (2008), 'Attended but Unseen: Visual Attention Is Not Sufficient for Visual Awareness', in *Neuropsychologia* 46: 864–9.

Koch, C., and Tsuchiya, N. (2007), 'Attention and Consciousness: Two Distinct Brain Processes', in *Trends in Cognitive Sciences* 11: 16–22.

Kouider, S., de Gardelle, V., Sackur, J., and Dupoux, E. (2010), 'How Rich Is Consciousness? The Partial Awareness Hypothesis', in *Trends in Cognitive Sciences* 14: 301–7.

Krauzlis, R. J. (2005), 'The Control of Voluntary Eye Movements: New Perspectives', in *Neuroscientist* 11: 124–37.

Lamme, V. A. F. (2003), 'Why Visual Attention and Awareness Are Different', in *Trends in Cognitive Sciences* 7: 12–18.

Lavie, N. (1995), 'Perceptual Load as a Necessary Condition for Selective Attention', in *Journal of Experimental Psychology: Human Perception and Performance* 21: 451–68.

Libet, B. (1985), 'Unconscious Cerebral Initiative and the Role of Conscious Will in Voluntary Action', in *Behavioral and Brain Sciences* 8: 529–66.

Loschky, L. C., and Larson, A. M. (2009), 'The Natural/Man-Made Distinction Is Made before Basic-Level Distinctions in Scene Gist Processing', in *Visual Cognition* 18: 513–36.

Mack, A. and Rock, I. (1998), *Inattentional Blindness* (Cambridge, MA: MIT Press).

Maddox, W. T., Ashby, F. G., and Waldron, E. M. (2002), 'Multiple Attention Systems in Perceptual Categorization', in *Memory and Cognition* 30: 325–9.

Marr, D. (1982), *Vision: A Computational Investigation into the Human Representation and Processing of Visual Information* (San Francisco, CA: W. H. Freeman), 8–38.

Naccache, L., Blandin, E., and Dehaene, S. (2002), 'Unconscious Masked Priming Depends on Temporal Attention', in *Psychological Science* 13: 416–24.

Navon, D. (1984), 'Resources: A Theoretical Soup Stone?', in *Psychological Review* 91: 216–34.

Neisser, U., and Becklen, R. (1975), 'Selective Looking: Attending to Visually Significant Events', in *Cognitive Psychology* 7: 480–94.

Norretranders, T. (1999), *The User Illusion: Cutting Consciousness Down to Size* (New York: Penguin Books).

O'Regan, J. K., and Noë, A. (2001), 'A Sensorimotor Account of Vision and Visual Consciousness', in *Behavioral and Brain Sciences* 24: 939–73.

Pashler, H. E. (1999), *The Psychology of Attention* (Cambridge, MA: MIT Press).

Pessoa, L., Thompson, L., and Noë, A. (1998), 'Finding out about Filling in: A Guide to Perceptual Completion for Visual Science and the Philosophy of Perception', in *Behavioral and Brain Sciences* 21: 723–802.

Posner, M. I., Walker, J. A., Friedrich, F. J., and Rafal, R. D. (1984), 'Effects of Parietal Injury on Covert Orienting of Attention', in *Journal of Neuroscience* 4: 1863–74.

Prinz, J. J. (2006), 'Beyond Appearances: The Content of Sensation and Perception', in T. S. Gendler and J. Hawthorne (eds), *Perceptual Experience* (Oxford: Oxford University Press), 434–60.

Pylyshyn, Z. W. (2003), *Seeing and Visualizing: It's Not What You Think* (Cambridge, MA: MIT Press), 201–79.

Ramachandran, V. S. (1992), 'Filling in Gaps in Perception: Part I', in *Current Directions in Psychological Science* 1: 199–205.

Rayner, K., Smith, T. J., Malcolm, G. L., and Henderson, J. M. (2009), 'Eye Movements and Visual Encoding during Scene Perception', in *Psychological Science* 20: 6–10.

Rensink R. A. (2000a), 'The Dynamic Representation of Scenes', in *Visual Cognition* 7: 17–42.

Rensink, R. A. (2000b), 'Seeing, Sensing, and Scrutinizing', in *Vision Research* 40: 1469–87.

Rensink, R. A. (2001), 'Change Blindness: Implications for the Nature of Attention', in M. R. Jenkin and L. R. Harris (eds), *Vision and Attention* (New York: Springer), 169–88.

Rensink, R. A. (2002), 'Change Detection', in *Annual Review of Psychology* 53: 245–77.

Rensink, R. A. (2004), 'Visual Sensing without Seeing', in *Psychological Science* 15: 27–32.

Rensink, R. A. (2009), 'Attention: Change Blindness and Inattentional Blindness', in W. Banks (ed.), *Encyclopedia of Consciousness* (New York: Elsevier), Vol. 1, 47–59.

Rensink, R. A. (2010), 'Seeing seeing', in *Psyche* 16: 68–78.

Rensink, R. A. (2013), 'Perception and Attention', in D. Reisberg (ed.), *Oxford Handbook of Cognitive Psychology* (New York: Oxford University Press), 97–116.

Rensink, R. A., and Enns, J. T. (1995), 'Preemption Effects in Visual Search: Evidence for Low-Level Grouping', in *Psychological Review* 102: 101–30.

Riddoch, M. J., and Humphreys, G. W. (1987), 'A Case of Integrative Visual Agnosia', in *Brain* 110: 1431–62.

Robertson, L. C. and Kim, M.-S. (1999), 'Effects of Perceived Space on Spatial Attention', in *Psychological Science* 10: 76–9.

Scholl, B. J. (2009), 'What Have We Learned about Attention from Multiple-Object Tracking (and Vice Versa)?', in D. Dedrick and L. Trick (eds), *Computation, Cognition, and Pylyshyn* (Cambridge, MA: MIT Press), 49–77.

Scholl, B. J., Pylyshyn, Z. W., and Feldman, J. (2001), 'What Is a Visual Object? Evidence from Target Merging in Multiple-Object Tracking', in *Cognition* 80: 159–77.

Simons, D. J., and Chabris, C. F. (1999), 'Gorillas in Our Midst: Sustained Inattentional Blindness for Dynamic Events', in *Perception* 28: 1059–74.

Sperling, G., and Dosher, B. A. (1986), 'Strategy and Optimization in Human Information Processing', in K. R. Boff, L. Kaufman, and J. P. Thomas (eds), *Handbook of Perception and Human Performance* (New York: Wiley), Vol. 1, 1–65.

Thorpe, S., Fize, D., and Marlot, C. (1996), 'Speed of Processing in the Human Visual System', in *Nature* 381: 520–2.

Treisman, A. M. (1969), 'Strategies and Models of Selective Attention', in *Psychological Review* 76: 282–99.

Treisman, A. M., and Gelade, G. (1980), 'A Feature-Integration Theory of Attention', in *Cognitive Psychology* 12: 97–136.

Tsotsos, J. K. (2011), *A Computational Perspective on Visual Attention* (Cambridge, MA: MIT Press).

Ullman, S. (1984), 'Visual Routines', in *Cognition* 18: 97–159.

VanRullen, R., Reddy, L., and Koch, C. (2004), 'Visual Search and Dual Tasks Reveal Two Distinct Attentional Resources', in *Journal of Cognitive Neuroscience* 16: 4–14.

Wolfe, J. M. (1999), 'Inattentional Amnesia', in V. Coltheart (ed.), *Fleeting Memories: Cognition of Brief Visual Stimuli* (Cambridge, MA: MIT Press), 71–94.

Wright, R. D. (ed.) (1998), *Visual Attention* (Oxford: Oxford University Press).

13

Can Sounds Be Red? A New Account of Synaesthesia as Enriched Experience

Ophelia Deroy

13.1 Introduction

Synaesthesia is often presented as a condition where people have 'a conscious experience of systematically induced sensory attributes that are not experienced by most people under comparable conditions' (Grossenbacher and Lovelace 2001: 36) or where 'experiences in one domain evoke additional experiences in another' (Marks and Mulvenna 2013: 1).

The label accounts for a series of strange cases where certain individuals report for instance seeing colours when hearing musical notes, or when seeing black letters on a page. These individuals do not present any other overt cognitive or perceptual deficit nor do they seem to make up their reports. The term 'synaesthesia' was introduced, after various other suggestions ('pseudoaesthesia', 'chromaesthesia') to distinguish this surprising accretion of experiences from systematic hallucinations (usually accompanied by cognitive and/or perceptual deficits) and false reports (the target individuals insisted they really perceived these extra-colours, and they were indeed much more consistent in their reports than one would expect from someone trying to make up a story or remember associations between, say, colours and sounds).

The name was later extended to other individuals having flavour experiences when seeing certain proper names, or feeling shapes in their hand when they eat—all sorts of unusual types of experiences which are not shared by the rest of us. The specific tokens of these strange experiences are also not shared among individuals who share the same kind of synaesthesia, as they have different additional experiences when presented with the same inducers. In other words synaesthesia is an idiosyncratic way of experiencing the world which puts individuals on 'private islands'.[1] But what sort of islands exactly?

[1] Duffy (2001: 5).

The reply given here can sound disappointing: the private synaesthetic islands are not just experiences that we cannot have, but also experiences that we cannot imagine having. It is the ignorance or rejection of this second fact—that they are human experiences that we cannot imaginatively reconstruct, and in this sense, share—which misleads researchers and philosophers dealing with synaesthesia.

Most often, the startling and private sensory blendings experienced by synaesthetes have been analyzed into experiences that are easier for us to imagine. They are presented as the juxtaposition or binding of two contents of experience that we can independently have and easily imaginatively associate. The experience of coloured-grapheme or coloured-hearing synaesthetes for instance is taken to look like seeing a black letter surrounded with a coloured halo, or a green after-image co-occurring with the sound of Middle C.

Something is wrong with this way of proceeding. If we constrain *a priori* the definition and study of a certain condition by the capacity we have to figure out or imaginatively reconstruct 'what it is like' to have this condition, we are performing a thought-experiment, rather than looking at an empirical challenge. We need to seriously consider the hypothesis that synaesthetic experiences are not experiences we could have, as non-synaesthetes, including through imagination. Synaesthetes might have experiences of coloured sounds, or letters that are both red and black, somehow, at the same time, while we cannot. We can only make sense of their experiences theoretically and from the outside.

The present chapter starts with a general description of synaesthetic experiences, and of the ways they have been scientifically approached (section 13.2). It then critically examines the dominant interpretation of synaesthesia as the joint experience of a normal and an atypical sensory content (section 13.3) and shows that there is no good reason to accept this as the only or best capture of the condition. Synaesthesia can—and I argue, should—be defined as cases where individuals enjoy a single, richer experience (section 13.4) which might be hard for us to imagine. The account makes more sense of both the synaesthetic reports and the empirical evidence; it also opens new ways to look at the perceptual status of synaesthetic experiences—including when they concern strange contents such as 'green sounds' and black letters which are also red.

13.2 Synaesthetic Experiences

Synaesthetic experiences are triggered by a large variety of objects, called '*inducers*', ranging from musical notes, linguistic items, flavours, tactile sensations—or even sport and orgasms. The mere presence of the inducer is not sufficient to trigger a synaesthetic experience, and it is most likely that the object needs to be at least attended.[2] Besides the neurotypical experience usually reported by

[2] In some rare cases, synaesthesia can be elicited by merely thinking or imagining a certain object (Dixon et al. 2000), but most known cases require the inducing object to be actually present in the

Table 13.1 Synaesthetic concurrents reported by D., a colour-hearing synaesthete (from Ortmann 1933). The two columns represent responses given ten years apart.

Inducer	Concurrent	Inducer	Concurrent
C	dirty red; black and red	C	dirty red
C#	no real colour; hint of green	C#	green and red
D	green, very dirty, almost black	D	green, rather dark
D#	green, so dirty	D#	a yellow-green
E	no real colour, dirty orange	E	yellow
F	no colour; dirty orange	F	orange
F#	orange and blue, dark	F#	orange and blue, deep
G	dirty blue	G	blue
G#	a blue-violet	G#	a blue-violet
A	dark purple	A	a purple, pretty
A#	dark brown	A#	a purple and brown, pretty

non-synaesthetes, synaesthetes experience a supplementary conscious component in a non-stimulated stream (e.g. colour). This extra component does not eclipse the typical experience and is experienced at the same time—the reason why it is known as a '*concurrent*'. Although it is most often visual, the concurrent can also be reported as tactile, gustatory, or auditory.

The terms 'inducers' and 'concurrents' are very useful as they can be used as terms of art. They were coined to refer, on the one hand, to the stimulus that elicits the reports, leaving it open where exactly in the processing of that stimulus synaesthesia gets grafted and how it becomes to be so grafted, and on the other hand, to the strange aspect of experience that synaesthetes would report. An illustration, coming from an exhaustive case study done by Ortmann (1933), is shown in Table 13.1. Ortmann played the same notes to D., a coloured-hearing synaesthete, on various occasions and recorded her colour responses ten years apart.

A legitimate concern when seeing such a list of inducers-concurrents is to know whether the concurrent is genuinely experienced—or simply evoked by association. The French poet Rimbaud, who wrote a famous poem on the colours of vowels, admitted making them up while writing.[3] He was certainly not a synaesthete. A robust way to test whether concurrents are consciously experienced relies not on subjective reports, but on testing people at different times or through large random series of inducers. Presumably, a person who can give the very same list of

environment. The mere presence of the trigger is however not sufficient, and there is now good evidence that it must be attended (e.g. Palmeri et al. 2002; Sagiv et al. 2006; Smilek et al. 2001). In other terms, there will be no pop-out effect or attention-capture, as previously claimed.

[3] See Harrison (2001).

concurrents after months or in large sets cannot do it only by memory. Her replies must therefore be based on conscious experiences.

Other evidence besides the consistency test now converges in establishing the veracity of synaesthetic reports, both at a behavioural and neurological level. At a behavioural level, the synaesthetic concurrent is shown to interfere with perceptual identification: for instance, if a colour-grapheme synaesthete for whom the letter B elicits a green concurrent is presented with a green B and a red B, she will be faster at naming the colour of the green B (which is consistent with her concurrent) than the second (whose colour clashes with her concurrent). Similar adaptations of the Stroop interference task are used for all sorts of synaesthesia: if a synaesthete feels a tactile concurrent on the left cheek while looking at certain objects, and is really touched on the cheek while this occurs, she will be faster at saying that she is (really) touched on the left cheek than on the right one.[4] Neurological evidence then shows unusual patterns of activation in synaesthetes—due to hyperconnectivity in the synaesthetic brain or eventually to neuronal hyperactivity.[5] More importantly, although cases vary and data need to be handled cautiously, many, but not all coloured-grapheme synaesthetes show, for instance, activation in V4 (the colour area) when presented with black graphemes suggesting that the synaesthetic experience can be due to other projections in the visual cortex.

Many researchers assume then that synaesthetic experiences are genuine cases of perception: they are triggered by physical objects and co-vary systematically with differences in the properties of these objects. Turning to the empirical literature especially, synaesthesia is often defined as cases where the 'stimulation of one sensory modality automatically triggers *a perception* in a second modality, in the absence of any direct stimulation to this second modality',[6] or the 'stimulation of one sensory modality reliably caus(ing) *a perception* in one or more different senses' or as an 'anomalous *sensory perception*'.[7] Yet this idea is immediately counterbalanced by the equally strong intuition that synaesthetic cases cannot really be counted as perception: perceiving p carries the assumption that p is real, and one cannot genuinely perceive green sounds, because sounds do not really have colours.

The classification of synaesthesia as perception has led to intense debates: Although they are caused by the presence of independent objects and co-vary with some of their properties, synaesthetic states do not seem to be capable of accurately representing properties of these objects. The way they represent the world is false: if Middle C is systematically represented as green, or if the synaesthete always

[4] See Mills (1999); Banissy et al. (2009). This said, Stroop interference might be a semantic interference in the 'naming' process. It mainly provides additional support to the idea that the concurrent is actually experienced, and shows that it is processed involuntarily (i.e. it is not modulated by strategic, top-down influences). See Auvray and Deroy (2014) for a discussion.

[5] See Rouw et al. (2011) for a review; see also Terhune et al. (2011).

[6] Harrison and Baron-Cohen (1997: 3), my emphasis.

[7] Respectively in Cytowic (1997) and Asher et al. (2009) emphasis my own.

represents the presence of greenness when Middle C occurs, this can never be a case of veridical perception as Middle C has no colour (nor does it possess any of the physical properties on which colour usually supervenes). Because synaesthetes systematically misrepresent certain objects, they have to be subjects to a hallucination,[8] an illusion,[9] or what Casey O'Callaghan suggests we call 'property hallucination'.[10]

Given this agreed inaccuracy of the green concurrent, many have wondered whether synaesthesia does not raise a challenge to representational theories of perceptual experience,[11] at least to some of the strong or externalist versions held for instance by Dretske or Tye where the phenomenal character of an experience has to be identical with or supervenes on the external object.[12] If the external object has no colour, the synaesthetic experience of colour cannot be identical with or supervene on the object.

At the moment, the only way to reconcile the idea that synaesthetic states are perceptual, despite the inaccuracy of the synaesthetically represented property, seems to involve accepting some disjunctive content of experience, where the representation of green, for instance, is true in case there is either a green-looking surface *or* Middle C in the environment. Spelled out in this way, both the synaesthete's experience of green when she hears Middle C and when she looks at grass are true, as they each satisfy one of the disjuncts in the accuracy conditions. However, a disjunctive account of perceptual contents looks like a costly solution, if it is supposed to apply to all the other experiences: every (typical, or non-synaesthetic) perceptual experience of a certain object O could have an endless number of disjunctive accuracy conditions, only a disjunct of which would ever be satisfied.

The details of these debates is not what matters for my present purpose, and not just because they are already discussed elsewhere. What they show is that the characterization of synaesthesia as a misrepresentation creates problems for otherwise robust theories of experience and perception—and can only be fixed at a high cost for these theories.

13.3 Dual Accounts of Synaesthesia

The difficulty of deciding on whether synaesthesia should count as a perception or not might come from the key claims—often assumptions—on which the debates are based:

The similarity claim: As the concurrent experienced in the synaesthetic case is reported using terms that are similar to the ones used for non-synaesthetic experiences, this means that the synaesthete is having an experience with the same character and content in both cases.

[8] E.g. like after-images, see Lycan (2006). [9] E.g. Gray (2001).

[10] O'Callaghan (forthcoming). According to Brogaard (2014), some cases of synaesthesia should count as a specific kind of 'visual seemings'.

[11] Gray (2001); Macpherson (2007); Sollberger (2012); Wager (1999, 2001).

[12] Dretske (1995); Tye (2000, 2002).

For instance, if a synaesthete uses the term 'green' to report on her experience both when looking at a green patch and when hearing Middle C, the idea is that she is in a similar (or overlapping) mental state in both cases, i.e. the state of having an experience of green. In both cases, she is in a mental state with the same character and content.

The separability claim: During the synaesthetic episode, a synaesthete experiences two separable experiences, each with their distinct character and content. The first corresponds to the experience of the inducer and its properties, and the other to the experience of a synaesthetic concurrent.

For instance, when a synaesthete hears Middle C, she is supposed to have two joint experiences, each with a distinct character and content, i.e. of Middle C and of the green concurrent.

Most accounts simply assume the similarity and the separability claims, and form the dominant 'dual accounts' of synaesthesia',[13] as we have called them elsewhere. Synaesthetic experiences are treated as a conjunction of two distinct experiences: one, sometimes labelled the 'synaesthetic experience' per se, would be enjoyed by the synaesthete only, whereas the other would be common or shared by synaesthetes and non-synaesthetes alike. MacPherson (2007), for instance, refers to an 'additional experience' joined to the otherwise normal experience common to us all. Psychologists also endorse this interpretation, saying for instance that in synaesthesia, 'stimulation of a sense ... triggers a *second* perception not normally associated with the stimulus'.[14]

Similarity and separability are distinct claims, but, as I said, they are often simply assumed and go hand in hand in the dual accounts. Similarity leads to the assumption that the experience of green in a coloured-hearing synaesthetic case resembles a classical visual experience of a green patch. It also leads therefore to the view that this green patch needs to be distinct from the rest of the auditory experience: how could a colour be part of the auditory experience? The synaesthete must have both a visual and an auditory experience at the same time.

In the most immediate interpretation of the separability claim, a synaesthetic experience can then be analysed as the experience of two separate objects:

The separate object claim: When a synaesthete hears Middle C, she experiences two objects that are really distinct, i.e. Middle C and a green patch (sometimes called 'photism').

'Really distinct' means that each element could be experienced by itself. In the case of synaesthesia, it means that the synaesthetic concurrent could be the object of a separate experience (a coloured photism experienced in one part of one's visual field, for instance). It just so happens that this experience is phenomenally co-present with the experience of the inducer, and the experiences of two separate objects unified in consciousness (e.g. Bayne and Chalmers 2003).

[13] Auvray and Deroy (2014). [14] Novich et al. (2011), emphasis is mine.

The separate object claim is quite intuitive when it comes to crossmodal cases: it is natural to think about a colour being distinct from a sound, and to interpret it as the object of a distinct experience (i.e. something that could possibly be experienced on its own).

However, another interpretation is possible, especially when it comes to intramodal cases, like coloured-graphemes. In those cases, for instance, the extra colour (such as red) is interpreted as being another distinct synaesthetic feature (e.g. a second colour, or a superimposed one) bound to the other features of the letter seen on the page. The separate feature claim is also strongly encouraged by accounts of synaesthesia in terms of binding—a concept which is used to explain how features are experienced as bound to a single object:[15]

The separate feature claim: When a synaesthete sees a letter A printed in black on a page, she experiences this letter with two distinct features, i.e. a real colour and a synaesthetic colour like red.

According to this interpretation, the synaesthetic red is experienced as a feature of the letter, or as belonging to the letter. In other words, the synaesthetic colour and the other visual properties of the printed letter share more than co-presence or phenomenal unity: they are also bound according to a form of object unity (see Bayne and Chalmers 2003; Deroy 2014a for discussion).

The feature account is not then committed to the idea that the synaesthetic addition and the inducer are such that they could be experienced separately: perhaps the synaesthetic colour cannot be experienced by itself, but can still be defined independently of other parts of the experience. A comparison with shape and colour can here be useful: one cannot experience shape without colour, but a shape can be defined independently of colour. We can define what a circle is without mentioning its colour. This is because shape can be defined relative to objective properties that do not intervene in the definition of colour, and vice versa. The same, in turn, applies in the separate feature claim: it might not be possible to have an experience of the synaesthetic feature independently of other features, but we can still define the inducer independently of the other features.

There are interesting differences between these two interpretations of the separability claim, as we shall see later. They still converge on the idea that the synaesthetic concurrent enjoys a form of independence. This core of the separability claim is driving most the current debates on synaesthesia,[16] together with the similarity claim.

[15] On accounts of synaesthesia evoking binding, see Mattingley et al. (2001); Mulvenna and Walsh (2006); on binding in general, see for instance Treisman (1996).

[16] See Wager (2001) for an exception. Wager's criticism of the separability claim remains, however, vague and based mostly on (not so robust) subjective reports of synaesthetes insisting that the concurrent is strongly connected to the experience of the inducer.

However, I want to suggest that its intuitive appeal rests on an initial confusion and weak arguments.

13.4 The Grounds for Dual Accounts

13.4.1 A method-content confusion

Going back to the first description of synaesthetic experiences, it is important to stress that the distinction between inducers and concurrents is first and foremost a methodological one: inducers correspond to the external stimuli on which experimenters have control, while concurrents correspond to what they ask the participants to report on. Synaesthetes, like D. in Ortmann's paper (see Table 13.1) are asked to report on a specific variation in their experience, like colour or tactile variations. Sometimes they are asked to select a visually experienced coloured patch on a screen that best matches their concurrent. In all cases, they are rarely asked or tested on the experience which corresponds to the inducer—which is then methodologically left out of the test.

It is, however, important that nothing in this method implies that the concurrent is distinct from the rest of the experienced content, be it like a distinct object or a distinct feature. The ability to report on a specific character of experience does not entail that what is reported enjoys a form of separability. In other words, the proper analysis of the experience *does not follow* from the way it gets tested and reported through the inducer/concurrent methodological tools.

Going one step further, the method of testing for inducer-concurrent is perfectly consistent with the non-separability of the concurrent. That is, it does not entail that the 'extra' reported by synaesthetes has the status of a distinct object or feature in the sense defined by the separability claim. The intuitive appeal of one interpretation is not sufficient to establish it as the right one. We need then better arguments in favour of this separability, and most of them, it seems, are found in the spatial display of the synaesthetic experiences.

13.4.2 The localization argument for object separability

An important argument for the separability of the synaesthetic concurrent comes from reports and studies suggesting that the concurrent can (at least for some synaesthetes, or in some circumstances) have a distinct localization. Although some synaesthetes report that their concurrent is not localized,[17] a majority say it is 'internal' or that they experience it 'in the mind's eye'. Only a few consider it is externalized (more on them later).

The majority of synaesthetes are not clear about where exactly the concurrent occurs when they talk about the 'mind's eye' but they seem to agree that that the

[17] Edquist et al. (2006).

concurrent occupies a distinct location from the other contents of experience. Now, if two things are differently located in space, then they are (possibly) distinct objects of experience—as they can be spatially segregated.[18] This claim, in turn, feeds the object separability claim.

However, more reliable information on the spatial aspects of the concurrent can be gathered from psychophysical studies than from subjective reports. Notice that the Stroop interference paradigm, used in most studies of synaesthesia, is closer to a co-location idea (as the colour words and the actual colours are experienced at the same place in Stroop tasks) than to the separation one. Besides Stroop interferences, three other series of tests have shown interferences in perceptual tasks. Real background colours make it more difficult for the synaesthete to identify a letter whose extra-colour matches the background: if Bs are green for the individual, then it will take him longer to distinguish the letter B, printed in black, on a green background than on a yellow or blue background.[19] This shows that the 'greenness' surrounding the letter actually spreads from the edges of the B into the background—and is not just located outside the letter. Two well-known grouping phenomena in which real colours influence grouping over time (as evidenced in apparent motion) or over space (as evidenced by global dominance in binocular rivalry) have also been found in synaesthetes.[20]

What this shows is that the synaesthetic concurrent is available in experience more or less at the same locus of attention as the experienced inducer. This goes against the argument for its spatial independence or separability. It is much more compatible with the claim that the synaesthetic concurrent is not spatially independent from the inducer—which is a rather controversial claim. I want to insist that it still makes better sense of the empirical evidence. The problem might be that it does not make sense of the subjective reports, which suggest a distinct location.

Do we need then to accuse the majority of synaesthetes of being confused about what their experience is? Isn't experience supposed to be transparent? Surely, one would think that they should be able to say whether the synaesthetic concurrent occurs at the same location as the inducer or not.

I think we can address this worry without accusing synaesthetes of being systematically confused in their reports. The first thing to note is that synaesthetes are quite diverse in their spontaneous reports—and the 'mind's eye' expression is one which is often suggested to them by experimenters or that they know through their knowledge of the experimental literature on synaesthesia. This might be the label they reach for when interrogated, but this might not perfectly capture their experience. Besides the

[18] It is possible that two spatial parts of the visual scene are experienced as parts of the same object—for instance as the head and the neck of a person. This said, the distinct spatial existence of these two parts means that each of them could figure as a content of a visual experience on its own, e.g. one could have the experience of a neck and a separate experience of a face.

[19] Smilek et al. (2001).

[20] Kim et al. (2006); Palmeri et al. (2002).

variety of claims, synaesthetes often report having difficulties putting their experiences into words. One should therefore not doubt the overall sincerity of synaesthetes when they try to give a linguistic capture of their experiences, but this does not mean accepting each single sentence as a true capture. Reports are also neither straightforwardly *believed* nor internally consistent. As an illustration, this is the way a colour-grapheme synaesthete describes her synaesthetic experience:

> My idea of an object . . . any object . . . has, maybe, a list of all possible features this object could have. You know, like if I were to give you a list of features that a chair would have . . . you know, four legs, a back, a seat . . . But there are these things . . . there are those chairs that you kind of kneel on, you have your butt on something . . . So, when I think of . . . when I think of The Chair Itself, to put it in Platonic terms, it's kind of an overlay of all of these different things. And some things are optional, and some things are not so optional. So it's the same way with my letters . . . you know, a colour is optional; a letter certainly doesn't *have* to have a colour . . . but that's just the way my letters are.
>
> (Karen, MIT synesthesia website, <http://web.mit.edu/synesthesia/www/karen.html>)

Going back to the question of localization, studies have also shown that synaesthetes are not consistent in their reports about the spatial location of the concurrent,[21] and do not show strong behavioural differences in the test, despite differences in their reports. They might also use the 'mind's eye' expression to express a different feature of the synaesthetic addition—something perhaps of the falsity or private character that they seem to realize. The number of 'mind's eye' reports is therefore not an objection to the conclusion drawn from experimental studies that the concurrent and inducer are experienced at the same locus of attention.

Does this turn all synaesthetes into so-called 'projectors'? The term 'projector' is a term of art, coined by experimenters to distinguish some synaesthetes who would insist that they experienced the concurrent as being localized in the real world, for instance on the page, where the letter is. They are, however, still capable of experiencing the real colour of the letter, for instance black. I don't want to dwell too much on the terminological distinction between projectors and the majority of associators or 'mind eye' synaesthetes. Although they nourish most of the philosophical literature, the status of projectors is still controversial. The advantage in visual search supposed to distinguish cases of reported projectors from others (i.e. 'associators') have not yet been robustly established. In larger studies, projectors do not show any behavioural difference compared to other 'associator' colour-grapheme synaesthetes.

A more serious objection to the lack of spatial separability comes from crossmodal cases. How could a colour be localized where the sound is (the localization of sound being a tricky question in itself)? It can even become problematic for colour-grapheme

[21] E.g. Edquist et al. (2006), Hupe et al. (2011), Ward et al. (2010).

cases: can synaesthetes experience the synaesthetic red and the real black exactly at the same place, at the same time? Wouldn't this be a great example of contradictory content of experience that philosophers argue about?[22]

There is however, as I want to argue, a possibility of making sense of the lack of spatial separability. Notice also that I am talking here of a lack of separability in experience—which is not the same thing as a clear experience of a precise shared location, nor as the impossibility of re-establishing a separation at the level of thought (just because the concepts used by individuals or the beliefs they hold lead them to think about two distinct objects).

The account I am proposing is that the concurrent might have only a strictly derivative spatial content in the overall experience. To understand what a derivative spatial content is, the easiest is to consider examples of multisensory interactions where certain perceptual contents 'borrow' the locations of others. For instance, in ventriloquist cases, the location of sounds is captured by the location of visual movements (think about the cinema when you experience sounds as coming from the mouth of the actors on the screen, when they actually come from around you). Now, in ventriloquist cases, sounds have their own spatial content: it just happens to be dominated by other (visual) spatial contents in certain situations of multisensory perception. If you close your eyes in the cinema, the sounds recover their proper spatial localization (i.e. they come from all around you or behind you, for instance). However, different cases of derivative spatial content exist in other modalities. For instance, in flavour perception, the retronasal smells (or aromas) which contribute to our overall experience of the foods we ingest are not ascribed to a proper spatial localization. Only orthonasal smells, experienced when we sniff a perfume, for instance, are localized 'out there'—and this is largely because of sniffing. No such information is coming from cases where a food is ingested and lets off aromas that are processed via retronasal olfaction.[23] Aromas do not then have their own spatial localization and yet get localized at the same place as tastants (i.e. on the tongue) as they come to contribute to flavour experiences.

The retronasal olfactory contribution to flavour perception can be thought as contributing an additional aspect to the overall flavour experience which is localized in the mouth[24]—but cannot be a separable object, experienced in its own location. As far as space is required to be a separable object of experience, it can be claimed that what we call retronasal aromas can never be experienced independently as separable objects of experience, although they happen to be 'somewhere' during flavour experiences. A similar claim can apply to synaesthetic concurrents:

[22] E.g. Crane (1988a and 1988b), Mellor (1988).

[23] Complexities regarding the role of the trigeminal components of odours in lateralization complement the picture, but fall beyond the scope of the present chapter.

[24] The same line can perhaps be applied for certain bodily feelings like tiredness, for instance, or nausea which, although they lack proper localization, inherit one from other sensory cues.

concurrents only borrow the spatial content of another experience. Synaesthetic concurrents have only a derivative spatial content, but no possibility of a separate spatial content that could warrant them the status of distinct objects.

13.4.3 The discriminability argument

A more general argument for the separability claim comes from the fact that synaesthetes are able to distinguish the concurrent from the rest of the experience. As Richard Gray (2001) puts it, in response to Wager's suggestion that the concurrent is not separate from the rest of the experience, 'synaesthetes are typically able to discriminate the colours they experience from the phenomenal character of the sounds they experience. It is, after all, for this reason they believe that they are undergoing unusual experiences.' The discriminability argument can come in support of either the object or feature separability claim, but I think it is better to focus on the latter—as we have now excluded the idea of two spatially distinct objects.

Let's start by noting that it is true that synaesthetic reports overall show that synaesthetes are able to discriminate their concurrent and report selectively on it when passing tests, for instance. However, discrimination is not a sign that a distinct feature is at stake. Brightness is for instance not experienced as a distinct feature of the object: it is experienced as a characteristic or dimension of an experienced feature. We often use perceptual reports like 'this sound is high-pitched', or 'this colour is bright'. It does not follow from the fact that we can report on these specific aspects of our experiences that we perceive brightness as a feature of coloured objects—analogous to shape, colour, etc. *Dimensions* are those subjective aspects of experience which constitute a feature, and explain the variations between different instances of this feature: for instance, hue and brightness are sets of values by which colours look different or similar.

Both dimensions like hue and brightness and features like shape/extension and colour fall short of being objects of experiences on their own, but there is an important difference between dimensions and features. As mentioned earlier, features can be conceptually distinguished: their definition does not need to refer to a common element. Conceptual distinction, as defined previously, means exactly this: that the definitions of a feature x and of a feature y are independent from one another. The definition of shape does not need to mention colour. By contrast, the definition of dimensions still draws on the fact that they capture all of the subjective variations of the same feature. Brightness is what can vary if you keep hue and saturation fixed, considering the same colour (more on this later).

Another illustration of the difference between dimensions and features comes from recombination through imagination: everybody agrees that is possible to combine imaginatively any value of shape and any value of colour that one has had the experience of, and picture a new coloured shape in one's mind. If one has had the experience of squares drawn in a specific shade of red and of circles drawn in a specific shade of blue, one can imagine a red circle and a blue circle. This follows from their conceptual distinction—and the combinatorial power which comes from having concepts. If one has a conceptual representation of A being x (e.g. a square being red) and a conceptual representation of C being y (e.g. a circle being blue), one must be able to form a representation of A being y and C being x (e.g. a square being blue and a circle being red).

The same is not true (at least not so evidently true) of dimensions. If one only had the experience of, say, the shade R12 (with red as value for hue, b1 as value for brightness, and s2 as a value for saturation) and a blue shade B34 (with blue for hue, b3 for brightness, and s4 for saturation), it does not follow that one could imaginatively recombine all these dimensions and say imagine an R34, with blue as hue and b3 and s4 as brightness and saturation respectively. I take it that it is why the missing shade of blue arises as a problem in Hume: from the fact that someone had a wide experience of the variations in brightness and saturation for the same hue (i.e. blue), it does not follow that he would be able to recreate a shade of the same hue, with a missing value of brightness and/or saturation (of course, Hume finally granted that they could—but this is another story . . .).

Dimensions do not therefore enjoy the conceptual independence—and perhaps the related privileges of a distinct cognitive representation, like recombination in imagination—enjoyed by sensory features (and of course, objects). They are still discriminable in the sense that they can be objects of reports and comparisons. Following this definition, synaesthetic concurrents can be discriminable but nonetheless akin to (non-separable) dimensions. The inference from discrimination to feature separability can be blocked.

To conclude on the previous two sections, the lack of separability claim fits better with the experimental evidence and is perfectly compatible with reports given by synaesthetes:

Lack of Separability Claim: The synaesthetic experience is not of a separate object, with its own location, which co-occurs in consciousness with the experience of another object, nor is it like the experience of an object with an additional feature which can be conceptually distinguished from the other features.

13.4.4 The similarity argument

Don't we have other reasons, though, to support the separate feature claim? After all, in their reports, synaesthetes compare the concurrent to *a feature* of experience, sometimes in another modality: for instance, they report experiencing colours when seeing graphemes or hearing notes. If the comparison is genuine, then we should conclude that the synaesthetic concurrent is experienced as a feature, exactly as it is experienced in the modality it is attributed to. Notice that what is at stake here is not just discriminability, but comparisons between experiences. The argument draws on the similarity claim stated above: the synaesthete's report of experiencing green when looking at grass and when hearing Middle C means that she is in a similar (or overlapping) mental state in both cases (i.e. experiencing green as a feature of a surface or a sound). But again, this interpretation can be questioned.

However, when a synaesthete reports visualizing green when hearing Middle C, she could be talking of a non-separable dimension no less than of a colour-feature. Terms used for the dimension of hue largely overlap with colour-terms: green refers both to the dimension of hue shared by several experiences of colour, and to a certain colour (i.e. a feature) which has not only this dimension but also a certain brightness and saturation. As we know from Travis's cases, colour terms might have different conditions of accuracy.[25]

The similarity between the concurrent and a feature can be the result of the methodology: synaesthetes are asked oriented questions such as 'which colour do you see when this note is played?' or, more frequently, asked to select a coloured patch which resembles his or her synaesthetic experience when he/she perceives a certain inducer. The resemblance might be driven only by a limited number of dimensions that are similar in the two experiences—for instance, hue and brightness.

There is a possible objection to the interpretation of synaesthetic "extra" as dimensions coming from crossmodal cases. Saying that an auditory synaesthetic experience resembles a visual experience relative to hue suggests that auditory experiences have *visual* dimensions, which seems like a contradiction.

The contradiction can however be avoided. A first strategy consists in thinking of the synaesthetic experience as a 'multimodal experience', as they are called, where a set of characters coming from different senses blur into a single unified object, and become dimensions of this object. Some dimensions of multimodal experiences can resemble unimodal experiences: for instance, the aromatic dimension of multimodal flavour experiences resemble some dimension present in orthonasal olfactory experiences. It does not mean that aromas are distinct features of flavour experiences and identical to either olfactory objects or some feature of olfactory objects. If synaesthetic experiences are multimodal unified experiences, they can have dimensions which resemble unimodal experiences—for instance their hue.

A second strategy consists in emphasizing that using the same term to characterize two dimensions in two modally distinct experiences does not imply that they are similarly experienced in the two cases. For instance, the use of brightness in the visual and auditory domains does not mean that there is a form of amodal or common way of experiencing brightness when hearing high-pitch violin sounds and seeing an intense yellow flash. The linguistic similarity could be a mere question of crossmodal analogy or correspondence, where one aspect of experience naturally evokes the other and calls for the same term.[26] In synaesthesia, using the term 'green' or 'bright' might amount to the same thing, and mean that the synaesthetic auditory experience

[25] E.g. Travis (1997).

[26] See Marks (1978), Spence (2011).

and the classical visual experiences are perceived as having analogous roles as dimensions, each within their own kind of experience.

The similarity claim does not look like the only solution we have to make sense of synaesthesia. The fact that synaesthetes use similar terms when they report on their synaesthetic and non-synaesthetic experiences does not mean that they are experiencing the same object or feature in both cases, and are in similar or overlapping mental states. This similarity can come mainly from communicative and methodological limitations, and is perfectly compatible with a weaker analogy claim, which states that:

The Analogy Claim: If the concurrent experienced in the synaesthetic case is reported using terms that are similar to the ones used for non-synaesthetic contents of experiences, this means that the synaesthete is experiencing contents that have analogous (but not necessarily identical) dimensions in both cases.

For instance, if a synaesthete uses the term green to report on her experience both when looking at grass and when hearing Middle C, it means that her experience has dimensions of hues or brightness that are analogous in both the synaesthetic and non-synaesthetic cases.

13.5 Phenomenal Enrichment

13.5.1 Extra-dimensions of experience

The non-separability and analogy claims bring us to the idea that synaesthetic concurrents are analogous to extra-dimensions of experience, that one can distinguish and compare across experiences and derivatively localize but which cannot be assimilated to separable objects or features. Most of the time, thinking of objects and features is sufficient for philosophers to think about perception and experience, and not much attention is paid to other aspects of experiences, like dimensions. Put at the centre of an account of synaesthesia, the concept of dimension can help us to capture synaesthetic experiences better.

Synaesthesia must correspond to the occurrence of an experience in a certain modality (the experience corresponding to the inducer) with something additional. As stressed earlier, the addition does not cancel the experience of the inducer—or of its features. But how shall we think of this addition? If the synaesthetic 'extra' cannot be separated from the overall content of the inducer's experience, it should rather be considered as an enrichment of the inducer's experience, rather than something conjoined to it. Drawing on Evans's notion of richness of experience, defined as the number of dimensions in which experiences vary,[27] synaesthesia is to be thought of

[27] Evans (1982) contrasts richness with the notion of fineness of grain, which is the number of values that experience can take on each of these dimensions.

as a form of phenomenal (or conscious) *enrichment*—as if experiences of inducers could vary for synaesthetes along more dimensions than for other perceivers.

Now, if this description is compatible with synaesthetes' reports, it becomes difficult to accept from our non-synaesthetic perspective: what does it mean to have subjective experiences of sounds which have one or more dimensions than ours, especially a dimension which is analogous to a visual dimension like hue? What is it like to have a synaesthetic experience? The reply is: something we cannot imagine.

The fact that we cannot imagine what it is like to be a synaesthete, whereas synaesthetes speak the same language as us and mean the same things as us when it comes to non-synaesthetic experiences, can be disturbing but is not a real objection against the present account. Take the different case of amusic individuals who cannot discriminate between high and low pitch. We cannot imagine what it is like to be amusic, for instance, if we are not—that is, we cannot imagine what it is like to have experiences lacking the dimension of pitch that ours have. Notice that it does not prevent some of these amusic individuals from expressing preferences about certain pieces of music, as they enjoy rhythm, for instance. Despite the fact that we cannot imagine or understand what the experience of amusic is—we can still clearly define what this experience is. The same applies to synaesthesia, with additional rather than missing dimensions: we cannot imagine or understand what the experience of a colour grapheme is—yet we can still clearly define what this experience is. When a synaesthete sees a character A printed in green, and then B printed in green, his experience of the hue of the letter varies along a synaesthetic hue dimension, while the non-synaesthetic hue dimension remains the same.

This description might be hard to accept. One cannot easily get round the idea of additional (nor of missing) dimensions. But the difficulty comes from our incapacity to imaginatively manipulate the dimensions of our experiences. It is not an objection to the definition of synaesthesia as phenomenal enrichment: synaesthesia must not be taken as a thought experiment, which, in cases of consciousness, uses our capacity to imagine a certain experience. It represents an empirical challenge.

Taking the idea of synaesthesia as a form of phenomenal enrichment seriously, it is then not crucial that we can represent ourselves as having synaesthetic experiences (as dual accounts do). What matters is that it makes sense of the empirical evidence collected about synaesthesia: phenomenal enrichment, as argued, is compatible (or even at times explains better) the subjective reports and the behavioural evidence accumulated about synaesthesia up to now. But is it equally compatible with our models of neural mechanisms and processes?

13.5.2 *Neurological and cognitive explanations of phenomenal enrichment*

Can we suggest a plausible process underlying enrichment? I want to argue that the notion of enrichment captures the subjective manifestation of a process not often discussed in philosophy, nor even in contemporary cognitive sciences, known as 'incorporation' or 'absoprtion'.

As detailed elsewhere (see Deroy 2014b), incorporation occurs, for instance, in so-called 'Perky cases'. These cases are named after the psychologist Cheves Perky, who was interested in the blur between contents of perception and contents of imagination. In the most often quoted of her experiments, she asked participants to imagine a banana, while facing and fixing a white wall. At the beginning of the task, the state the participants were in was a canonical state of visual imagery. After they could form a mental image of a banana, a faint picture of a banana would gradually appear on the wall, and cause a change in their experience: participants reported a change in the orientation of the banana they were visualizing, consistent with the orientation of the banana projected on the wall.[28] Although some participants reported having been surprised to experience a change in the banana orientation during the session, they still considered it was something they imaginatively generated and that the second image was something they *could* change or control. Various follow-ups and interpretations of Perky cases have been given, which are not all reviewed here.[29] People might or might not have consciously detected the banana on the wall and their imagery state can be then enriched either by the concurrent *unconscious* perceptual processing or a conscious perceptual state. In another experiment, she asked people to imagine the New York skyline while an image of a red tomato would progressively appear on the wall. They reported experiencing the skyline under the sunset.

These examples show what 'incorporation' or 'absorption' amounts to: the integration of some dimensions, features, or objects that are not presently perceived into the content of an occurring perceptual experience.

As noted by Tellegen and Atkinson, 'Phenomena of this kind, while apparently overlooked by contemporary academic treatments of attention, perception, and memory, have been described and discussed widely in literature on meditation, expanded awareness, peak experiences, mysticism, esthetic experience...altered states of consciousness, and in the literature on drug effects' (Tellegen and Atkinson 1974: 274). Tellegen and Atkinson suggest defining absorption as a mode of attention, that is what they call a 'total' attention 'involving a full commitment of available perceptual, motoric, imaginative and ideational resources to a unified representation of the attentional object' (Tellegen and Atkinson 1974: 275)—an account that can be reconciled with the availability of the 'synaesthetic extra' at the same locus of attention as the inducer. Later, Rader and Tellegen (1987) also confirmed that individuals reporting synaesthetic experiences scored higher on the Absorption Scale.

[28] Perky (1910).

[29] See Segal and Gordon (1969) for further experimental evidence, and Deroy (2014) for a longer analysis.

This account can also easily be reconciled with the current state of neurological investigation regarding hyperconnectivity or lack of inhibition in synaesthesia. It is already worth emphasizing that people who are more prone to 'synaesthetic induction' under hypnosis (Cohen Kadosh et al. 2009; Cohen Kadosh and Terhune 2012) are the most suggestible—with suggestibility being measured in terms of susceptibility to absorption and decrease in inhibition.

Furthermore, the idea of enrichment via a process similar to incorporation leaves open several origins for the concurrent (see also Deroy 2014b): what is sure is that the concurrent is consciously experienced once incorporated into the perceptual state, but it could come from imagery or other neural nonconscious processes whose workings are never capable of generating a conscious experience in and of themselves.

13.6 Conclusions and Consequences for the Perceptual Status of Synaesthetic Experiences

Synaesthetes are not subjects who both hear and see green,[30] see green halos located 'out there', and hold the deluded belief that sounds have colours. They are subjects for whom the experience of Middle C has *something analogous to* seeing a tomato. Their experiences are phenomenally richer than typical experiences—where such subjective similarities between experiences of sounds and tomatoes, or the black letter A and a tomato, do not surface.

This definition is important in several respects, notably because synaesthesia can be defined as a phenomenal kind—which explains why many different neurological profiles could be placed under that label (see Simner 2012). Synaesthesia finds its unity as a *phenomenal* psychological kind.[31] It is a type of conscious experience, and does not necessarily correspond to a single etiology or neurological basis: different types of processes whereby some dimensions of other sensory/imagistic contents are involuntarily absorbed into the content of the experience elicited in a stimulated stream.

To summarize, synaesthesia is a condition where, necessarily, S-experiences occur:

S-experiences: An experience is synaesthetic if and only if it is (i) a vivid experience triggered by a certain set of stimuli, (ii) phenomenally differs from the experience normally induced by this kind of stimuli, be it in other subjects or in similar situations of stimulation, by being (iii) richer than these experiences.

This new definition is also important to start a new reflection on the perceptual status of synaesthetic experiences. As mentioned at the beginning of this chapter, the

[30] E.g. Gray et al. (2002, 2006).

[31] See Auvray and Deroy (2014), Deroy and Spence (2013), and Simner (2012) for discussion.

existence of synaesthetic experiences has been difficult to reconcile with current accounts of perception. Which status should we now grant to experiences of coloured-hearing, colour-graphemes, or other synaesthetic experiences, now conceived as phenomenally enriched experiences? Addressing this question requires thinking about the accuracy conditions we want to grant to dimensions of experience.

Dimensions (such as brightness, hue, saturation for colour) are primarily defined as the subjective axes which delineate the spaces on which conscious perceptual experiences can be compared to one another. They explain judgements of difference and similarities between experiences. Going one step further, the idea is that they do not explain judgements of similarities and differences about objects or features: a variation in the experienced brightness of a surface as one turns it towards the illuminant will not be experienced as a change in the colour property of the object, but as a change in how this colour *looks*. More precisely, it will be experienced as a change in how bright this colour looks.

The dominant interpretation is that dimensions are therefore 'merely subjective'—which seems to suggest that they cannot be evaluated for accuracy. A correlate of this view comes from the evidence that brightness perception does not target a single or constant property of objects (i.e. for instance, their illuminance property). It depends on a complex evaluation of ratios and relations in the visual scene,[32] noticeably the relative size of the different areas and structural relations between them, as shown in the various illusions represented in Figures 13.1, 13.2, and 13.3.

Is this sufficient to conclude that our perception of brightness cannot be evaluated for accuracy conditions? A distinction can be drawn between mere subjective aspects of experience and aspects that have complex and non-linear correlation with objective properties. The latter can correspond to what O'Callaghan (in prep.)

Figure 13.1 The innermost patches are physically the same but the one on the left is perceived as darker than the one on the right. This effect is due to what is known as 'brightness assimilation': their perceived brightness goes in the same direction as their perceived *immediate* backgrounds, i.e. the outer patches. The left outer patch is perceived as darker than the right one. These two *distant* outer patches, which are also physically the same, however *exhibit brightness contrast*, and are perceived as going in opposite directions compared to their background: the left one appears darker on a brighter background and the right one appears brighter on a darker background.

[32] See Ghosh and Bhaumik (2010) for a review. See also O'Callaghan (forthcoming) for a similar analysis of pitch.

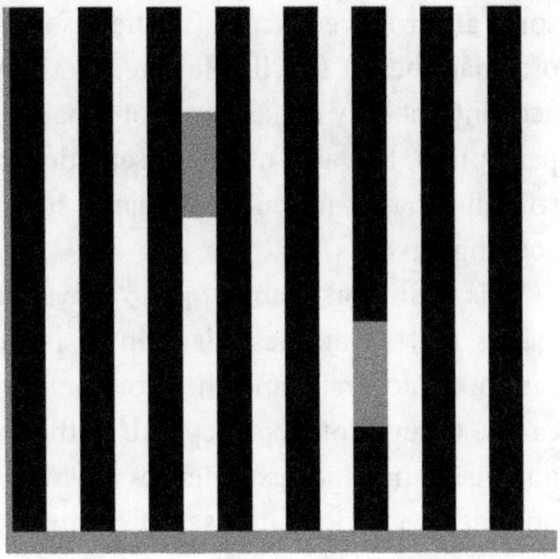

Figure 13.2 The White effect: a grey patch on white coaxial bar is perceived darker than a physically similar patch situated on the black bar.

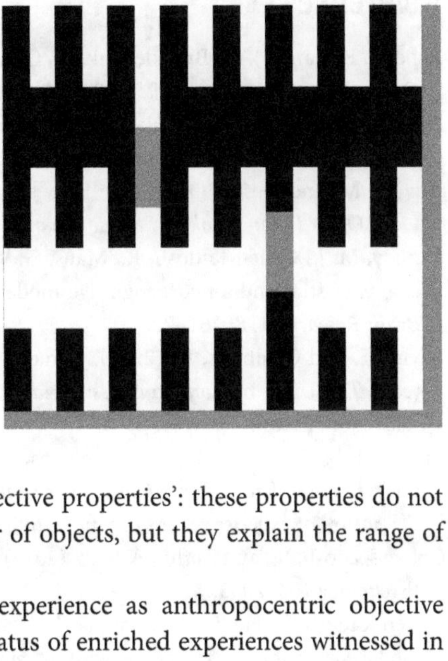

Figure 13.3 Flanking white and black bars next to the patches reduce the 'White effect'. This 'Howe effect' depends on the height of the flanking bars and their relative position vis à vis the patches.

has suggested calling 'anthropocentric objective properties': these properties do not interest physicists or predict the behaviour of objects, but they explain the range of reactions they elicit in us.

The understanding of dimensions of experience as anthropocentric objective properties can illuminate the perceptual status of enriched experiences witnessed in synaesthesia. Instead of looking for accuracy between a synaesthetic content and a single physical property of the object, it is possible to consider that the supplementary synaesthetic dimensions (e.g. hue, brightness, etc.) capture another set of complex relations between properties of objects.

Recent evidence suggests that there is a non-linear correlation between synaesthetic experiences and a variety of external features—for instance, angularity and phonological properties of letters. The failure to linearly correlate the variations in brightness or synaesthetic enriched experiences with *quantitative variations* in the physical stimuli should, however, not be taken as the sign that they do not represent some anthropocentrically (in the case of brightness) or idiosyncratically (in the case of synaesthesia) specifiable interrelations between properties of the stimulus. This account not only makes sense of synaesthetically enriched experiences being cases of perception, but also of the observation that they largely occur for anthropocentric stimuli—that is, for cultural objects such as letters, musical notes, sport movements, cooking flavours, etc.

This definition enables one to move away from the tension between psychological claims that synaesthesia is akin to perception, and philosophical concerns that it cannot be accurate, and therefore pertains to illusion or hallucination. Synaesthesia can be thought of as perceptual, in the sense that it consists in having an additional dimension in which experiences get compared, a dimension which in turn represents nonlinear variations in a set of complex properties of physical objects that are only interesting to the synaesthete.

References

Asher, J. E., Lamb, J. A., Brocklebank, D., Cazier, J. B., Maestrini, E., Addis, L., Sen, M., Baron-Cohen, S., and Monaco, A. P. (2009), 'A whole-genome scan and fine-mapping linkage study of auditory-visual synesthesia reveals evidence of linkage to chromosomes 2q24, 5q33, 6p12, and 12p12', in *American Journal of Human Genetics* 84: 279–85.

Auvray, M. and Deroy, O. (2014), 'How synaesthetes experience the world', in M. Matthen (ed.), *Oxford Handbook of Philosophy of Perception* (Oxford: Oxford University Press).

Banissy, M. J., Cohen Kadosh, R., Maus, G. W., Walsh, V., and Ward, J. (2009), 'Prevalence, characteristics and a neurocognitive model of mirror-touch synaesthesia', in *Experimental Brain Research* 198: 261–72.

Bayne, T. and Chalmers, D. (2003), 'What is the unity of consciousness?', in A. Cleeremans (ed.), *The Unity of Consciousness: Binding, Integration and Dissociation* (Oxford: Oxford University Press).

Brogaard, B. (2014), 'Seeing as a non-sensory relation: The case from synesthesia and visual imagery', in R. Brown (ed.), *Consciousness inside and out: Phenomenology, neuroscience, and the nature of experience. Studies in Brain and Mind* (Amsterdam: Springer Press), 377–94.

Cohen Kadosh, R., and Terhune, D. B. (2012), 'Redefining synaesthesia? ' in *British Journal of Psychology* 103: 20–3.

Cohen Kadosh, R., Henik, A., Cantena, A., Walsh, V., and Fuentes, L. J. (2009), 'Induced cross-modal synaesthetis experience without abnormal neurinal connections', in *Psychological Science* 20: 258–65.

Crane, T. (1988a), 'The Waterfall Illusion', in *Analysis* 48: 142–7.

Crane, T. (1988b), 'Concepts in perception', in *Analysis* 48: 150–3.

Cytowic, R. E. (1997), 'Synaesthesia: Phenomenology and neuropsychology. A review of current knowledge', in S. Baron-Cohen and J. E. Harrison (eds), *Synaesthesia: Classic and contemporary readings* (Oxford: Basil Blackwell), 17–39.

Deroy, O. (2014a), 'Multisensory integration and the many unities of consciousness', in D. Bennett and C. Hill (eds), *Multisensory integration and the unity of consciousness* (Cambridge, MA: MIT Press), 105–24.

Deroy, O. (2014b), 'Synaesthesia: An experience of the third kind?', in R. Brown (ed.), *Consciousness inside and out: Phenomenology, neuroscience, and the nature of experience. Studies in brain and mind* (Amsterdam: Springer Press), 395–407.

Deroy, O., and Spence, C. (2013), 'Why we are not all synesthetes (not even weakly so)', in *Psychonomic Bulletin and Review* 20 (1): 1–22.

Dixon, M. J., Smilek, D., Cudahy, C., and Merikle, P. M. (2000), 'Five plus two equals yellow', in *Nature* 406: 365.

Dretske, F. (1995), *Naturalizing the mind* (Cambridge, MA: MIT Press).

Duffy, P. L. (2001), *Blue cats and chartreuse kittens: How synesthetes color their worlds* (New York: Henry Holt and Company).

Edquist J., Rich A. N., Brinkman C., and Mattingley J. B. (2006), 'Do synaesthetic colours act as unique features in visual search?' in *Cortex* 42: 222–31.

Evans, G. (1982), *The varieties of reference* (Oxford: Oxford University Press).

Ghosh, K., and Bhaumik, K. (2010), 'Complexity in human perception of brightness: A historical review on the evolution of the philosophy of visual perception', in *OnLine Journal of Biological Sciences* 10: 17–35.

Gray, J. A., Chopping, S., Nunn, J., Parslow, D., Gregory, L., Williams, S. C. R., Brammer, M. J., and Baron-Cohen, S. (2002), 'Implications of synaesthesia for functionalism: Theory and experiments', in *Journal of Consciousness Studies* 9: 5–31.

Gray, J. A., Parslow, D. M., Brammer, M. J., Chopping, S., Vythelingum, G. N., and Fytche, D. H. (2006), 'Evidence against functionalism from neuroimaging of the alien color effect in synesthesia', in *Cortex* 42: 309–18.

Gray, R. (2001), 'Synaesthesia and misrepresentation: A reply to Wager', in *Philosophical Psychology* 14: 339–46.

Grossenbacher, P. G., and Lovelace, C. T. (2001), 'Mechanisms of synesthesia: cognitive and physiological constraints', in *Trends in Cognitive Sciences* 5: 36–41.

Harrison, J. E. (2001), *Synaesthesia: The strangest thing* (Oxford: Oxford University Press).

Harrison, J. E., and Baron-Cohen, S. (1997), 'Synaesthesia: An introduction', in S. Baron-Cohen and J. E. Harrison (eds), *Synaesthesia: Classic and contemporary readings* (Oxford: Basil Blackwell).

Hupe, J. M., Bordier, C., and Dojat, M. (2011), 'The neural bases of grapheme-color synesthesia are not localized in real color-sensitive areas', in *Cerebral Cortex* doi:10.1093/cercor/bhr236.

Kim, C. Y., Blake, R., and Palmeri, T. J. (2006), 'Perceptual interaction between real and synesthetic colors', in *Cortex* 42: 195–203.

Lycan, W. (2006), 'Representational theories of consciousness', in E. N. Zalta (ed.), *The Stanford Encyclopedia of Philosophy*, at <http://plato.stanford.edu/archives/win2006/entries/consciousness-representational/>.

Macpherson, F. (2007), 'Synaesthesia, functionalism and phenomenology', in M. de Caro, F. Ferretti, and M. Marraffa (eds), *Cartographies of the mind: Philosophy and psychology in intersection series: Studies in brain and mind* (Netherlands: Springer), 65–80.

Marks, L. E. (1978), *The unity of the senses: Interrelations among the modalities* (New York: Academic Press).

Marks, L. E., and Mulvenna, C. M. (2013), 'Synesthesia, at and near its borders', in *Frontiers in Psychology* 4: 651.

Mattingley, J. B., Rich, A. N., Yelland, G., and Bradshaw, J. L. (2001), 'Unconscious priming eliminates automatic binding of colour and alphanumeric form in synaesthesia', in *Nature* 410 (6828): 580–2.

Mellor, D. H. (1988), 'Crane's waterfall illusion', in *Analysis* 48: 147–50.

Mills, C. B. (1999), 'Digit synaesthesia: A case study using a Stroop-type test', in *Cognitive Neuropsychology* 16: 181–91.

Mulvenna, C. M., and Walsh, V. (2006), 'Synaesthesia: supernormal integration?', in *Trends in cognitive sciences* 10 (8): 350–2.

Novich, S. D., Cheng, S., and Eagleman, D. M. (2011), 'Is synesthesia one condition or many? A large-scale analysis reveals subgroups', in *Journal of Neuropsychology* 5: 353–71.

O'Callaghan, C. (forthcoming), 'Cross-sensory synaesthesia', in O. Deroy (ed.), *Sensory blending: New essays on synaesthesia* (Oxford: Oxford University Press).

O'Callaghan, C., 'Pitch' (unpublished ms).

Ortmann, O. (1933), 'Theories of synesthesia in the light of a case of colored Hearing', in *Human Biology* 5: 155–211.

Palmeri, T. J., Blake, R., Marois, R., Flanery, M. A., and Whetsell, W. (2002), 'The perceptual reality of synesthetic colors', in *Proceedings of the National Academy of Science of the United States of America*, 99: 4127–31.

Perky, C. W. (1910), 'An experimental study of imagination', in *American Journal of Psychology* 21: 422–52.

Rader, C. M., and Tellegen, A. (1987), 'An investigation of synesthesia', in *Journal of Personality and Social Psychology* 52 (5): 981.

Rouw, R., Scholte, H. S., and Colizoli, O. (2011), 'Brain areas involved in synaesthesia: A review', in *Journal of Neuropsychology* 5: 214–42.

Sagiv N., Heer, J., and Robertson, L. (2006), 'Does binding of synesthetic color to the evoking grapheme require attention?', in *Cortex* 42: 232–42.

Segal, S. J., and Gordon, P. E. (1969), 'The Perky effect revisited: Blocking of visual signals by imagery', in *Perceptual and Motor Skills* 28: 791–7.

Simner, J. (2012), 'Defining synaesthesia', in *British Journal of Psychology* 103: 1–15.

Smilek, D., Dixon, M. J., and Merikle, P. M. (2001), 'Synaesthetic photisms guide attention', in *Brain and Cognition* 53: 364–7.

Sollberger, M. (2012), 'Rethinking synaesthesia', *Philosophical Psychology* 26: 171–87.

Spence, C. (2011), 'Crossmodal correspondences: A tutorial review', in *Attention, Perception, and Psychophysics* 73: 971–95.

Tellegen, A., and Atkinson, G. (1974), 'Openness to absorbing and self-altering experiences ("absorption"), a trait related to hypnotic susceptibility', in *Journal of abnormal psychology* 83 (3): 268–77.

Terhune, D. B., Tai, S., Cowey, A., Popescu, T., and Cohen Kadosh, R. (2011), 'Enhanced cortical excitability in grapheme-color synesthesia and its modulation', in *Current Biology* 21: 2006–9.

Travis, C. (1997), 'Pragmatics', in B. Hale and C. Wright (eds), *A companion to the philosophy of language* (Oxford: Blackwell), 87–106.

Treisman, A. (1996), 'The binding problem', in *Current Opinion in Neurobiology* 6 (2): 171–8.

Tye, M. (2000), *Consciousness, color, and content* (Cambridge, MA: MIT Press).

Tye, M. (2002), 'Representationalism and the transparency of experience', in *Noûs* 36: 137–51.

Wager, A. (1999), 'The extra qualia problem: Synaesthesia and representationalism', in *Philosophical Psychology* 12: 263–81.

Wager, A. (2001), 'Synaesthesia misrepresented', in *Philosophical Psychology* 14: 347–51.

Ward J., Jonas C., Dienes Z., and Seth A. (2010), 'Grapheme-colour synaesthesia improves detection of embedded shapes, but without pre-attentive "pop-out" of synaesthetic colour', in *Proceedings in Biological Sciences* 277: 1021–6.

14

Technical Issues in Naive Sense-Datum Theory

John M. Nicholas

14.1 Introduction

It is our brains that make colours. It is not the things we see. If our visual states are representations, they are representations *by* colours, not representations *of* colours.

What could motivate such views? One answer is that significant numbers of vision scientists, neurologists, physicists, colour theorists, and the *Commission internationale de l'éclairage* have offered grounds for the belief that the bearers of colours are brain-based sensations or percepts, not objects external to the body. While they are coy about what they take sensations or percepts to be, they employ the vocabulary unabashedly. On the other hand, philosophers are almost uniformly dismissive of opinions like that. Usually, they associate them with traditional sense-datum theories (SDT), often tut-tutting about them as not just mistaken but as a vice. I believe that those scientists are right, that the philosophers are wrong, and that the tut-tutting about the SDT thesis is wrong-headed.

In this chapter, I shall examine some aspects of the Naive Sense-Datum Theory (NSDT) of the title.[1] After a brief commentary on the usual arguments against SDT, I shall flag some of the arguments that motivate the acceptance of sensations or percepts as the bearers of colours. I shall assume the cogency of the arguments in question, and not mount a defence of them here. Rather, I wish to give some illustrations of what I term 'technical puzzles'. These are puzzles, both difficulties and novelties, that face a sense-datum approach, when we pick up the ball and run with it, so to speak. I don't want to dive into the philosophical Sargasso Sea of pros and cons for the philosophers' Argument from Illusion. Nor is my approach propelled by epistemological or metaphysical bells and whistles, like foundationalism or logical atomism, but rather by what I take to be suggested by evidence from the recent

[1] Coining 'Naive' and 'Naivete' as technical, if loose, terms, I shall use neither the diaeresis nor the acute accent of the English words 'naïve' and 'naïveté'.

scientific literature. I prefer to ask what happens, from the scientific point of view, if we take SDT to be true. What new questions arise, and how does our scientific knowledge constrain how SDT might be developed?

Why *Naive* Sense-Datum Theory? I shall explain the Naivete of the Sense-Datum Theory (or family of theories) rather unsystematically as I go along, by identifying particular Naive assumptions as they surface in the discussion. Very roughly, Naive SDTs are those which are the simplest, most commonsensical ways of instantiating SDT's core theses. In most cases, what is Naive is the sort of thing that we might carry over from Direct Realism, allowing for the new context. However, part of my goal is to consider some ways in which NSDT might be forced to become less Naive.

One Naive assumption which I think will not be given up is that sense data are in a physical space in or at the brain. Consequently, I shall describe what little comfort NSDT currently gleans in the light of contemporary models of the brain and the functions of its parts. At the same time, my commentary will equally serve to stress part of the shortfall in the capacity of contemporary models of consciousness to explain the way our experience is. Further, as an illustration of a major retreat from Naivete, I shall propose that SDT will be in better shape if it takes our visual experience to be two-, not three-dimensional, and shall urge that two-dimensionality is not as implausible as most readers likely believe. In conclusion, I will suggest that SDT may have to give up a central plank of its position, bringing it closer to its cousin and deadly adversary, Intentionalist Representationalism.

14.2 Preliminaries: Orientation for the Reader

What are the allegations against SDT? Its opponents often offer four strategic arguments which are, in rough and ready terms (Huemer 2001): (1) SDT implies a 'veil of the appearances' and, thus, justifies scepticism about the world beyond the sense data, which is contrary to epistemic intuition; (2) SDT is committed to dualism or immaterialism and is, therefore, scientifically or naturalistically unacceptable; (3) arguments from illusion and hallucination, the core arguments in favour of SDT are unsound and, hence, SDT is unfounded; and; (4) SDT implies an 'homunculus', sometimes conceived of as a locus 'where it all comes together', meaning perceptual, affective, intellectual, and executive functioning. The SDT's supposition of an homunculus implies a vicious infinite regress and, thus, SDT is unacceptable.

(1) is unjustified. The argument usually comes with the supposition that enumerative induction, the correlation of experienced properties, is our only resource for inference. It is not; we have powerful methods of hypothetical inference available, too.

(2) is incorrect. Currently, there is no warrant for claiming that the properties of sensations are not reducible by physical theory. It is not even clear yet what the details of the explananda are to be. In any case, reduction is not a necessary condition

for physicality. For example, the acceptance of electric inverse square forces in the late eighteenth century, with the work of Cavendish and Coulomb, did not require that they be reducible to mechanics, inertia, and gravitation. They were, relative to the context, 'neo-physical', one might say, but readily integrated into the larger physics. SDT need not assume that sense data are not physical, at least not without further ado.

(3) is unfair; SDT is grounded in a much wider range of evidence than just illusions and hallucinations. Further, the grounding is inductive, for the most part hypothetical. Once in a while, in developed sciences, rich-enough models and suitable data do permit plausibly sound deductive reasoning from phenomena. The case of SDT is mainstream science, not an exceptional case, like, say, Newton's derivation of the exponent of the gravitational distance law from the advance of the perihelion of the moon is argued to be. The Argument from Illusion, supposedly a deductively sound argument, was a reach from the outset.

Something in certain respects like (4), but with a weaker conclusion may be plausible, but no infinite regress is implied. There is no inner 'seer'. I shall say more about the alleged implication to dualism, and the alleged homunculus regress below.

What grounds steer us to taking sensations, percepts, or sense data, rather than the relevant external objects to be the bearers of colours? I take these three considerations to be fundamental:

(i) To attribute phenomenal colours to distal stimuli would be to add an 'idle wheel' to the explanation of colour vision. We have well-established ideas about what contributions distal stimuli make to the process of colour and other vision, and they do not include the generation of colours (i.e. those attributes that at the very least conform to the structure of colour similarity spaces, etc.) at those distal stimuli. Stimuli which characteristically cause us to see, say, red, may as well be brown or tartan for all that it would contribute to the visual process, whose pivotal outcome is the generation of an electromagnetic luminance profile at the retina. Given the redundancy of phenomenal colour to our scientific understanding of distal stimuli, we have no particular reason to attribute colours to them, although, as F. H. Bradley rightly pointed out to Bertrand Russell, SDT does not prohibit the existence of colours in physical things other than living brains, even if they are not experienced. SDT does not insist that colours only exist if someone or something is conscious of them, even in the brain. Without further evidence, such a claim would be premature.

(ii) Colours have particular properties and relations (similarities, unique/binary character, variability with frequency of uniqueness by subject, for example). Distal stimuli have no physical grounding for those attributes (Nassau 2001, Hardin 1988, Hardin 1990, Pautz 2007).

(iii) In addition to partially understanding why the roles of light sources, transmissive media, and reflecting surfaces in causing colours and their vision are exhausted by their generating luminance spectra, we also partially comprehend how colours are produced—in or at the brain.

Consider Jameson and Hurvich's construction of chromatic response functions (Jameson and Hurvich 1955: 551) in the context of their colour Opponency Model. For a given subject, the response function represents the weighting of chromatic components, R(ed), G(reen), B(lue), Y(ellow), in binary hues, in terms of energies delivered to the retina. Other things being equal, each frequency in the spectral range will yield a characteristic *binary* hue with relative weightings for R/Y, Y/G, G/B, and B/R as dictated by the given curves. The curves are empirically determined by hue cancellation, assuming (1) that there are two parallel chromatic opponent channels, RG and BY, and (2) that the measure of a given opponent is given by the (energy) intensity of its complementary that is required to annihilate it. In those special cases where each of one pair of opponents takes a zero value, there appears a *unique* hue which is one of the second opponent pair. If red and green are annihilated, then either unique blue or unique yellow will appear, depending on wavelength.

The Jameson and Hurvich Opponency Model is, admittedly, a preliminary and imperfect model of hue formation, but it is an important first step in our understanding of the calculus of the generation of hues—behind the retina. Direct Realists with even modest scientific proclivities may be troubled by the locus of hue formation being in the brain, not in the distal stimulus. Intentionalist Representationalists may be troubled by the process being the formation of the hues themselves not the formation of neural symbolism to serve as the vehicle for intentional content. I presume that Intentionalists will interpret the Opponency Model as describing the formation of a neural encoding whose intentional content is of binary colours blended in proportion to the retinal energies implicated in the hue cancellation experiments. Nobody doubts that intentional content can be carried by encodings, for example, writing, without any characteristic phenomenology. What is not obvious is how the presentational character of phenomenology can be achieved without instantiation of the qualitative properties in question. It would be useful to know, for example, what principled basis underlies the distinction between modes of presentation that are 'presentational' and those modes of presentation that do not 'present' in any essential way at all.

14.3 Naive Sense-Datum Theory

In order to make clear what NSDT asserts, it will help the reader if I first identify a *criterion* for Naive Direct Realism. Naive Direct Realism is the doctrine that:

(NDR) The Phenomenal Array is the Visual Field.

What does 'the Visual Field' refer to? The expression is used in conflicting ways in different specialty literatures but, in this chapter, it will denote the array of *distal stimuli*, at any given time, outside our bodies, which causally contribute to our seeing them. It is a part or several parts of the environment. This follows fairly standard usage in perceptual psychology.

What does 'the (visual) Phenomenal Array' refer to? It refers to what almost all of us, at a given time, believe to be the Visual Field, that is, the array of distal stimuli given to us in experience, causing our perception. The NDRist asserts that what, at any given time, she believes to be the external world given in experience is, indeed, the external world. Some readers may find it curious that a doctrine of Direct Realism could employ any notion like the Phenomenal Array, but I wish to stress that all the term denotes here is what is given to us in experience, which we usually believe to be the world outside our bodies. Indeed, 'the Phenomenal Array is the Visual Field' seems to me to be a natural and economical way of picking out Naive Direct Realism.

On the other hand, according to the doctrine of the NSDTist, the Phenomenal Array is not the Visual Field, but is located in the physical space of the brain. Our mistaken belief that the Phenomenal Array is the world outside our bodies does not lead us into much trouble on a day-to-day basis, apart from in the philosophical seminar room, and in some particular contexts in, say, the colour sciences. In fact, it is a sign of a not-disordered mind in the NSDTist (never mind the rest) that outside the seminar room and away from the desk, they share the NDRist's mistake. It is a serviceable belief and functions well because Natural Selection has made that possible. It is unlikely that many, if any, other animals share this mistaken belief, if only because they have no opinion at all on the ontology of the Phenomenal Array.[2] The same goes for humans, when they are not thinking explicitly about the matter.

The brief formulation of NSDT is:

(NSDT) The Phenomenal Array is an array in the brain.

In introducing NSDT this way, I implicitly aim to forestall some widespread misconceptions about what is essential to SDT. One of the misconceptions is that sense data are unfamiliar, exceptional, and essentially strange or 'spooky'. The appeal to the idea of the Phenomenal Array constitutes a reminder that sense data (the component parts of the Phenomenal Array) are as familiar in our experience as items like tables and chairs, the colours of burning coals and blue skies, cottages and the Chrysler Building. Recall that NSDT presupposes that most of us, most of the time, if we actually have the relevant beliefs, believe that what is given to us in (visual) experience is the world outside our bodies. As believers, we are all

[2] Strictly, as I have put it above, animals and humans who do not hold a position on the matter either have no Phenomenal Array or the issue is not well-defined. For reasons of brevity and simplicity, I shall continue to address those readers who do hold a position.

spontaneous Naive Direct Realists. The disagreement between NDRists and NSDTists is not that the latter wish to introduce new-fangled (or old-fangled!), mysterious entities; it is just that they want to claim that the familiar things and properties given in experience are somewhere other than where the former suppose them to be. They are in the brain. As we shall see, admittedly, those familiar things may not quite have the character we judge them to have.

I shall label the supposition that we mistake the experienced part of the world for the world outside our bodies 'Prichard's Diagnostic'.[3] Prichard's Diagnostic allows us a new perspective on the question of whether SDT implies immaterialism. A full dress review of the issue is beyond the scope of this brief chapter, but I think it worth making explicit the circumstantial case, which follows from Prichard's Diagnostic, that it does not. If we mistake the Phenomenal Array for the Visual Field, and we judge that external objects bear the properties which our sense data do, then we may plausibly conclude that there is nothing in the qualitative character of sense data that is manifestly non-physical. For when we mistake 'what it's like' for attributes of objects in the external world, we have no sense of anomaly when we also attribute physical variables to them. We see a yellow tulip, and do not doubt for a minute that it instantiates not only phenomenal yellow but also momentum, energy, gravitational mass, electric charge, and so on. Further, there is nothing non-physical, as of the current state of physics, in qualia that we perceive in their *intuitable* character. Otherwise, we could never readily make the mistake of identifying the Phenomenal Array with the external world, while taking the external world to be exclusively physical. The attributes instantiated in the Phenomenal Array are not alien; they are the properties which we believe we see the physical world to have, even if we cannot currently explain them by appeal to their microscopic physical constituents.

Why the properties in the Phenomenal Array should suddenly become outlandish when thought to be in the brain when not deemed outlandish when thought to be in tables, chairs, and flowers escapes me. While the different context does change the specific details of what physico-chemical resources are available for the grounding of phenomenal qualities—neurological resources in the brain, solid state resources in, say, a metal bar—there does not seem to be a greater generic explanatory gap in the brain case. (There is, however, a difference of detail, as we saw in the failure of external things to have the kind of make-up which grounds the known properties and relations of colours).

If we did discern phenomenal qualities to be manifestly non-physical, then presumably Direct Realists and Disjunctivists (in the veridical case) would be Immaterialists, too. But none of us need be immaterialists, at least not on the grounds that there is something 'spooky' about what is experienced. Further, if it is very hard to conceive of

[3] H. A. Prichard (1950: 61) stressed the possibility that we mistake our sense data for external bodies in his critique of Russell's doctrine of 'knowledge by acquaintance'. He opposed Russell's taking acquaintance to be a kind of knowledge.

how atoms and molecules can give rise to colours, sounds, tastes, and bodily sensations the difficulty afflicts Direct Realists and Disjunctivists as much as it does Sense-Datum Theorists. They too have Hard Problems, though theirs are in the physics of external bodies, while ours are in the physics, chemistry, and biology of brains.

14.4 How and Where Can the Phenomenal Array Be in the Brain?

14.4.1 Disposing of the homunculus fallacy critique

NSDT supposes what the likely majority of neurologists and philosophers deny: that there is a unitary cerebral site in which multi-modal binding or co-location of experienced sensory attributes is distributed in space and is available to awareness and attention in a unitary way. It is the physical locus of the Phenomenal Array, and I will refer to it as the 'Sensorium'. Roughly speaking, NDRists may be understood to be claiming that the (visual) Phenomenal Array is the array of facing surfaces of distal stimuli, and that the Sensorium is the external physical space occupied by them. NSDTists insist that the Phenomenal Array occupies the Sensorium, which is a unitary site in the brain. Is the prospect of a Phenomenal Array in a cerebral Sensorium feasible?

The idea is usually opposed for being a so-called 'Cartesian Theatre'. 'Somehow it stands to reason' Antonio Damasio has conceded:

> that what is together in the mind is together at one place in the brain where different sensory aspects mingle. The usual metaphor has something to do with a large Cinemascope screen equipped for glorious Technicolor projection, stereophonic sound, and perhaps a track for smell too. (Damasio 1994: 94)

But as Dennett and Kinsbourne have observed:

> it is obvious that it is a bad idea, not only because, as a matter of empirical fact, nothing in the functional neuroanatomy of the brain suggests such a general meeting place, but also because positing such a Center would apparently be the first step in an infinite regress of too-powerful homunculi. (Dennett and Kinsbourne 1992: 197)

I shall address two of the three parts of this critique: the *homunculus* and the *one place*.[4] Let's take the *homunculus* first. Gareth Evans has given an economical account of 'the homunculus fallacy', as:

[4] The third part of the critique concerns the scope of the powers of the supposed viewer in the model, and is too large a topic to take on in this chapter.

> when one attempts to explain what is involved in a subject's being related to objects in the external world by appealing to the existence of an inner situation which recapitulates the essential features of the original situation to be explained... by introducing a relation between the subject and inner objects of essentially the same kind as the relation existing between the subject and the outer objects. (Evans 1985: 397)

A Cartesian Theatre, with inner projectors, screens, and images requiring a viewer in the brain whom we suppose to have vision in the same way as does the person whose vision is to be explained, would perhaps satisfy Evans's criterion for the homunculus fallacy. However, *such a conception is absolutely not implied by the Sense-Datum Theory*. In logical terms, it is extraordinarily hard to see why the accusation of homunculus fallacy is taken to get off the ground. NSDT does not satisfy Evans's criterion. To begin with, barring some astonishing empirical surprise in future research, it is not at all plausible that the presumably physical process of forming the (visual) Phenomenal Array and bringing awareness and attention to bear on it involve, to begin with, cerebral sources of electromagnetic radiation, partial absorption and re-emission by surfaces in the Array, and the detection of luminance profiles in retinas in, say, the neo-cortex, leading to whatever process embodies the Phenomenal Array/Awareness/Attention system. Even if there were a first regressive step, it would not imply the infinite regress.

In the light of the above, an unfamiliar refinement of common usage seems desirable in the technical formulation of SDT. Let's say that the perceiver is 'consciously aware' of only the sense data composing the Phenomenal Array, and 'sees' the distal stimulus. Being aware is not the same sort of process as vision or seeing. Conscious awareness of sense data is only a part—a module or sub-system, perhaps—of the functional architecture which constitutes the seeing of external things. (Of course, it is this nesting of the awareness sub-system within the seeing system which gives rise to the homunculus regress argument, but only when it is gratuitously assumed that awareness is a kind of seeing, rather than just a part of it.) One is consciously *aware* of sense data; one *sees* distal stimuli. One does not *see* sense data; one is not consciously *aware* of distal stimuli. There are no external things in the Phenomenal Array, only brain parts or their immediate effects. It may be responded that it is unintuitive that we should end up saying that we are not *aware* of external things. However, given that what we are (visually) aware of has colours, and that it is hard to see how those colours are grounded in external things, then, I think that it is right to conclude that what we are aware of is not external things. We are not aware of external things when we see them.[5]

[5] Sense datum advocates have, for dubious reasons, sometimes elected for the apparently homuncular option. Frank Jackson's fundamental 'analytic thesis' (Jackson 1977: 27–8, emphasis added) was that 'to *see* a reasonable-sized, opaque material object is to *see* something distinct from that object, the relevant immediate object of perception...'. This is outer seeing explained by inner seeing. It does not alter the logical point that SDT does not require such a commitment.

14.4.2 Is there one place where it all comes together?

Particularly in the case of vision, as Damasio has allowed, it is tempting to suppose that the retino-geniculo-striate pathway should assemble a visual framework in the occipital lobe and then fill in details in a feed-forward 'cascade' through the association cortices, presumably targeting some ulterior site in the parietal cortex, the temporal cortex, the frontal cortex, or some arrangement within the parahippocampal complex (Damasio 1989a). Some authors pick out frontal and parietal cortices as the preferred targets of primary cortex output (Zeki 2001). Relatively enlarged neuronal receptive fields anterior to the occipital lobes, and increased multimodality reinforce that impulse (Driver and Noesselt 2008; Macaluso 2006; Macaluso and Driver 2005; Macaluso et al. 2002). It would not be unnatural to look for the Phenomenal Array in these locales.

Some researchers have been quite plain about the need for assembly of a unitary construction. For example, highlighting the role of the corpus callosum in permitting this assembly, Tootel et al. (1998: 819) have identified visual field maps in the extrastriate cortex of one hemisphere, which 'begin' approximately where complementary representations in the opposed cortex 'end'. They accept that:

> communication across the interhemispheric 'seam' in higher visual areas presumably is related to the construction of a *unitary visual percept*, uniting the two hemifield maps present in the lower-tier areas. (Tootell et al. 1998: 822, emphasis added)

Similar unifying conceptualizations have appeared in discussions of somatosensory cortical areas. Thus, Manzoni et al. (1989) have described in mammals the predominance in the primary somatosensory area, SI, of neurons which have receptive fields of the roughly mid-line axial and paraxial trunk, with little or no representation of peripheral limbs, roughly mimicking the visual system's divisions. In the simplest model that they discuss, the corpus callosum permits:

> a *unitary body representation* generated by fusing together two somototopically matching maps, one of the contralateral hemibody mediated by thalamo-cortical input and one of the ipsilateral hemibody replicated by the corpus callosum. (Manzoni et al. 1989: 251, emphasis added)

While the above authors envisage a pooling of disjoint components into a 'unitary visual percept' or a 'unitary body representation', they do not offer much comfort for NSDT. Both assemblies are merely unimodal, one visual and the other somatosensory, while NSDT needs exhaustive multimodality for its Phenomenal Array. A Naive account of our perception of, say, a hand which is shaped and coloured, making a rustling sound in motion, smells of hand cream, stings from a paper cut, and so on, suggests a colocation of all the sensory modalities where applicable.

On the other hand, Damasio has argued against the assumption held by many neurological researchers that perceptual processes culminate in 'a place where it all comes together', although the starting point for his 1989 proposals (Damasio 1989a) seems to be one shared by NSDT's conception of the Phenomenal Array: experience is not 'parcellated', that is, it is 'coherent' and 'in-register' (Damasio 1989a: 29):

> The brain must have devices capable of promoting the integration of fragmentary components of neural activity, in some sort of ensemble pattern that matches the structures of entities, events, and relationships thereof. (Damasio 1989a: 29)

Usually, Damasio has reported, it has been assumed that 'a representation of integrated reality' in perception is formed in anterior temporal and anterior frontal multimodal 'integrative' cortices,

> on the basis of a unidirectional cascade of processors, which provides, step by step, a refinement of the extraction of signals, first in unimodal streams and later in a sort of multimedia and multitrack apparatus where integration occurs. (Damasio 1989a: 29)

If this assumption were borne out, Damasio has insisted, then substantial bilateral lesions to anterior temporal and frontal cortices would undermine the coherence and multimodality of experience. Further, even the fine structure of perception and recall based on projections from earlier unimodal sites would be compromised (Damasio 1989a: 31). But these things do not come about. Significant damage to anterior temporal cortices leaves a subject's quality of experience (and covert sensory knowledge) comparable to that of controls. Substantial ablation of prefrontal cortices leaves perception normal, although it does impinge on attention and some other higher-order functions (Damasio 1989a: 33). Damasio has concluded that the feed-forward convergence model has overwhelming difficulties.

In its stead he has proposed the doctrine that (Damasio 1989a: 26, emphasis added):

> perceptual experience depends on neural activity in *multiple regions activated simultaneously*, rather than in a single region where experiential integration would occur.

Damasio has substituted for the unidirectional feed-forward convergence model one that is rich with feed-back linkages from convergence zones in the more rostral cortices to 'earlier', caudal areas. The convergence zones store 'binding codes' at the levels of property, object, and event in response to perceptual inputs. When they discharge, they enable projections back to caudal cortices at which 'representations are reconstituted and evoked', and where the cycle can be restarted. Despite that, according to Damasio, the model has no need for 'an ultimate integration' area (Damasio 1989a: 40). It is not wrong to say that there is convergence as neural processes proceed from caudal to more rostral, but there is also massive feed-back to caudal areas. What convergence there is seems to be, disappointingly for NSDT, a convergence of *encoding* rather than of the assembly of representations of properties, objects, or events. It is nothing that might be mistaken for the outside world.

It is not obvious, however, that the representations 'reconstituted' in caudal areas can be conscious on this account in a way that fits the bill of the Sense-Datum Theorist. Damasio's proposal was that consciousness occurs when there is sufficient simultaneous activation of multiple remote sites to which attention ('simultaneous enhancement of a pertinent set of activity against background activity') is brought to bear (Damasio 1989b: 128). While widely separated sites might be made 'coherent' and 'in-register' by their being simultaneous or being 'phase-locked' (Damasio 1989b: 124), there is nothing which fits NSDT's bill. The Phenomenal Array as a unitary physical artefact seems to have no plausible basis in that proposal. Non-parcellation seems to be a property of a hierarchy of convergence zones, *scripts* or *recipes*, as it were, for the simultaneous or phase-locked activation of a repertoire of *disjoint* neural ensembles each dedicated to its own perceptual attribute (Damasio 1989b: 128–9). How this gives rise to what we are aware of in our phenomenology is unclear, to say the least, and, if anything, implies 'parcellation' because distinct sense attributes are reconstituted unbound or disjointly in space. How they get bound in the phenomenology is nowhere addressed. Mere scripts for assembly do not in themselves suffice for assembly per se.

Semir Zeki has proposed something in a number of ways similar: distributed *conscious* instantiations of *individual sensory attributes*. His work on the localization of dedicated processing for particular sensory attributes in the extrastriate cortex has led him to promote a doctrine of 'microconsciousnesses'. He conceives of the distribution of what is experienced as being in a neural archipelago as opposed to in a unitary site. The functional specializations of V4 and V5 provide Zeki with what he calls the 'cornerstone' for a theory of multiple microconsciousnesses. The separation or autonomy of the input paths, the differential consequences of lesions in the respective areas (achromotopsia in V4, akinetopsia in V5), and the autonomy or 'juxtaconvergence' (Shipp and Zeki 1995) of outgoing paths to other areas, point, according to Zeki, to the conclusion that 'the consciousnesses of elementary visual attributes are distinct from one another' (Zeki 2003: 214).

Zeki's microconsciousnesses are very surprising, because, again, it is very hard to conceive of a phenomenology—in normal experience—which comes in only one modality at a time. He has defended his view by appeal to the functional segregation by modality in the extrastriate cortex, a double dissociation argument on V4 and V5,[6] and a rather far-reaching interpretation of Riddoch Syndrome—a variant on blindsight.

[6] Mathematical simulations by Malcolm Young and his colleagues call into question the decisiveness of double dissociation arguments in the case of cortical functions. See Young and Scannell (2000). See also Young et al. (2000). Characteristic loss of functionality with cortical lesions may suggest a cortical locus for function which is illusory, as in the Sprague Effect, which I discuss below.

Zeki has written:

> One conclusion from the clinical evidence is that a microconsciousness for colour or visual motion is generated at a distinct processing site, and *therefore* that a processing site is also a perceptual site. (Zeki 2003: 214, emphasis added)

Zeki's conviction that there can be disjoint consciousnesses of instances of single modalities of perception is an alien notion for those who experience a phenomenology of what I take to be the usual kind, and it is certainly alien to NSDT.[7] NSTD implies a unitary Phenomenal Array, not an archipelago of arrays that are, respectively, devoted to colour, motion, figure, orientation, sound, or somatic sensation. Similar observations apply to Nancy Kanwisher's hypothesis that rejects the (Naive) notion of 'a single unitary consciousness system' and affirms, along with Zeki, that 'each conscious perceptual content is represented in the same set of neurons that analyze the perceptual information in the first place' (Kanwisher 2001: 109). She has proposed that particular classes of multi-modally bound *percept* (e.g. face, house) occur at widely separate locales in the brain (e.g. fusiform face area, hippocampal place area). On this account, one might suppose, a face seen against the background of a house would seem to involve components which are spatially remote in a way not reflected in the phenomenology. If I am aware of (the percept of) a face close up and moving from left to right across the central visual meridian, am I supposed to conclude that the right side of the face is in the fusiform gyrus of my left cortex while its *motion* is in left V5, and, correspondingly, that the left side of the face and its motion are segregated appropriately in the other cortical hemisphere? This is hard to understand: at least, Naivete says so. (DRists too, we can note, have a spatially distributed array of disjoint 'percepts', but their combination into a unitary Phenomenal Array has an initially plausible rationale that reflects the centrality of the retinal viewpoint and the physical optics involved.) In the face of these problems of assembly of remote shards of consciousness, Sense-Datum Theorists might permit themselves some satisfaction at seeing accusations of 'spooky stuff' or 'mystical' happenings going elsewhere for a change.

Zeki and ffytche (1998) observed from their fMRI studies of Riddoch Syndrome patient, G.Y., that the variability between the patient's aware and unaware conditions in response to motion stimuli matched discernible neural variation. They concluded that the transition from the unconscious to the conscious awareness of motion varies with the level of activity uniquely in area V5, and reasoned that if V5 were required to

[7] Zeki also stresses the lack of synchrony in our experience of different attributes as counting against 'a single, unified consciousness' (Zeki 2003: 214). See also Zeki and Bartels (1998). For Zeki, what I call 'the problem of remote assembly' appears in both spatial and temporal dimensions. Zeki appeals to a hierarchical structure in order to ground what he calls 'macroconsicousness' (Zeki 2003: 217).

relay to some 'master integrator' then activity should have been discovered also at that ulterior site. No such cortical activity was detected.

Zeki and ffytche *did* see other activity, but it was in the *medulla*, not the cortex. Their educated guess was that the activity was in the ascending reticular formation, although the resolution of their fMRI did not permit precise confirmation of that. They gave no hint that subcortical activity might be linked to a 'master integrator'. Other researchers have proposed that 'cortico-centrism' may be leading us astray, as we now see.

14.4.3 Subcortical laminar maps

Some philosophers are fond of pointing out that having a representation of a spatial array of objects does not require the representation to be a spatial array of representations of the respective objects. However, while it is not obligatory, it is at least optional. Taking up the option commits no philosophical error or fallacy. The brain frequently elects for it. It widely uses retinotopic and spatiotopic maps, as well as other topographical representations. The most startling is the dorsal lateral geniculate nucleus (LGNd) in the thalamus. The congruence of the distinct retinal maps of magno-, parvo-, and koino-cellular projections (from hemifields of both eyes) in the respective layers of each LGNd is so precise that target mappings are aligned, as one author put it, 'like one of the toothpicks in a club sandwich' (Walls 1953, cited in Sherman and Guillery 2006: 327). However, those mappings bring into registry only a proper subset of variables in only the visual modality.

But consider the superior colliculi. Each colliculus has the wide range of modalities we are looking for and, like the lateral geniculate nucleus, employs the device of careful alignment of laminar structures to bring different dimensions of sensory experience into close registry—one of the key elements of the Naive SDT to which I give some credence. Unlike the LGN, the superior colliculi offer a wider synthesis. Laminar structures bring into registry retinotopic, somatosensory, and auditory spaces. This is arguably what is required for the entire Phenomenal Array.

Sprague (1966) has observed that cats whose primary visual and extrastriate cortex had been removed on one side unsurprisingly lost the capacity to detect and orient towards targets in the contralateral visual field. After the removal of the contralateral superior colliculus or after sectioning of the anterior commisure which connects the two superior colliculi, those competences returned, very surprisingly.

This seeming redundancy of the cortex may appear to be a challenge for those who propose cortical sites for neural correlates of consciousness, or at least those of core consciousness. The Sprague Effect, together with the more or less normally conducted lives of decorticated rodents, arguable signs of consciousness in hydranencephalic human infants devoid of much or all cortex, and the striking preservation of consciousness and functionality of patients subject to partial decortications (while conscious!) prompt Bjorn Merker (2007) to propose that the resources for consciousness lie subcortically rather than cortically.

Merker focuses on the superior colliculus (SC), which is one of the most studied sites in the brain. Conventionally, SC is understood to be a lynchpin in the brain's system for orientation of the head, the eye, and in the appropriate mammals, the ear. Importantly, it contributes to the regimentation of saccades. It takes early delivery of information from the optic tract and is remarkable for its capacity for 'intermodal integration', which serves to remedy some of the profound complexities which arise for animals like us that have mobile receptor arrays, like our eyes and cats' and dogs' ears.

The crucial structure in this locus is what Merker calls the 'selection triangle' which embodies the interaction of target selection, motivational state, and ultimately the selection of action. In terms that an advocate of SDT can only warm to, Merker proposes that the 'conscious mode of function' associated with SC grounds the interactions in the selection triangle in 'the general form of a *neural analog reality simulation*'. He envisages:

> an analog (spatial) mobile 'body' (action domain) embedded within a movement-stabilized analog (spatial) 'world' (target domain) via a shared spatial coordinate system subject to bias from motivational variables, and supplying a premotor output for the control of the full species-specific orienting reflex. (Merker 2007: 76)

In addition, in terms reminiscent of Prichard's Diagnostic, Merker emphasizes 'the synthetic nature of what we typically take to be physical reality itself' (Merker 2007: 73). This synthetic scene has a coordinate system 'lodged in the head representation of the simulated analog *visual* body, say in close proximity to its analog eye region' (Merker 2007: 71). He judges that:

> [t]here is reason to believe that the implicit 'ego center' origin of this coordinate space is the position that we ourselves occupy when we are conscious, and that the analog body and analog world of that space is what we experience as and call our tangible, concrete body and external world... (Merker 2007: 72)
>
> In its peculiar nesting of a body inside a world, around an ego-center in a shared coordinate space subject to motivational bias, this interface possesses the essential attributes of phenomenal consciousness. (Merker 2007: 73)

As resonant as it seems to NSDT, Merker's view might over-reach. Given that we are considering the prospects for Naive SDT, could the superior colliculus be the locus of the Phenomenal Array? It is certainly true that SC has the capacity to bind auditory and somesthetic with visual, including chromatic (White et al. 2009), projections, so it meets the necessary condition of multimodality. In addition, SC achieves multimodality by the superposition of laminae corresponding to the respective modalities. That is to say, it does it by assembling spatial maps and bringing them into registry—a difficult task, given that different modalities come from sources with different metrics. Consequently, we can see in SC the resources for a spatial Phenomenal Array.

Consider the difficulties. First, there are two superior colliculi, left and right, connected by the callosal anterior commisure. Is one SC the unique locus of the whole Phenomenal Array? If not, then how are the two overlapping halves of the sensory fields brought into registry? I discuss this problem more generally below. Second, what confidence do we have that in decorticated cats, the functionality of the gaze and visual orientation is not an *unconscious* system, as the dorsal stream is argued to be (Goodale and Milner 2004)? The cats are not in a position to report on any experience.

One human case of likely Sprague Effect, now deceased, was able to report the initial loss and then some restoration of conscious functionality, after coincidentally a cyst invaded his left superior colliculus. This shut down the inhibitory projections to the right colliculus causing its reactivation. However, his initial visual disruption was not from lesions to the visual cortex but to the pre-frontal cortex (Weddell 2004). Consequently, because primary and extrastriate cortices were intact, we cannot preclude the possibility that his consciousness still derived from the cortical level. If that were so, we cannot confidently eliminate the possibility that the cats and mice who function semi-normally without cortex do so without any phenomenology.

In the light of the issue of cortico-centrism, the development of Damasio's own thought has been intriguing. Parvizi and Damasio (2001) have proposed a *constitutive* role for the (subcortical) ascending reticular formation in mammalian consciousness. Two classes of evidence motivate them. The first is that damage to the upper brainstem causes coma and vegetative state. The second is that the reticular formation conditions 'wakeful and attentive states'. They observe:

> Such evidence supported a general account of the relationship between brainstem and consciousness that can be summarized as follows: (a) the brainstem contains the reticular formation which is the origin of the ascending reticular activating system; (b) the engagement of the ascending reticular activating system activates the cerebral cortex; (c) the process of activating the cortex underlies wakefulness and attention; and (d) wakefulness and attention are indispensable constituents of consciousness, or, as some might say, constitute consciousness.
>
> (Parvizi and Damasio 2001: 136)

Further, the authors distinguish two problems in investigating consciousness. The first is the problem of understanding how the brain yields a 'mental pattern' in any sensory modality. They loosely describe such mental patterns as 'images'.

> This first problem of consciousness is the problem of how we form a temporally and spatially unified 'movie-in-the-brain', a metaphorical movie, of course, with as many sensory tracks as the brain's sensory systems. Solving this first problem in neuroscientific terms consists in discovering how the brain makes neural patterns in its neural circuits and turns those neural patterns into the explicit mental patterns of the whole range of possible sensory images, which stand for any object, any relationship, concrete or abstract, any word or any sign.
>
> (Parvizi and Damasio 2001: 137)

However, they deny that there is any 'homunculus', preferring to have the 'owner and observer' of the 'movie' be merely a character in it.

Damasio seems to suppose that the limits within which the metaphor of the internal movie theatre applies exclude any audience for the movie. He gives no explicit guide to the employment of the metaphor, but it is not unnatural to suppose that he conceives of something like a screen, even if without a viewer. If that is right, then NSDT may be onto something. The surprise is that Damasio has sidestepped his own arguments against a cortical screen and proposed a subcortical one.

14.4.4 The problem of decussation and the left–right division of the cortex (and other sites)

Whether or not one embraces an archipelago model such as Zeki's or Kanwisher's, there is in any case a glaring need for assembly at a distance. It is due to the separation, for each sensory modality, of substantially distinct streams assigned to different *cortical hemispheres*. With that comes the division of a sensory target into rough halves which are represented in the cortex contralateral to each. Where relevant the same applies to subcortical structures.

Vision provides a dramatic case. After stimulation of the retina, projections via the optic nerves are segregated at the optic chiasm. This occurs in such a way that the projections from the right retinal hemifields of both eyes, 'nasal' for the left and 'temporal' for the right, which capture the left visual field, project to the right side of the brain. Similarly, the left eye's temporal hemifield and the right eye's nasal hemifield project via the optic chiasm to the left brain. The main projections are to the primary visual cortex, via the dorsal lateral geniculate nucleus (LGNd) of the thalamus, in what is commonly referred to as the retino-geniculate-(striate)-cortical pathway.

This division of the Visual Field into two near halves, overlapping at the central meridian roughly close to two degrees of arc, cannot be more important for the Naive Sense-Datum Theorist. For if we assume that there is a unitary neural site in which the visual, auditory, and somatosensory sensory inputs are brought into registry, so that our phenomenology may be taken at face value, there has to be substantial processing which can recombine the divided halves. Naturally we must ask what the corpus callosum contributes to the unification of the two halves to make up the Phenomenal Array. Here the preliminary answers are tantalizing but incomplete. Peculiarly, the primary visual cortices are *almost* completely 'acallosal'; for the most part, they lack connections via the corpus callosum. The exception is a set of spatiotopically ordered reciprocal connections between the interfaces of V1 and V2 in each cortex, and these are exclusively of the central meridian by which the two hemifields overlap. Clearly, there is communication between left and right visual cortex, but it is not at all clear how exactly it is to be useful. The connection is simple in that it is 'homotopic', so that projections are between mirror-image structures left and right. However, if I would like to know how my new jacket will look, I would hope that my tailor would be more informative than just telling me how well the buttons on the right side match with the button holes on the left side. Clearly, if the Naivete of NSDT is to be vindicated, some additional operations will be required so that the two full halves of the Phenomenal Array can be brought into proper juxtaposition along their common 'seam'.

Because the corpus callosum is not a good candidate for the locus of assembly, we might entertain the idea that the whole assembly is in one hemisphere. If this were the case, there would likely be idiosyncratic pathologies which reflect the failure to link up the halves appropriately. Simple lack of registry between the left and right eyes would not do. On the other hand, hemianopia and hemineglect have some of the properties that might be symptomatic of the failure of interhemispheric callosal connections. Further, the well-known asymmetry of the hemispheres in this regard favours the right parietal cortex as the locus, since right parietal lesions with left visual field loss of competence is the statistical norm, though with exceptions. Expert opinion leans towards interpreting hemineglect as a failure of attention rather than of vision (Mesulam 1999). For NSDT, a crucial issue would be the finding of empirical means for distinguishing degradation of attention or awareness from failure of formation of the Phenomenal Array.

14.5 Are the Sensorium and Phenomenal Array Three-Dimensional?

Must the Phenomenal Array be a simulacrum of the seen external environment? If it is, then it may well be expected to be *three-dimensional*, although it could scarcely be uniformly scaled across dimensions. Further, there is no plan or side elevation view of our environment with us in it. It is not so much Super Mario as Doom that sets out the phenomenology, dictated initially by our retinocentric perspective. A 3D Array is not an inappropriate starting guess, because we preserve, in our Naivete, what it is reasonable to take from Direct Realism. Direct Realists have no problem on that front. The Direct Realist Phenomenal Array is the trivial simulacrum; it is the very array of visible parts of the world *itself*, and it is, accordingly, spatially three-dimensional. There is plenty of volume in the world for the facing surfaces that we see and are aware of on the DR account. But the brain offers a tighter space for the SDTists' objects of awareness.

Let's consider a simple, if artificial, visual experience. Consider Figure 14.1, which I will discuss again below for different reasons. Viewers usually see in (a) a central square nearer than the surround, and in (b) a square behind the surround or 'vignette'. The effects are, however, a little labile, and, in either graphic, the square can momentarily shift from nearer to further or conversely. Suppose, then, that there is a cerebral *volume* in which the components of the Phenomenal Array in this momentary effect are segregated into separate planes. Three planes are implicated, for the nearer square, for the surround, and for the further square, although only two at a time with the surround being in common. Consider first the simple hypothesis that the generation of the planar surround and detached planar square are surface effects of some neural array, made available to the awareness and attention of the subject. (This is a Naive assumption; it is the sort of thing that a Direct Realist with a scientific bent might consider for colour or lightness on a body's surface.) Then there should be a local neural surface to ground the front square, another to ground the remote square, and, presumably, one for the surround in the periphery. Note that when the forward square vanishes, the space appears empty all the way through the middle of the surround up to the remote square which has now appeared.

The Sensorium, the space in which the Phenomenal Array is constructed, will rarely if ever be full, in the sense of being everywhere occupied by elements of some Phenomenal Array. In the case of Figure 14.1, it is mostly empty of sense data. Natural scenes often involve many more visual planes This is instructive because it points to the Sensorium's being sufficiently densely occupied with neural structure that elements of the Phenomenal Array can be generated presumably almost anywhere within it. If that is so, then we learn something about the capacities of awareness and attention. They are insensitive to certain classes of neural arrangements, as, for example, the inactive neural surface which initially yielded the nearer centre square. Such an insensitivity should absolutely not be confused with transparency. This scenario seems to suggest that sometimes activated neural arrays generate elements of a Phenomenal Array to which awareness and attention respond, and other times, not suitably activated, they are undetected. The processes of selective detection would present a significant investigative problem.

Perhaps we should say, given the above assumptions, that the neural underpinnings of the elements of the Phenomenal Array are *always* 'invisible' to awareness and attention. For it is striking that, if what we are aware of is an array requiring a volume in the brain, then we do not experience something like the graphical representations of structures of neurons that we see in neurology texts or in Ramon y Cajal's exquisite drawings, even allowing for the fact that the living cells have not been stained or do not phosphoresce. What we are aware of is very different in character from those complex discrete structures. Perhaps it is not the neuronal arrays, neuronal bodies, axons, arborizations, and so on, themselves, that constitute the Phenomenal Array. Conservatively, supposing that contemporary physics (rather than 'neo-physical' variables) suffices, we might suppose electric fields—at least, classically conceived—to be starting candidates to explain continuous expanses in the Phenomenal Array.[8]

[8] On such an assumption, how the phenomenal might be ploughed back into the neuronal might be illuminated by the recognition of the influence of ephaptic potentials on synchronization in ambient neurons. See Weiss and Faber 2010 and Anastassiou et al. 2010).

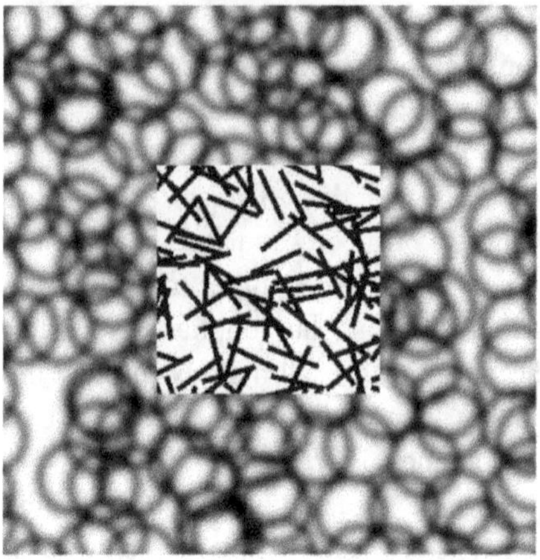
(a)

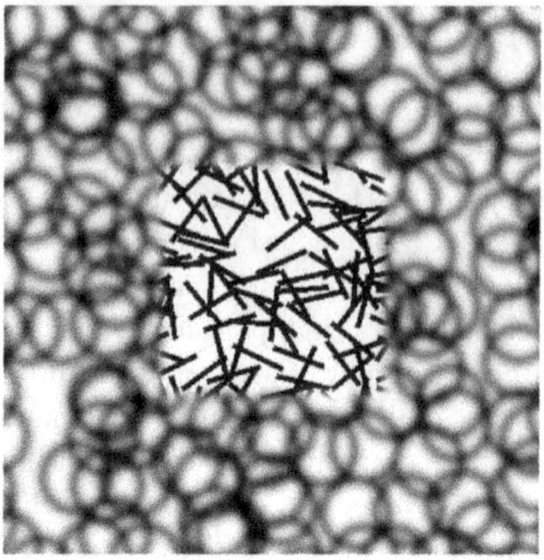
(b)

Figure 14.1 Courtesy of Optical Society of America, from Marshall et al. (1996: 682).

14.5.1 Is the phenomenal array two-dimensional?

A voluminous Sensorium containing multiple planes of visual sense data as well as other phenomenal qualities is not the only possibility at the level of Naive assumptions. Could the Sensorium and Phenomenal Array be two-dimensional? This is a highly counter-intuitive view, and no doubt for many readers preposterous. I think it is not preposterous, and that it is sufficient for the details of our phenomenology. First, note that at any given fixation only the segment of the visual Phenomenal Array corresponding to the foveal region of the retina offers the sharply delineated figure–ground separations and occlusions characteristic of focused vision. The foveal region contributes to the Phenomenal Array roughly one–two degrees of apparent arc, which is about the area of the tops of two thumbs held together at arm's length. Only a very small portion of the Phenomenal Array is so tidily formed at each fixation. The antidote to that is, of course, that we re-fixate relentlessly. What are the crucial variables in the phenomenology of depth vision? Let's see what the crucial variables are in the different responses one has to (a) and (b) in Figure 14.1 (Marshall et al. 1996: 682. See also Mather and Smith 2000).

There are several attributes in play here. One is surface blur, and the central square and the surround differ in blur. Another is edge blur. We see, typically although not without exception, the centre square in (a) in front of the plane of the surround. In (b), we seem to be focused on the inner square behind the outer plane. Why? The crucial difference does not depend on colour, texture gradient, stereopsis, vergence, or even surface blur (that is held constant), but on *which of the inner objects owns the sharp boundary.*[9] In more natural targets, many other factors enter into the formation of the Phenomenal Array and its apparent depth structure. In addition, movement introduces parallactic variation which, like stereopsis within relatively near distances, dominates other cues. Stereopsis permits quantitative estimates of depth, as does accommodation, but I propose that the net effect in the construction of the phenomenology is no different in principle from the static case given in Figure 14.1. Quantitative estimates of depth arising from parallax in movement do not result in the experience of depth per se, but in the appropriate rate of displacement of the distant surface against a foreground target.

Even if the Phenomenal Array were 3D, its appearance, I propose, would be indistinguishably replicated by a 2D surface with the appropriate combination of sharp contours, contour blur, surface blur, texture gradients, and luminance variation in the foveal zone. Having the production of colours or brightness, say, on a surface rather than in a 3D volume in the brain reduces the need for remote neurological influences in the formation of sensations, and is conformable to the brain's efficient use of *laminar* structures in the cortex generally, and in 'binding' devices such as the superior colliculus and the lateral geniculate nucleus.

If this proposal is correct, which I am sure many readers will doubt,[10] then our judgements that we are aware of depth in the Phenomenal Array might well be taken to be what Titchener called *Stimulus Error*: we allow our phenomenological reports to be biased by what we know to be true of the world outside us. As E. G. Boring put it '[w]e commit the stimulus-error if we base our psychological reports upon objects rather than upon the mental material itself, or if, in the psycho-physical experiment, we make judgments of the stimulus and not judgments of sensation' (Boring 1921: 451). That we might make such a Stimulus Error is a natural consequence of what I will call the Grand Stimulus Error, that of judging that the Phenomenal Array is the world outside our bodies.

14.6 Concluding Observations

In this brief commentary on NSDT, I have tried to illustrate some ways in which we might give up some Naivete in the face of SDT's interpretation of facts of perceptual psychology or of neuroscience. Thus, most prominently, my suggestion that the Phenomenal Array is 2D requires stepping back from the Naive (and Direct Realist) assumption that it and the Sensorium are voluminous. The merits of the suggestion

[9] I am very struck by the discrepancy, on fixation, between the utter immobility of the central target and the slight movement of the surround, perhaps reflecting microsaccadic displacements. Perhaps the discrepancy can be added to the factors that enhance the delineation of sharp contours.

[10] See, however, Jonathan Lowe's chapter in this volume.

must ultimately be decided by empirical work in the context of rich and detailed modelling, but, if it is true, then it moves the explanatory goal posts closer; the brain's widespread exploitation of laminar mappings, especially in the universally laminar neo-cortex, seems to offer a more congenial environment for something like screens, rather than theatres with deep stages and sets—with or without an audience. And there is well-known precedent in the philosophical literature for such a claim.

In addition, I have indicated that SDT's interpretation of examples involving depth perception might require us to think more explicitly than hitherto about the division of labour between phenomenal qualities on the one hand, and awareness and attention on the other. In the 3D understanding of the Phenomenal Array, it seems likely that we have to describe and explain a selectivity in the capacity of awareness to detect some artefacts of the brain while ignoring others in the same space.

If there is some encouragement for SDTists in all this, there is also the prospect of even more radical and surprising transformations of central SDT commitments. Consider well-known effects of variation of attention on the qualitative character we experience. Ned Block lists (perceived-) contrast, colour saturation, spatial frequency, gap size, speed, and flicker rate as perceptual qualities which focal attention can alter (Block 2010: 33). He classifies these perceived attributes as 'perceptual qualities', by which he means 'the relevant phenomenological qualities of the perceptual states that ground the perceiver's knowledge of objective contrast, saturation, etc.' (Block 2010: 34).

This dependency of phenomenology on attentional factors might be accounted for in more than one way within SDT models. One version would be, let us call it, 'perfect' or invariant attention with variation in Sense-Datum. Another would be imperfect or variant attention with no variation in the Sense-Datum. Another would be a hybrid of the two.

If we were to have evidence that favoured the second or third version, then the SDTist may well be compelled to concede a point of principle to the Intentionalist Representationalist. Usually, SDT is committed to the assumption that the qualities that things appear to have in experience are actually instantiated in the sense data. If one phenomenology is different from another because of a variation in attention, and not uniquely because of variation of the Sense-Datum, then at least one of them is an experience of apparent phenomenal qualities which are not there. Indeed, if awareness and attention are always in some degree imperfect, there may be a case for saying that although there really are sense data with determinate phenomenal qualities, what is generally experienced in the phenomenology are qualities that are not present in the Phenomenal Array.[11]

[11] I wish to thank Sam Coleman for acute and very helpful comments on an earlier draft of this chapter, and to thank an anonymous referee for valuable suggestions.

References

Anastassiou, C.A., Perin, R., Markram, H., and Koch, C. (2010), 'Ephaptic coupling of cortical neurons', in *Nature Neuroscience* 14: 217–24.

Block, N. (2010), 'Attention and mental paint', in *Philosophical Issues* 20: 23–63.

Boring, E. G. (1921), 'The stimulus error', in *American Journal of Psychology* 32: 449–71.

Damasio, A. R. (1989a), 'Time-locked Multiregional Retroactivation: A systems level proposal for the neural substrates of recall and recognition', in *Cognition* 33 (1–2): 25–62.

Damasio, A. R. (1989b), 'The brain binds entities and events by multiregional activation from convergence zones', in *Neural Computation* 1: 123–32.

Damasio, A. R. (1994), *Descartes' error: emotion, reason, and the human brain* (New York: Putnam).

Dennett, D. C., and Kinsbourne, M. (1992), 'Time and the observer', in *Behavioral and Brain Sciences* 15: 183–247.

Driver, J., and Noesselt, T. (2008), 'Multisensory interplay reveals crossmodal influences on "sensory-specific" brain regions, neural responses, and judgments', in *Neuron* 57: 11–23.

Evans, G. (1985), *Collected papers* (Oxford: Clarendon Press).

Goodale, M. A., and Milner, A. D. (2004), *Sight unseen: An exploration of conscious and unconscious vision* (Oxford; New York: Oxford University Press).

Hardin, C. L. (1988), *Color for philosophers: Unweaving the rainbow* (Indianapolis, IN: Hackett).

Hardin, C. L. (1990), 'Color and Illusion', in W. G. Lycan (ed.), *Mind and Cognition: A Reader*, 1st edition (Cambridge, MA: Blackwell Publishers), 555–67.

Huemer, M. (2001), *Skepticism and the veil of perception* (Lanham, MD: Rowman and Littlefield).

Jackson, F. (1977), *Perception: A representative theory* (Cambridge: Cambridge University Press).

Jameson, D., and Hurvich, L. M. (1955), 'Some quantitative aspects of an opponent-colors theory. I. Chromatic responses and spectral saturation', in *Journal of the Optical Society of America* 45: 546–52.

Kanwisher, N. (2001), 'Neural events and perceptual awareness', in *Cognition* 79: 89–113.

Macaluso, E. (2006), 'Multisensory processing in sensory-specific cortical areas', in *Neuroscientist* 12: 327–38.

Macaluso, E., and Driver, J. (2005), 'Multisensory spatial interactions: A window onto functional integration in the human brain', in *Trends in Neurosciences* 28: 264–71.

Macaluso, E., Frith, C. D., and Driver, D. (2002), 'Directing attention to locations and to sensory modalities: Multiple levels of selective processing revealed with PET', in *Cerebral Cortex* 12: 357–68.

Manzoni, T., Barbaresi, P., Conti, F., and Fabri, M. (1989), 'The callosal connections of the primary somatosensory cortex and the neural bases of midline fusion', in *Experimental Brain Research* 76: 251–66.

Marshall, J. A., Burbeck, C. A., Ariely, D., Rolland, J. P., and Martin, K. E. (1996), 'Occlusion edge blur: A cue to relative visual depth', in *Journal of the Optical Society of America* 13: 681–8.

Mather, G., and Smith, D. R. (2000), 'Depth cue integration: Stereopsis and image blur', in *Vision Research* 40: 3501–6.

Merker, B. (2007), 'Consciousness without a cerebral cortex: A challenge for neuroscience and medicine', in *Behavioral and Brain Sciences* 30: 63–81; discussion: 81–134.

Mesulam, M.-M. (1999), 'Spatial attention and neglect: Parietal, frontal and cingulate contributions to the mental representation and attentional targeting of salient extrapersonal events', in *Philosophical Transactions of the Royal Society of London* B 354: 1325–46.

Nassau, K. (2001), *The physics and chemistry of colour*, 2nd revised edition (New York: Wiley).

Parvizi, J., and Damasio, A. (2001), 'Consciousness and the brainstem', *Cognition* 79: 135–59.

Pautz, A. (2007), 'Intentionalism and Perceptual Presence', in *Philosophical Perspectives* 21: 495–541.

Prichard, H. A. (1950), *Knowledge and perception: essays and lectures* (Oxford: Clarendon Press).

Sherman, S. M., and Guillery, R. W. (2006), *Exploring the thalamus and its role in cortical function* (Cambridge, MA: MIT Press).

Shipp, S., and Zeki, S. (1995), 'Segregation and convergence of specialised pathways in macaque monkey visual cortex', in *Journal of Anatomy* 187: 547–62.

Sprague, J. M. (1966), 'Interaction of cortex and superior colliculus in mediation of visually guided behavior in the cat', in *Science* 153: 1544–7.

Tootell, R. B., Mendola, J. D., Hadjikhani, N. K., Liu, A. K., and Dale, A. M. (1998), 'The representation of the ipsilateral visual field in human cerebral cortex', in *Proceedings of the National Academy of Sciences* 95: 818–24.

Walls, G. L. (1953), 'The lateral geniculate nucleus and visual histophysiology', in *University of California Publications in Physiology* 9: 1–100.

Weddell, R. A. (2004), 'Subcortical modulation of spatial attention including evidence that the Sprague effect extends to man', in *Brain and Cognition*, 55 (3): 497–506.

Weiss, S. A., and Faber, D. S. (2010), 'Field effects in the CNS play functional roles', in *Frontiers in Neural Circuits* 4: 1–10.

White, B. J., Boehne, S. E., Marino, R. A., Itti, L., and Munoz, D. P. (2009), 'Color-related signals in the primate superior colliculus', in *Journal of Neuroscience* 30: 12159–66.

Young, M. P., and Scannell, J. W. (2000), 'Brain structure-function relationships: Advances from neuroinformatics', in *Philosophical Transactions of the Royal Society of London* B 355: 3–6.

Young, M. P., Hilgetag, C. C., and Scannell, J. W. (2000), 'On imputing function to structure from the behavioural effects of brain lesions', in *Philosophical Transactions of the Royal Society of London* B 355: 147–61.

Zeki, S. (2001), 'Localization and globalization in conscious vision', in *Annual Review of Neuroscience* 24: 57–86.

Zeki, S. (2003), 'The disunity of consciousness', in *Trends in Cognitive Science* 7: 214–18.

Zeki, S., and Bartels, A. (1998), 'The asychrony of consciousness', in *Philosophical Transactions of the Royal Society of London* B 265: 1583–5.

Zeki, S., and ffytche, D. H. (1998), 'The Riddoch syndrome: Insights into the neurobiology of conscious vision', in *Brain* 121: 25–45.

Index

Ability hypothesis, 42
Abramov, I., 45, 283, 285
Absolute processes, 79, 80–5, 87
Access consciousness *see* Consciousness, access-
Achromatopsia, 205, 287–8, 410
Acquaintance, 4–6, 7, 16, 106, 116, 121–4, 126–7, 165, 169, 174, 187, 219, 220
  knowledge by, 219, 405
  quasi-, 98
  real, 16–17, 122–4, 125, 127–38, 141
  semi-, 134–6
  structural, 135
Adverbialism, 224, 235
After-image, 2, 17, 160, 163–4, 167–9, 171, 377, 380
Akinetopsia, 410
Allen, K., 186
Allport, A., 347, 349
Alston, W., 150
Anastassiou, C. A., 417
Andermann, F., 191
Anscombe, G. E. M., 11, 163
Anterior cingulate cortex (ACC), 319–20
Anti-physicalism (immaterialism), 16, 121–2, 138, 401, 405
Antirealism (*see also* Realism), 258–60, 262–3, 265–6, 270, 272–3
Aristotle, 20, 34, 48, 61, 365
Armstrong, D., 73, 74, 84, 86, 98, 119, 121, 126, 190, 289
Arnauld, A., 214–15, 225, 233
Arnheim, R., 365
Asher, J. E., 379
Atkinson, G., 392
Attention, 5, 25–6, 94, 123, 124, 183, 199, 204, 209, 244, 247, 249–50, 300, 305, 392, 406–7, 409–10, 414, 416, 417, 420
  as condition for synaesthesia, 377–8, 384–5
  bias due to, 40, 44
  covert, 353
  grounding demonstrative reference, 42
  overt, 353
  taxonomy of processes of, 349–71
  visual, 347–71
Attentional binding, 355–6, 360, 362, 364–6, 370
Attentional blink, 357
Attentional filtering (gating), 25, 353–5, 359–61, 362, 365, 368–70
Attentional holding, 356–8, 366, 369
Attentional individuating (indexing), 358, 367
Attentional sampling, 25, 352–3, 361
Attridge, G., 274
Audition (hearing), 1, 2, 35, 48, 49, 52–3, 55, 59–60, 195, 239, 243, 247, 376, 389, 412, 414–15
  synaesthetic concurrent, 378
  experience, 195, 303, 325, 381, 389
  imagery, 325
  qualities of, 1, 44, 55
  stimulus, 50–1, 54–6, 58
Augustine, 216
Austin, J. L., 177
Auvray, M., 379, 381, 393
Avant, L. L., 43
Awareness, 5, 7, 47, 69, 71, 79, 95–6, 147, 165, 171, 181, 188, 191
  act of, 164–5, 167, 204, 250, 331, 341, 407, 416–17, 420
  awareness of (*see also* Experience, self-intimation of), 227, 228, 246–50
  C-, 243, 247, 249
  cognitive, 184, 209
  conscious, 2–3, 23, 70–1, 76–8, 181, 192, 198–9, 278, 341, 407, 411
  direct, 98
  higher-level, 305
  immediate, 10, 22, 181, 184–7, 204, 207, 210
  introspective (*see also* Introspection), 23, 34
  non-conceptual, 5, 22, 182–4
  object of, 148, 150, 156, 160–3, 165–7, 169–70, 172, 174–5, 177, 416
  of colour difference/sameness, 278, 289
  of self, 182
  partial, 363
  perceptual, 185, 188, 208, 250
  relational model of, 96–8
  sensible, 174
  sensory, 147, 148, 151–2, 160, 162, 164, 166, 168–9, 171, 175, 178, 182, 190, 197–8, 242, 316, 367, 406
  subjective, 35–7, 40–5, 47, 49, 51, 204
  tactual, 153
  unconscious, 217
  visual, 161, 201, 205–6
Aydede, M., 301, 307
Ayer, A. J., 5, 156, 166

Baars, B. J., 328, 360
Bach-y-Rita, P., 58
Bahrami, B., 359

Balog, K., 37, 106, 107, 112, 117, 122, 123, 131, 136
Baldwin, T., 149, 159, 160, 165, 171
Ballard, D. H., 353
Banissy, M. J., 379
Barlow, H. B., 353
Baron-Cohen, S., 54, 379
Bartolomeo, P., 354
Bayne, T., 218, 226, 381, 382
Becklen, R., 362, 366
Behaviourism, 93, 107, 108, 109
Bela Julez stereogram, 199
Belief, 162, 219, 327
  about phenomenal qualities, 124, 131, 133
  dispositional, 331
  hallucinatory (*see also* Hallucination), 7
  implicit/explicit, 331
  in external world, 271
  introspective, 133
  perceptual, 8, 128, 133, 184, 187, 197, 199, 202, 209, 216, 316, 404
Bennett, J. F., 12
Berger, J., 34, 43
Berkeley, G., 48, 239, 240, 266, 271
Berlin, B., 45
Bhaumik, K., 394
Binding (*see also* Attentional binding), 26, 281, 351, 356, 358, 360, 361, 364, 368, 369, 370, 377, 382, 406, 410, 419
  codes, 409
  feature, 355
  part, 355
  position, 356
  reflexive, 355, 363
Binocular rivalry, 362, 384
Bisiach, E., 354, 362
Blindsight, 3, 69, 97, 224, 329, 331, 410
  super, 332–3
Blackburn, S., 89
Block, N., 12, 13, 14, 24, 33, 73, 106, 112, 114–17, 122, 138, 201, 218, 300, 305, 324, 327–32, 334, 361, 363, 365, 366, 420
Bohm, D., 86, 87, 92
BonJour, L., 216
Boring, E. G., 419
Braun, D., 311
Braun, J., 352, 362, 364
Breitmeyer, B. G., 36
Brentano, F., 8, 227, 325
Brewer, A., 287
Brewer, B., 236, 279, 280
Bridgeman, B., 361
Broad, C. D., 80, 148, 149, 150, **174**
Broadbent, D. E., 348
Brogaard, B., 380
Burge, T., 301
Busch, N. A., 367
Byrne, A., 4, 6, 11, 39, 150, 161, 163, 188, 300
Campbell, J., 6, 181, 188, 236
Canberra plan, 139
Carnap, R., 93, 98
Carpenter, R. H. S., 353
Casati, R., 60
Carruthers, P., 326, 327
Cartesian theatre, 406, 407
Cartwright, R., 171
Cassam, Q., 166
Causation, 90–1, 182, 307
  condition of perception, 235
  physical, 84
  qualia of, 90
Ceivism, 244–5
Chabris, C. F., 366
Chalmers, D. J., 11, 13, 14, 19, 36, 37, 42, 96, 107, 117, 118, 123, 128, 137, 139, 218, 328, 381, 382
Change blindness, 218, 357, 366, 369
Changeux, J.-P. 361, 367, 368, 369
Charles Bonnet syndrome (*see also* Hallucination), 8, 191
Cheesman, J., 40
Chisholm, R. M., 5, 149, 150, 153, 159, 160, 163, 169
Chokron, S., 354
Chong, S. C., 363
Chuard, P., 280
Chun M. M., 218, 347, 350, 352
Churchland, P., 116
Clark, A., 6, 38
Clarke, T., 153
Coates, P., 6, 10, 12, 182, 184, 195, 197, 208, 236
Cognitive penetration, 326
Cohen, J., 282
Cohen, M. A., 347, 360, 363, 369
Cohen Kadosh, R., 393
Coleman, S., 3, 79, 97
Colour, 1, 14, 15, 22, 23, 25, 37, 48, 50, 52, 74, 82, 87, 90, 98, 103, 112, 117, 148, 167, 169, 174, 175, 176, 178, 181, 183, 187, 189, 190, 191, 198, 199, 202, 204, 205, 206, 208, 209, 216, 238, 240, 242, 274, 281, 283, 302, 326, 349, 353, 379–80, 381, 382, 383, 387, 400, 405, 411, 417
  anomia, 288
  as universals, 167
  as-we-see-it, 216–17, 241, 242
  Augustinian, 216–17, 241
  binary, 403
  blindness, 203, 206, 207
  categories, 46
  centre, 286–7
  composite, 202
  concepts, 117, 186, 276, 279–80
  constancy, 162, 183, 218, 284, 286, 288
  contrast, 261

dreaming, 81
experience of, 42, 46, 111, 116, 176, 201, 202, 203, 204, 206, 217, 218, 227, 239, 241, 247, 284, 301, 361, 363–4, 371, 388–9
generation of, 402–3, 419
impressionism, 187–8
intransitivity of indiscriminability of, 24, 289–95
memory, 275, 287
mental, 34, 35, 39, 42–7, 49, 276
objective, 210
ontology of, 276
opponent-process theory of, 205, 277, 285, 403
particles, 78–80
perception, 41, 204, 276, 278, 280, 282, 289, 291, 292, 295, 353, 357
phenomenal, 10, 202, 204, 206, 210, 267, 269, 277, 402
physical, 41, 52, 200–1
primitivism, 188
process, 84
response, 274–80, 287–8, 291, 292, 295, 378
sensation, 54, 55, 241
simultaneous contrast, 42–3
space, 37–8, 45, 282, 402
spectrum, 93
-stuff, 81, 84–5, 87
synaesthetic (*see also* Synaesthesia), 382
vision *see* Vision, colour
Concept, 9, 108, 110, 118, 125, 209, 210, 219, 257, 259, 279, 314, 326, 339, 388
descriptive, 132
demonstrative, 98, 219, 279–80
empirical, 116
formation, 365
geometrical, 199
hybrid, 132
indexical, 125
low-level, 10, 182
mathematical, 272
mental, 121
neurological, 19
non-conscious, 340
phenomenal *see* Phenomenal concept
physical, 13, 15, 16, 17–19, 21, 108, 272
physical-functional, 121, 122
possession, 279–80
radically opaque, 131, 133, 139
recognitional, 23
sortal, 9, 257, 260, 262, 263, 265
spatial, 61, 199
topic neutral, 17
transparent, 126
vague, 333
Common factor, 190, 191
conception of experience, 195
view, 6
Conceptualism, 276, 280
Concurrent, 26, 378–90, 393
Conjunction detection, 356
Consciousness, 2–3, 9, 12–17, 19–21, 25, 27, 66, 75, 77, 87, 93, 95, 117, 175, 178, 182, 192, 209, 216, 236–8, 243–4, 248, 315, 323, 330, 333, 339, 342, 360, 410, 414
access-(A), 24, 26, 174, 324, 327–9, 331–2, 338, 341, 361, 366
altered states of, 392
background, 363
higher-order thought (HOT) theory of *see* Higher-order thought theory
micro, 410–11
neural correlates of, 412
object, 366
perceptual, 84, 182–3, 185, 192, 204–5, 226, 365
phenomenal (P-), 3, 5, 11, 14, 26, 69–70, 111, 150, 178, 183, 273, 324, 326, 361, 413
problem of, 14–19, 68–70, 107, 401, 414
relational analysis of, 71, 76, 95–7
sensory, 24, 167
stream of, 35
subjectivity of, 24
unconscious, 217
unity of, 381, 388, 411
Content, 12, 77, 187
as a set of possible worlds, 313–14
conceptual, 327, 340
conscious, 333, 338–42
contradictory, 386
gappy, 310–13
general, 310, 314
geometrical, 272
high-level, 326
imperative, 24, 300, 306–9
indicative, 24, 300, 308
individual, 193–5, 210–11
intentional, 9, 11, 39, 150, 403
mental, 226–7
nonconceptual, 9, 12, 23, 257–61, 266–7, 272–3, 279
non-representational, 272
object dependent, 229
of experience, 4, 8, 71, 104, 112, 185, 210, 226–9, 237, 272, 299–300, 302–3, 309–10, 313–17, 360, 368, 370, 377, 380–1, 383–4, 386, 390, 392–3
of imagination, 392
of thought, 24, 106, 219, 231, 314, 324, 327, 333, 337–42
perceptual, 163, 193, 231, 257–60, 263, 265–7, 272–3, 380, 386, 392, 411
phenomenal, 105, 270
qualitative, 70, 93, 104–5

Content, (*cont.*)
representational, 11, 14, 161, 193, 210, 222, 258, 266, 272, 276, 277, 279, 306, 310, 313–16, 337, 356, 360
representationalism, 317
Russellian, 279, 311–12
sensory, 10, 26, 167, 227, 340, 377, 393
singular, 193, 310–13
spatial/causal, 166, 386–7
synaesthetic, 395
unconscious, 338–41, 368
visual, 267, 272, 360, 384
wide/narrow, 227–31
Coslett, H. B., 357
Crane, T., 11, 189, 294, 386
Critical realism, 5, 182, 236
Crowne, D. P., 353
Cutter, B., 300, 316
Cytowic, R. E., 54, 379

Damasio, A. R., 406–9, 414–15
Damnjanovic, N., 138
Dark structure, 368
Da Silveira, R., 234
Darwin, C., 247
Davidoff, J., 288
De Brigard, F., 347, 361, 366, 369
Definite description, 152
Dehaene, S., 360, 367, 368, 369
Demircioglu, E., 17
Demonstrative, 42, 153
perceptual, 151, 257, 259–60, 263
reference, 187, 195–6
Dennett, D., 111, 118, 324, 328, 333, 360, 362, 406
De Rosa, R., 233
Deroy, O., 379, 381, 382, 392, 393
Descartes, R., 83, 91, 214–15, 225, 231–4, 242, 271
deVries, W. A., 81
de Weerd, P., 218
Diaphaneity (*see also* Transparency), 175, 177
Diaz-Leon, E., 138
Dienes, Z., 40
Direct realism, 6–10, 12, 22, 104, 150, 172, 181, 184–6, 190–6, 205, 210, 214–17, 221–5, 229–36, 241–6, 249, 401, 404, 406, 416–17, 419
about thought, 215
metaphysical objection to, 192
naive, 403–5, 419
phenomenological vs. metaphysical, 245–6, 250
real, 22
Disjunctivism, 6, 23, 105, 181, 186, 230, 310–11, 380, 405–6
about pain experience, 310
Display sentence, 97
Dixon, M. J., 377
Dokic, J., 60
Dorsal simultanagnosia, 357
Dosher, B. A., 352
Drake, D., 5, 182
Dretske, F., 121, 316, 380
Driver, J., 355, 408
Dualism, 16, 27, 75, 106, 112, 401, 402
Cartesian, 83, 232
conceptual, 16, 122, 124
property, 17, 84
Ducasse, C. J., 5
Duffy, P. L., 376
Dummett, M., 289

Eddington, A., 85, 137
Edge-detection, 283
Edquist, J., 383, 385
Egan, A., 184
Ekroll, V., 42
Eliminativism, 77, 95
Emergence, 72–3, 75, 82, 84, 86, 91
Enns, J. T., 355, 364
Epiphenomenalism, 79–80, 83, 88, 115
qualia, 88
quality, 82, 84, 90
Esfeld, M., 189, 208
Essence, 125, 139, 141, 340
scientific, 140
Evans, G., 60, 166, 173, 195, 279, 390, 406–7
Experience 1, 3–4, 6, 11, 22–3, 25, 42, 67–8, 77, 87, 94–5, 98, 103, 107–14, 116, 119, 124, 127, 130, 137, 141, 150, 162, 182, 200, 205, 210, 218, 220, 229–30, 235, 237–8, 288, 301, 303, 307, 309, 312, 314–15, 319, 386, 409, 411
accuracy conditions for, 316–18
aesthetic, 22, 209
affectively valenced, 309
ambient, 363, 370
assembled, 364–6, 368
auditory *see* Audition, experience
cognitive (*see also* Phenomenology, cognitive), 227
coherent, 366–7, 370, 369–70
content of *see* Content, of experience
dimensions of, 394–5
extra dimensions of, 390–1
fragmentary, 25, 362–6, 368, 370
hallucinatory *see* Hallucination
itch, 305
multimodal, 389
of colour *see* Colour, experience of
of pain *see* Pain
perceptual, 2, 5–11, 13, 22, 151, 159, 171, 181–99, 204, 207–8, 210, 221, 226, 234, 239, 241, 243–6, 250, 341, 347, 350, 380, 392

privacy of, 106, 218
pure, 71
self-intimation of, 227–8, 248–50
sense/sensory, 148, 151, 161, 163–75, 178, 223–4, 301, 327, 365, 412
subjective, 104, 202–3, 209
synaesthetic *see* Synaesthesia
transparency of *see also* Transparency, 26
virtual, 370
visual, 9, 14, 23, 25, 36, 58–9, 103–4, 129, 157, 158, 161, 168, 175–8, 182, 199, 201, 218–19, 222, 234, 249–50, 270–2, 281–2, 298, 303, 305–6, 310–11, 313, 318, 322, 326, 341, 347–8, 354, 360–4, 367–71, 381, 384, 401, 404
Explanation
a posteriori, 4, 112, 115
causal, 271
conceptual, 13, 15
mechanistic, 71
physical, 13, 67, 77
qualitative, 88, 91
reductive, 13, 72, 74, 189, 401
scientific, 69, 75, 112, 115, 189
Explanatory gap, 13–15, 99, 106, 108–12, 114–15, 405
External function, 350–1
Externalism, 8, 12, 226–7, 229, 231, 273, 307, 338, 380
radical, 232

Faber, D. S., 417
Farah, M. J., 356, 357
Faul, F., 42
Fei-Fei, L., 362, 363, 364, 365
Feigl, H., 85, 86, 93, 95, 98, 137, 215, 220
ffytche, D. H., 8, 411, 412
Fields, H., 319
Filling-in, 218, 362
Fine, K., 125
Firth, R., 25
Fish, W., 6, 7, 181, 191
Foster, J., 14, 156
First-person perspective, 24, 55–6, 111, 193–5
Franconeri, S. L., 349
Functionalism, 107, 197, 325, 333–4, 336
analytic, 132, 137
Fungibility, 67, 76
Fusiform face area, 411

Galileo, 21, 242
Geithner, C., 46
Gelade, G., 356, 365
Ghosh, K., 394
Gilchrist, A., 46
Gist, 26, 362, 363
Goff, P., 19, 126, 131, 138, 139
Gollisch, T., 234
Goodale, M. A., 322, 368, 414
Goodman, N., 25, 38, 51, 290
Gordon, J., 45
Gordon, P. E., 392
Graff, D., 291
Grahek, N., 298
Grain problem, 78–9, 80
Grantham, D., 60
Gray, J. A., 393
Gray, R., 380, 387
Grice, H. P., 5, 6, 34, 193
Griffin, D. Ray, 137
Grimes, J., 218
Grossenbacher, P. G., 376
Gurwitsch, A., 248–9
Gustation, 49, 51, 53, 57–8, 61, 184, 378

Hall, R., 307
Hallucination, 2, 6–9, 11, 105, 185, 190–5, 199, 202, 209, 230, 232, 298–9, 310–12, 316–17
argument from, 191, 401
indiscriminability of, 182
property, 380
veridical, 314–15
Hamwi, V., 275
Hanson, N. R., 259
Hard problem, 106–11, 113–14, 406
Hardin, C. L., 41, 45, 46, 203, 206, 285, 402
Harman, G., 11, 39, 105, 121, 299
Harrison, J. E., 54, 378, 379
Hartshorne, C., 85, 93
Hassel, H., 90
Hatfield, G., 348
Hawken, M., 285, 286, 287, 288
Hawthorne, J., 316
Heil, J., 89, 140
Held, R., 60
Heisenberg, W., 76
Henderson, J. M., 353
Heywood, C., 286, 287, 288
Hicks, G. Dawes, 149–50, 159–60, 163, 174, 176
Higher-order thought (HOT) theory, 69, 70, 71, 95, 97, 324, 334
quotational, 97
Hilbert, D., 188
Hill, C., 122, 237
Hobbes, T., 215, 220, 247
Hobson, K., 185
Hollingworth, A., 353
Holomovement, 92
Homunculus, 246, 401, 415
fallacy, 27, 406–7
regress, 402, 407

Hooker, C. A., 84
Hornsby, J., 171
Howe effect, 395
Huemer, M., 401
Hume, D., 73, 74, 85, 90, 158, 165, 219, 388
Humphreys, G. W., 356
Hupe, J. M., 385
Hurvich, L. M., 277, 403
Husserl, E., 9–10, 325
Hylomorphism, 365

Idealism, 130, 164, 215, 233, 237–8
Identity, 96, 140, 232, 289
  a posteriori, 14
  assumption, 290
  brute/primitive, 117, 139, 140
  criteria of, 264–5
  mind-brain, 17, 95, 104, 112–16
  of looks, 290–1
  of mental and physical, 112, 202
  numerical, 155
  object, 261–5
  property, 112–13
  scientific, 112, 114–15
  theory of truth, 171
Illusion 173, 250, 311, 380, 396, 402
  argument from, 22, 105, 149, 153–4, 156–8, 164, 167, 176–7, 400–2
  perceptual, 172
  visual, 22, 58, 161, 203, 394
  waterfall, 294, 317
Illusory conjunctions, 356
Inattentional blindness, 218, 354, 362, 371
  types of, 365–7
Incorporation (absorption), 392–3
Inducer, 376–8, 381–5, 389–92
Induction, 87, 401
Inkstand, 150–2, 154
Integrative agnosia, 356, 363
Intentionalism, 11, 150–1, 163–4, 171–3
  non-reductive, 96
  strong, 11–12
  weak, 11–12
Intentionality, 9, 85, 161–3
  mark of, 162
  of experience, 4, 163, 237
  of perception, 10
  of visual awareness, 161
  phenomenal, 89
  proto-, 89
Internalism, 77, 226, 238, 242
  quality, 77
Interocular suppression, 354
Introspection, 8, 9, 17, 23, 25, 33–4, 39, 93, 113, 129, 136, 150, 170, 174–5, 184, 192, 199, 209, 219, 236, 258, 266, 271, 275, 277, 281–2, 300, 366
  judgement based on, 44, 49, 113, 133, 138
  knowledge from, 129, 150
Intuition, 33–4
  of distinctness, 118
  pump, 95, 118
Inverted spectrum, 36, 46, 68, 94, 200–1
Itti, L., 348, 354
Iwasaki, S., 363, 366

Jackendoff, D., 339
Jackson, F., 11, 13, 14, 42, 75, 98, 117, 139, 140, 150, 186, 218, 407
James, W., 19, 20, 71, 95, 233, 237, 325
Jameson, D., 277, 403
Jennings, C. D., 347, 348
Jensen, M. S., 357
Johnston, M., 7–8, 77, 156, 169, 181, 186, 187, 201–2, 219, 316
Juan, C-H., 353
Just noticeable difference (JND), 21, 37–50, 52, 54–5, 61, 274, 279, 289, 294
  bridge, 51–3, 56–61

Kahneman, D., 357, 358
Kant, I., 9, 72, 165, 187, 200, 261
Kanwisher, N., 356, 411, 415
Kay, P., 45, 46, 275
Keefe, R., 290
Keller, A., 34
Kelly, S., 279
Kentridge, R., 286, 287, 288, 347, 361, 369
Kercel, S. W., 58
Kim, C. Y., 384
Kim, M.-S., 355
Kind, A., 9, 237, 241
Kinsbourne, M., 406
Kirk, R., 13
Klein, C., 307
Klincewicz, M., 49
Koch, C., 322, 347, 362
Kok, P., 45
Kouider, S., 363, 366
Kovakovitch, K., 316
Knowledge argument, 13, 75, 110–11, 116–17, 137
Krauzlis, R. J., 353
Kriegel, U., 3, 20, 71, 89, 97, 323
Kripke, S., 114, 131, 189, 201, 218
Kuehni, R. G., 38, 46, 203
Kuhn, T. S., 259

Ladyman, J., 208
Lam, V., 189, 208
Lambie, J., 182
Lamme, V. A. F., 347
Landis, C., 375
Langsam, H., 150

Langton, R., 189
Larson, A. M., 363
Lateral geniculate nucleus (LGN), 284, 285, 412, 415, 419
Lavie, N., 364
Leibniz, G. W., 13, 72
Leibniz's Law, 16, 107–8, 111, 232
Leibniz law problem, 16, 107, 110, 113–14, 118
Lenay, C., 204
Levin, D. T., 218
Levin, J., 116, 132–4, 136
Levine, J., 3, 6, 13, 122, 218, 326–7
Lewis, D., 42, 121, 126, 189, 219
Libet, B., 361
Loar, B., 15, 108–9, 111–12, 122, 336
Locke, J., 59, 216, 222, 242, 247, 248, 264, 340
Logue, H., 6, 181, 188
Logvinenko, A. D., 46
Loschky, L. C., 363
Lovelace, C. T., 376
Lowe, E. J., 6, 191, 197, 261, 267, 419
Lutra, R., 333
Lycan, W., 11, 71, 104, 301, 380

Macaluso, E., 408
Macbeth's dagger, 8, 202, 298–9
Mach, E., 99
Mack, A., 362, 364, 367
Mackie, J. L., 6, 216, 222, 246, 339
Macpherson, F., 6, 8, 34, 191, 326, 380, 381
Maddox, W. T., 356
Maffi, L., 45, 46
Malebranche, N., 216, 225
Mandik, P., 276, 280
Manford, M., 191
Manifest image, 81, 84, 103
Manzoni, T., 408
Marcel, A. J., 36, 182
Marks, L. E., 376, 389
Marois, R., 218
Marr, D., 350
Marshall, D., 189
Marshall, J. A., 418
Martin, C. B., 89, 140
Martin, M. G. F., 6, 7, 127, 181, 191, 236
Martinez, M., 307
Mary (*see also* Knowledge argument), 75, 106, 108, 111–12, 116–18, 121, 123
Matching, 38, 51, 52, 275
Materialism (*see also* Physicalism), 17, 219
Mather, G., 418
Mattingley, J. B., 382
Maxwell, G., 137, 199, 215, 220
McCamy, C., 274
McClelland, T., 75
McDowell, J., 6, 171, 187, 279
McGinn, C., 6, 14, 18, 94, 187–8, 218, 222, 316
McIntyre, R., 10
McLaughlin, B., 122
Mealor, A. D., 40
Meehl, P. E., 83
Meister, M., 234
Mellor, D. H., 386
Memory, 275, 287, 379, 392
  iconic, 347, 363
  long-term, 339, 357, 367
  visual short-term, 349, 358, 366, 369
  working, 332
Mental paint, 104, 105, 301
Menzies, P., 186, 188
Merikle, P. M., 40
Merker, B., 412–13
Mesulam, M.-M., 416
Metamerism, 41, 57
Millar, A., 6, 182
Mills, C. B., 379
Milner, A. D., 322, 368, 414
Modality, 25, 35, 38–9, 41, 47–9, 51–2, 54, 56–61, 85, 215, 322, 379, 388, 390, 410, 412, 414–15
  chemoreceptive, 57
  individuation of, 37–61
  multi, 408–9, 413
Mode of presentation, 37, 226
  phenomenal, 109
Mollon, J. D., 353
Moltmann, F., 153
Molyneux's question, 59–60
Monism:
  categorial, 82–3
  neutral, 20, 71, 78, 164
  Russellian, 137–38
Montague, M., 218, 226, 227, 281
Moore, G. E., 4, 5, 21–2, 147–78, 236–8, 242–4, 325
Muhlenberg, G., 79
Multiple relation theory of appearing (MRTA), 21–2, 148–50, 156–7, 160–4, 166–75
Mulvenna, C. M., 376, 382
Munsell test, 202, 287
Murdoch, I., 214
Mylopoulos, M., 54

Naccache, L., 367
Nagel, T., 2, 20, 36, 42, 66–70, 74, 76–8, 95, 99, 218
Naïve realism (*see also* Direct realism), 6, 105, 181, 188
Nassau, K., 402
Naturalism, 14, 33–4, 74, 76, 96, 140, 303–4, 401
Navon, D., 349
Neander, K., 97
Neisser, U., 362, 366
Nemirow, L., 42

Neuroscience, 13, 18, 27, 80, 88, 93, 99, 178, 314, 315, 319, 414, 419
Noë, A., 218, 361
Noesselt, T., 408
Nominalism, 126–7
  blobby, 126
Non-reductionism, 67, 69, 76, 78, 119
Noren, S. J., 81
Norretranders, T., 368
Novich, S. D., 381
Nudds, M., 60

Obama, 314, 330–1
Object-specific preview benefit, 357
O'Callaghan, C., 380, 394
Ockham's razor, 139–40, 350
Öğmen, H., 36
Olfaction, 34, 44, 48–9, 51, 53, 57, 61, 234, 386, 389
Ontic structuralism, 86
Ontology, 4, 16, 21, 79–80, 116, 121, 139–40, 182, 315
  common-sense, 257
  fundamental, 81
  non-particulate, 80
  of colour, 276
  of perceptual experience, 194
  of phenomenal array, 404
  of physics, 94
  physical, 80, 85, 124
O' Regan, J. K., 361
Ortmann, O., 378, 383
Overflow, 365
Owen, A. M., 330

Pain, 2, 4, 12, 14, 18, 36–7, 38, 88–90, 93–6, 103–5, 123, 126–7, 129, 134, 136–8, 140, 165, 182, 192, 227, 298–316, 318
  concept of, 17–18, 121, 130, 133
  essence of, 125–6, 139
  experience of, 24, 218–19, 300, 302, 304, 308–10, 313–15
  negative affect of, 24, 301–4, 308–9
  neurophysiological basis of, 319–20
  phantom limb, 24, 299
  sensory aspect of, 319–20
Palmer, S., 301
Palmeri, T. J., 384
Panpsychism, 19–20, 66, 68–70, 77, 83, 90, 137
Panqualityism, 20, 66, 77, 87, 89, 96
Papineau, D., 12, 14, 15, 83, 97, 112–13, 115, 117–18, 122–3, 131, 136
Parker, A., 198
Particle, 13, 66, 72, 78–81, 84, 86–9, 91–2, 340
Part-whole relation, 154, 313
Parvizi, J., 414
Pashler, H. E., 348
Pautz, A., 169, 302, 402
Peacocke, C., 201, 279
Perception, 1, 4, 8–9, 21–3, 25–7, 34–5, 39, 50, 55, 90, 92, 96, 99, 150–1, 161, 164, 167, 169, 185–6, 202, 214–16, 222, 225, 230–1, 236–7, 244–6, 257–61, 266, 273, 325, 356–7, 379–80, 390, 392, 396, 408–9
  aesthetic conception of, 208–10
  brightness, 394
  causal theory of, 22, 182, 195–6, 210, 404
  colour, 41, 276–80, 282, 289, 292, 295, 353
  conscious, 47, 220–1, 223–4, 226, 235, 238, 243–4, 246, 250, 282
  depth, 267, 419–20
  directness of, 22
  flavour, 386
  function of, 22, 185, 196–201, 204, 206–7, 217
  enactive account of, 197–8
  error theory of, 184
  gist, 363
  intentionality of, 10
  judgements of, 151–4
  machine, 235
  mode of, 11
  motion, 285, 353
  multisensory, 386
  navigational picture of, 196–208, 210
  object dependence of, 229
  objects of, 5, 10, 153, 156, 171, 187, 192, 194–5, 215, 222, 229, 231–4, 237, 264, 407
  relativity of, 105
  reliability of, 265
  representational powers of, 279
  scene, 347, 369
  sense, 147–50, 158, 167, 171, 175, 177–8, 214–15, 218, 223, 379
  shape, 365
  tactile, 1, 59–60
  unconscious (subliminal, nonconscious), 34, 217, 224, 235, 244
  veridical, 4–5, 7, 171, 181, 184–5, 190–1, 194, 230, 235, 380
  visual, 7, 188, 267–8, 270, 272, 281, 310, 352, 361, 369
Perceptual taking, 10, 182
Pereboom, D., 14, 19, 72, 75, 77, 98
Perky, C. W., 392
  cases, 392
Perry, J., 122
Pessoa, L., 218, 362
Phenomenal array, 403–20
Phenomenal certainty, 124, 127–31, 133–6
Phenomenal character, 2–4, 7, 9, 11–12, 23, 107, 181, 188–9, 269–70, 272, 300–1, 308–9, 315–18, 363, 380, 387
  primitivism about, 319

Phenomenal consciousness *see* Consciousness, phenomenal
Phenomenal concepts, 15–17, 18, 21, 37, 105–6, 108–11, 113–17, 121, 128–30, 132
  direct, 123, 130–1, 133, 137
  quotational model of, 97, 106, 123
  radically opaque, 139
Phenomenal concept strategy (PCS), 15–17, 105–6, 111, 113, 116–17, 119, 121–4, 130, 132
Phenomenal enrichment, 26, 390–1
Phenomenal insight, 128–34, 136, 141
Phenomenal intentionality research program, 89
Phenomenality (*see also* Consciousness, phenomenal), 19, 67–71, 75, 80, 95–6, 109, 122, 323
Phenomenal judgement, 130
  infallibility of, 130
Phenomenologists, 242, 325
Phenomenology, 13, 25, 49, 60–1, 95, 134, 230, 306, 315, 326–8, 335, 337, 342, 403, 414–16
  cognitive, 24, 94, 226, 323–7, 341–2
  colour-shape, 322, 325
  impure cognitive, 326–7
  of experience, 8
  of perception, 9, 94, 191, 194, 207, 326
  of veridical experience, 23
  sensory, 24, 94, 323–6, 333–41, 410–11
  sound, 325
  visual, 201, 322, 418–20
Photism, 381
Photoreceptor, 41, 349, 353, 361
Physicalism, 14, 16–18, 20, 23, 66, 70, 75–6, 78, 83–4, 90, 106, 109, 111, 116–17, 121–4, 130, 133, 137–8, 215, 219
  acquaintance, 122, 130–1
  Acquaintance argument against, 136–41
  austere, 20–1
  counterintuitiveness of, 110
  PCS (*see also* Phenomenal concept strategy) 122, 130, 132–3, 137, 139
  real, 220
  reductive, 17
  relational, 93
  Russellian, 19, 75
  Strawson-style, 137–8
  topic-neutral, 107
  type b, 75
Physics, 78
  causal completeness of, 83
  structural character of, 86
Pitt, D., 2, 342
Place, U. T., 95, 105
Platchias, D., 8, 191
Plato, 80
Pointer, M., 274
Point of view, 55, 67–70, 178
  subjective, 194
Posner, M. I., 354
Power, 140, 242
  causal, 79, 88–90, 92, 207
  chemical, 92
  combinatorial, 388
  explanatory, 34
  of conceiving, 15
  of qualia, 94–5
  of visual discrimination, 206
  representational of perception, 279
  transductive of the organs, 61
Pre-frontal monitoring, 97
Prichard's diagnostic, 405, 413
Prichard, H. A., 164, 405
Primary visual cortex (V1), 284–8, 322, 415
Prinz, J., 326, 337–40, 347, 361, 365, 366, 369
Projectivism, 183–4, 187, 210
Proper names, 106, 152, 376
Property:
  absolutely intrinsic, 72–3, 75
  anthropocentric objective, 395
  apparent, 174
  behavioural, 115
  categorical, 140
  causal-functional/similarity, 132
  causal role, 137
  colour, 48, 183, 187–9, 200–1, 206, 277, 280–1, 286, 394
  comparatively intrinsic, 72–3
  cluster, 316
  complex, 189, 317–19
  conscious, 282
  configurational, 92
  dispositional, 18, 74, 85, 87, 140
  essential, 123, 125
  ethical, 140
  experiential, 137
  extrinsic, 72–3
  formal, 271
  fragmentary, 364–5
  functional, 71, 134, 329, 333
  fundamental, 19, 73, 75–6, 78, 88–9
  fundamental intrinsic, 189–90
  geometrical, 54–5, 130
  gradable determinable, 303, 308–9
  hallucination, 380
  high-level, 13, 66, 74, 77, 326
  identity, 113, 115, 117
  intentional, 3, 11, 77
  intrinsic, 70, 72, 77, 186–90, 196, 198, 200–1, 204, 207–8, 210
  irreducible, 76
  local physical, 307
  locational, 301, 310
  logical, 86
  low-level, 326

Property: (*cont.*)
macrophenomenal, 67, 75
macroscopic, 72
manifest, 108
microphenomenal, 67
mind-independent, 197
mental, 34, 36, 48, 121, 139–40, 224, 307
monadic, 12, 203
moral, 140
natural, 140
necessary, 124
neural, 108, 110, 114
non-locational, 300
non-physical, 107, 110
objective, 4, 189, 201, 203, 205, 382
olfactory, 48
optical, 285–6
perceptible, 39–40, 44, 46–8
phenomenal, 16–17, 66–9, 75, 77, 116, 121, 138, 276–7, 281, 289, 323, 334, 337
physical, 4, 10, 12–13, 41, 48–50, 68, 77–8, 109, 111, 121, 123, 132–4, 138, 183, 205, 242, 307, 358, 361, 380
physical-functional, 109
physiological, 305, 314, 320
private, 106
projective, 271
protophenomenal, 137
public, 98
qualitative, 7, 20, 74, 77, 80, 107, 403
relational, 19, 73, 85, 208, 270
representational, 26, 129, 161
represented, 306
response-dependent, 74
scientific, 189–90
semantic, 307, 339
sensible, 7–8, 22, 181, 186, 189–90, 197–98, 210
spatial, 48–9, 59, 198, 271
structural, 134, 137, 361
subject-indexed, 303
subjective, 98
syntactical, 324
temporal, 49
thick, 114–15
valuational, 301, 303, 307, 310
wavelength, 286
Propositional attitude, 162, 171, 327
Proto-object, 26, 355–6, 358, 359
Proust, M., 250
Pylyshyn, Z. W., 358

Qualia, 20–1, 68–71, 73–5, 77, 82, 90, 103–7, 115, 405
absent, 68
causal, 90
complexes, 96
consciousness of, 97
construction of, 92–4
epiphenomenal, 88
fundamental, 95
identification of, 219
intersubjective accessibility of, 97–8
intrinsic, 72
inverted, 68
micro-, 79, 89
objectivity of, 98–9
of magnetic attraction, 90
privacy of, 99
unconscious, 88, 323
unexperienced, 20, 73
Qualitative character, 1, 34–7, 39–40, 43, 75, 217, 239, 405, 420
experiential, 218–19, 224, 227, 239, 242
Qualities, 10, 21, 69, 71, 73–4, 77–8, 80, 84–5, 88, 91–2, 95, 99, 112
causal, 82, 87, 89, 93–5
colour, 199–200, 202, 216–17, 241
conservation of, 94
dynamic, 81
eliminativism about, 77
experiential, 106–7, 111, 141, 162, 409
explanatory, 88
external, 189, 198, 200, 206, 210, 238
field, 86–7
hallucinatory, 7–8
internalism, 77
intrinsic, 22, 200, 220
inverted, 46
irreducibility of, 74–6, 86, 91, 93, 111, 113
mental, 21, 34–49, 52, 54–6, 58–61, 93, 104, 106
objective, 184, 200
of manifest world, 104
of visual field, 280, 282
particularized, 167
perceptual, 3, 8, 155–6, 420
phenomenal, 1–6, 9–12, 14–16, 20–25, 27, 103–5, 107–8, 110–11, 114–16, 119, 121–4, 127–38, 181–92, 200, 202, 205, 209–11, 405, 418, 420
physical, 78, 94, 96, 98, 200, 206
powerful, 89
primary, 173, 199
primitive, 79
private, 106
relations, 90–2
secondary, 103, 105, 114
sensible, 7–9, 152, 161, 162–72, 174–5, 177, 196–7, 199, 207, 210
sensory, 3, 24, 68–73, 85, 300–1, 309, 363
simple, 110
tertiary, 90
unconscious, 7, 21, 51, 73, 88, 96
visual, 44, 201

Quality space (QS), 21, 33–5, 38–40, 42–5, 47, 49–50, 53–5, 60–1
asymmetry, 46
for colour, 39, 43, 46
gustatory, 57–8
olfactory, 48, 57
overlap of, 51–4
species, 56
theory (QST), 34–5, 38–42, 44, 47–9, 52, 57
Quiddity, 140

Rader, C. M., 392
Raffman, D., 279, 291
Raftopoulos, A., 23, 257–7, 273
Ramachandran, V. S., 362
Ramanath, R., 46
Rayner, K., 357
Realism (*see also* Direct realism, Critical realism), 23, 257–60, 265, 267, 270–3
about experience, 217–20, 230, 232, 237
about mental representations, 231
about secondary qualities, 105
common sense, 152
indirect, 5, 96, 98, 216, 222, 225, 234–6, 246
phenomenal, 66
physicalist, 119
quality, 76
scientific, 211
structural, 199, 208
Real nature, 109, 122–7, 129–31, 134, 137–41
of external world, 259
of physical colour, 199–201
Regier, T., 275
Reid, T., 158, 214–15, 236–41, 271
Reduction, 17, 66, 71, 80, 104–5, 401
of perception to function, 197
of seeing to judging, 162
Reductive explanation, 13, 74, 105
Reflectance, 13, 41, 43, 81, 188, 190, 199
Rensink, R., 347, 348, 350, 352, 353, 354, 355, 356, 357, 358, 359, 362, 363, 364, 366, 367, 368, 369
Repetition blindness, 356
Representation, 26, 35, 214
accuracy conditions of, 315
body, 408, 413
cognitive, 388
coherent, 358–9
colour, 280, 295
conceptual, 280, 388
higher-order (HO), 69, 96
high-level perceptual, 326
mental, 34, 77, 214–15, 221–22, 225–26, 231–34, 236, 247, 312, 328, 339, 356, 417
mis-, 300, 305, 312, 380
modes of, 12
non-conceptual, 279, 316–17
of experienced valuational properties, 307
perceptual, 14, 171, 184, 221–5, 230, 234, 236, 238, 244–5, 258, 283, 337, 347, 350, 354, 357, 364, 366–7, 380, 409, 412
pictorial, 281
poised, 317
property, 316, 355, 410
resemblance theory of, 340
self-, 71, 249
sensory, 305, 316, 320
temporary, 358
topographical, 412
unconscious, 235, 337, 339
under-, 305
unified, 392
vehicles of, 277, 412
virtual, 369
visual, 369, 400, 408
Representationalism, 11, 105, 150, 171, 221, 222, 401 (*see also* Intentionalism)
eliminativist, 77
self-, 96
strong, 315
strong property, 317
weak, 315–16
weak property, 316–17
Retinal blind spot, 361
Revelation, 124, 127, 129, 181, 187, 190, 196–7, 200, 206, 209–10, 219
dual, 138–41
picture, 186
semi-, 134–6
structural semi-, 135
Richardson, R. C., 79
Riddoch, M. J., 356
Riddoch syndrome (*see also* Blindsight), 410–11
Rigid designator, 126
Ro, T., 54
Roberson, D., 275, 289
Roberts, D. D., 57
Robertson, L. C., 355
Robinson, H., 6, 7, 12, 104, 105, 111, 116, 117, 149, 156, 191
Rock, I., 362, 364, 367
Rosenthal, D., 3, 20, 34, 41, 47, 59, 66–71, 73, 77, 95–7, 98, 99, 276
Roska, B., 234
Rouw, R., 379
Russell, B., 4–5, 16, 18, 20, 85, 86, 99, 106, 137–8, 147–8, 152, 154, 162–5, 176–7, 215, 220, 402, 405
Ryle, G., 105

Sainsbury, M., 314
Saffran, E. M., 357
Sagi, D., 362, 364
Sagiv, N., 378

Sartre, J.-P., 227, 249
Sasaki, Y., 39
Scannell, J. W., 410
Scepticism, 23, 159, 215–16, 230, 265–6, 401
Schloss, K., 301
Scholl, B. J., 359, 367
Schroer, R., 132–4, 136
Schwenkler, J., 59
Scientific image, 79–80
Searle, J., 112, 115, 117, 218, 322, 323
Seibt, J., 81, 82
Segal, G., 227
Segal, S. J., 392
Self, 106, 122
Sellars, R. W., 5, 85, 91, 93, 98
Sellars, W., 5, 6, 9–10, 12, 66, 74, 77, 78–85, 87, 88, 91, 95, 182, 197, 200, 259
Sensation, 3, 4, 6, 10, 12, 44, 103–6, 152, 236, 243, 244, 246–7, 319, 402, 419
  acts of, 164, 248
  bodily, 2, 33, 38, 305–6, 307–8, 319, 406
  colour, 54–5, 174, 184, 192, 204, 221, 225–7, 231, 236–9, 241–2, 400
  intentionality of, 163–4, 227
  perceptual, 23
  privacy of, 165
  somatic, 319, 411
  tactile, 238–41, 377
  taste, 49
  unpleasant, 320
  visual, 234, 235, 237, 239, 241, 250
Sense-datum, 4–5, 25, 27, 106 122, 147–52, 155–6, 159, 164–5, 167, 174–5, 177, 416, 420
  'early' theory, 166
  fallacy, 164
  inference, 159–60
  language, 159, 166
  naive theory (NSDT), 400–1, 403–20
  non-physical, 155, 161
  traditional theory (TSD, SDT), 4–5, 11, 21, 26, 122, 147–51, 157–9, 161, 163–5, 167–71, 173, 176–7, 400
Sensory substitution, 58–9, 204
Seth, A., 40
Shankar, M. U., 40
Shapley, R., 285, 286, 287, 288
Shepherd, G. M., 57
Shifted spectrum, 202
Shipp, S., 410
Shoemaker, S., 46, 68
Siegel, S., 7, 161, 191, 326
Siewert, C., 325
Simner, J., 393
Simons D. J., 218, 366
Sivic, L., 274
Smart, J. J. C., 17, 95, 107, 116, 119
Smilek, D., 378, 384
Smith, A. D., 181, 191
Smith, D. R., 418
Smolin, L., 87
Sollberger, M., 380
Somato-sensory cortex (SSC), 319–20
Spelke-object, 263–4
Spence, C., 389, 393
Sperling, G., 352
Spirit of the woodland, 139–40
Sprague, J. M., 412
Sprague effect, 410, 412, 414
Stalnaker, R., 13, 14, 112, 115–17, 122
Stereopsis, 418–19
Stevenson, R. J., 49
Stimulus error, 419
Stoljar, D., 15, 19, 37, 75, 137
Strawson, G., 19, 89, 137–8, 140, 186, 220, 227, 228, 231, 236, 247, 248, 323, 325, 326, 331–2
Strawson, P. F., 166–7,, 173, 264
Stroop task, 379, 384
Structural realism *see* Realism, structural
Stuff-ing, 84–7, 91, 92, 94
Subject, 2–12, 21–26, 89, 96, 98, 108, 114, 123–4, 126–8, 129–35, 155, 162, 165–6, 173–4, 181–93, 195–7, 201–6, 221–2, 224–5, 231–6, 241, 243–6, 249, 271, 299
  epistemic position of, 170, 174, 186–7, 198–9, 208, 210, 219, 259, 262–3, 279, 291
  navigational actions of, 199
Subjective character, 3
Subjectivity, 24, 66–70, 78
Superior colliculus (SC), 27, 353, 412–14, 419
Supervenience:
and fundamental intrinsic properties, 190
  of badness on local physical properties, 307
  of causal power on quality, 89
  of colours on physical properties, 188
  of phenomenal character on intentional content, 11
Synaesthesia, 26, 56, 376–96
  colour-grapheme, 379, 391, 394
  colour-hearing, 377, 394
  colour-sound, 55–6
  dual account of, 380–90, 393
  total, 55–6

Tactition, 48, 59–60
Taste, 1, 2, 49, 57, 73, 81, 94, 99, 178, 181, 184, 218, 239, 243, 247, 303, 309, 335, 406
Taylor, A. J., 57
Taylor, J. H., 138, 140
Telepathy, 98
Tellegen, A., 392
Terhune, D. B., 379, 393
That-it-is-for-ness, 3, 95, 97

Theory of appearing *see* Multiple relation theory of appearing
Third-person perspective, 14, 25, 118, 194–6
Thorpe, S., 363
Thought, 2, 11, 12, 33, 106, 122–3, 166, 181, 192, 208, 219, 222, 228–9, 231–2, 235, 248, 337
  conscious, 10, 24, 192, 226, 227, 229, 314, 316, 323–42
  demonstrative, 259
  direct realism about, 215, 231–3
  dispositional, 331
  experience (*see also* Phenomenology, cognitive), 245, 247
  non-conscious occurrent, 323, 333–4
  perceptual, 151, 183–4
  syntactical structure of, 324
  Tibbles, 261–2
Tootel, R. B., 408
Transparency, 107, 300, 384, 417
  metaphysical, 243
  of experience, 186, 238, 300, 301, 384
  of perception, 8–9, 23, 124, 188, 195, 196, 236–45
  phenomenological, 243
  strong, 241
  weak, 103–5, 114, 241
Travis, C., 4, 188, 389
Treisman, A., 347, 356, 363, 365, 382
Trope, 126–7, 153, 167
Tsotsos, J. K., 349, 360, 361
Tsuchiya, N., 347, 362
Tye, M., 8, 11, 12, 14, 104, 123, 184, 189, 193, 203–4, 237, 300, 306, 313, 314, 316, 317, 380

Ullman, S., 358
Unger, P., 79
Unique hue, 45–6, 202–4, 403
Universal, 7, 126, 151, 167
  aristotelian, 126
  colours as, 167
  platonic, 126–7

Valberg, J. J., 6, 7, 12, 186, 191, 197
Van Cleve, J., 233, 237
Van Gulick, R., 334
VanRullen, R., 352, 356, 363
Veillet, B., 326
Ventral simultanagnosia, 357
Vision, 35, 47–8, 52–3, 55, 58–60, 153, 155, 158, 193, 197–8, 201, 215, 239, 241–3, 245, 258, 283, 306, 322, 339, 347, 353, 355, 400, 407–8
  achromatic, 206
  colour, 41, 155, 203–6, 276, 284–5, 287–8, 402–3, 415
  computational theories of, 322
  conscious, 277, 279–82
  depth, 418
  focused, 418
  form, 288
  monocular, 267
  three-hundred and sixty degree, 369
Visual extinction, 354
Visual field, 23, 43, 92, 94, 280–1, 283–5, 331, 339, 347–9, 354, 359, 365, 381, 403–5, 408, 412, 415–16
  geometry of, 267–73
Visual neglect, 354, 362, 416
Visual system, 41, 91, 98, 178, 184, 205, 206, 234, 271, 277–8, 306, 408

Wager, A., 380, 382, 387
Walsh, V., 376, 382
Ward, J., 385
Watanabe, T., 39
Weatherson, B., 189
Weber, A. I., 48
Webster, M. A., 45, 46
Weddell, R. A., 414
Weiss, S. A., 417
Werner, J. S., 277
What-it-is-like-ness, 2–3, 24, 42–3, 68, 79, 95, 98, 181
White, A., 170
White, B. J., 413
White effect, 395
Whitehead, A. N., 87
Wiggins, D., 264
Williamson, T., 290
Winawer, J., 275
Wittgenstein, L., 185, 326
Wolfe, J. M., 366
Woodruff Smith, D., 10
Wooten, B. R., 277
Woozley, A. D., 222
Wright, C., 290
Wright, R. D., 348, 356
Wright, W., 201

Yolton, J., 222
Young, B. D., 34, 46, 48, 49, 57
Young, M. P., 410

Zahavi, D., 227
Zeki, S, 286, 287, 408, 410–12, 415
Zemach, E. M., 97
Zombie, 36
  argument, 13, 137
  conceivability of, 15, 36, 94–5, 110–12, 121, 133

The manufacturer's authorised representative in the EU for product safety is Oxford University Press España S.A. of el Parque Empresarial San Fernando de Henares, Avenida de Castilla, 2 – 28830 Madrid (www.oup.es/en or product.safety@oup.com). OUP España S.A. also acts as importer into Spain of products made by the manufacturer.

www.ingramcontent.com/pod-product-compliance
Lightning Source LLC
LaVergne TN
LVHW011903200926
848484LV00002B/513
* 9 7 8 0 1 9 8 7 1 2 7 1 8 *